Contemporary Endocrinology

Series Editor
Leonid Poretsky, Division of Endocrinology
Lenox Hill Hospital, New York, NY, USA

Contemporary Endocrinology offers an array of titles covering clinical as well as bench research topics of interest to practicing endocrinologists and researchers. Topics include obesity management, androgen excess disorders, stem cells in endocrinology, evidence-based endocrinology, diabetes, genomics and endocrinology, as well as others. Series Editor Leonid Poretsky, MD, is Chief of the Division of Endocrinology and Associate Chairman for Research at Lenox Hill Hospital, and Professor of Medicine at Hofstra North Shore-LIJ School of Medicine.

Alyson K. Myers

Editor

Diabetes and COVID-19

Considerations and Clinical Management

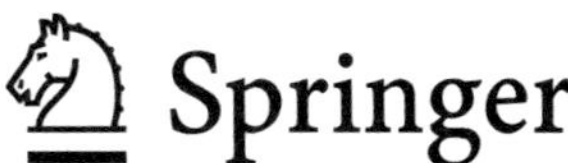 Springer

Editor
Alyson K. Myers
Division of Endocrinology, Department of Medicine
Montefiore Einstein
Bronx, NY, USA

ISSN 2523-3785   ISSN 2523-3793   (electronic)
Contemporary Endocrinology
ISBN 978-3-031-28538-7   ISBN 978-3-031-28536-3   (eBook)
https://doi.org/10.1007/978-3-031-28536-3

This Springer imprint is published by the registered company Springer Nature Switzerland AG
The registered company address is: Gewerbestrasse 11, 6330 Cham, Switzerland

I would like to dedicate this book to three Hunter High School teachers who fostered and encouraged my interest in the sciences: Drs. Marjorie Goldsmith and Judith Klein, as well as Ms. Brandeis.

I would also like to dedicate this book to Mr. Jules Taylor, his widow Emmlynn Taylor, my cousin Doodles, as well as the millions who we have unfortunately lost to COVID-19.

Foreword

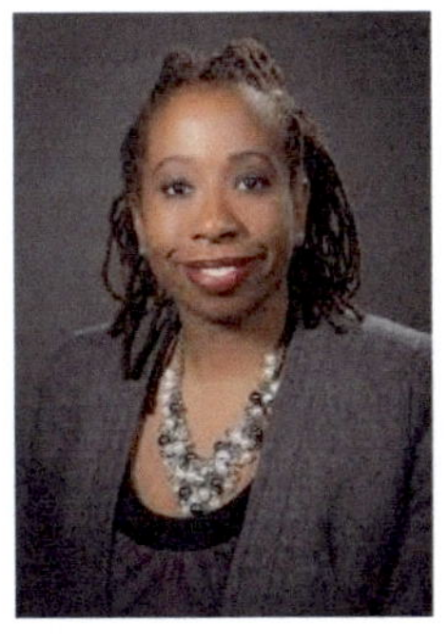

Diabetes is recognized as a major risk factor for increased morbidity and mortality among patients with COVID-19, particularly among minority populations. This volume specifically addresses the patients with diabetes and COVID-19 providing practical and cutting-edge information at the fingertips of the busy practitioners, the specialists, the researchers as well as the students and trainees.

The book is edited by Alyson Myers, MD, a renowned Endocrinologist, Associate Professor and Associate Chair of Diversity, Equity, and Inclusion in the Department of Medicine at Montefiore-Einstein School of Medicine. Dr. Myers has a highly credible work in the field as an imminent scholar with seasoned experience and firsthand knowledge of the serious complications of COVID-19 among people with diabetes.

This book is a culmination of scientific work driven by personal conviction to enhance the care provided to the vulnerable populations COVID-19 patients with diabetes.

Dr. Myers assembled a group of prominent experts in the field addressing the various aspects of COVID-19 and diabetes interface. The book is well organized for easier comprehension in a logical order. It spans topics from the epidemiology and predictors of complications and increased mortality in COVID-19 to in-depth discussion of the pathophysiology of the disease.

Pathophysiology of COVID-19 is addressed comprehensively as common pathogenetic pathways, and also by organ system such as the lung, the kidney, and most pertinently for diabetes, diabetic foot ulcers, and diabetes comorbidities.

This in-depth presentation of the pathophysiology provides rationale for the therapeutic interventions outlined in the following section of the book; the comprehensive management of diabetes in COVID-19 section then becomes easy to understand and follow. This section on management includes very highly practical tips for the practicing endocrinologists as well as the hospitalists and other inpatient care providers ensuring effective, safe, and high-quality care for patients with COVID-19 and diabetes.

The book also provides a dedicated chapter on the utility of diabetes technology including continuous glucose monitoring, remote monitoring, telehealth with specific focus on health disparity, an area that Dr. Myers champions.

The book addresses also, in a dedicated chapter, long-haul COVID presentations in people with diabetes, providing the latest and emerging knowledge in this evolving area of scientific inquiry.

Finally, on a personal note, I must say that I am so proud of Alyson and her achievements. I have served as her Professor during her studies in the College of Medicine at SUNY-Downstate Health Science University, and I continued to serve as her mentor throughout her career with multiple co-authorship on scientific papers. This book is only part of Dr. Alyson Myers great accomplishments and yet many more to come, addressing health equity and eliminating health disparity.

College of Medicine, Department of   Samy I. McFarlane
Medicine, Division of Endocrinology
Downstate Health Science University
Brooklyn, NY, USA
smcfarlane@downstate.edu

Preface

March 8, 2020 was the first time I saw COVID-19. A woman over age 60 with diabetes who was connected to numerous lines and a respirator, lay still in an ICU room. I peered at her through the glass, scared of contracting this novel corona virus. She unfortunately succumbed to her illness as did so many that we cared for during that first surge. Unfortunately, diabetes was one of the pre-existing conditions that was associated with increased mortality from COVID-19. Thankfully, with subsequent surges we have seen fewer deaths.

COVID itself can cause new-onset diabetes in patients some of whom had no predictable risk factors. It can also worsen hyperglycemia in patients with prior diagnosis of diabetes, which can be a dilemma for the patient as well as inpatient and outpatient providers.

In order to cover all aspects of the relationship between COVID and diabetes, I enlisted the help of colleagues in both the United States and Europe who had experience in treating patients with diabetes. A multi-disciplinary approach was needed to manage these complex patients, thus the authors represent a variety of disciplines including pharmacology, endocrinology, nephrology, infectious disease, podiatry, vascular surgery, pulmonary/critical care, and general medicine. In addition, the authors represent different positions in medical care: medical students, residents, fellows, physicians, nurses, nurse practitioners, and pharmacists.

In the process of editing this book, I was fortunate to work with a dynamic group of people who were eager to participate. One of the biggest challenges is that with each new variant, there has been changes in medications as well as vaccines. The FDA no longer recommends the use of the first vaccines as well as some of the treatments that gained emergency use approval in 2020 or 2021.

Bronx, NY   Alyson K. Myers

Acknowledgment

- Dr. Leonid Poretsky for his ongoing mentorship.
- My co-workers from my first attending job at North Shore University Hospital where I was the Medical Director for inpatient diabetes. This would have never happened if it was not for the vision and leadership of Dr. Tracy Breen. I was further supported by my inpatient diabetes team: Ann Marie, Marie, Patricia, Aren, Nick, Sharon, Melissa, and Kaila. I am especially grateful to my fellow endocrine attendings and others who were deployed during that first horrific COVID surge in March 2020. The environmental services, security, dietary, support staff, nursing, hospitalists, respiratory therapists, physical and occupational therapists, and critical care teams were all invaluable.
- Lastly, I could not have survived COVID without my personal support team: my parents and the rest of the crew. Thanks for being who you are.

Contents

List of Contributors

Mersema Abate Donald and Barbara Zucker School of Medicine at Hofstra/ Northwell, Hempstead, NY, USA

Grazia Aleppo Division of Endocrinology, Metabolism and Molecular Medicine, Department of Medicine, Northwestern University Feinberg School of Medicine, Chicago, IL, USA

Inthuja Baskaran Department of Medicine, Center for Health Innovations and Outcomes Research, Northwell Health, Manhasset, NY, USA

Fuad Benyaminov Department of Medicine, North Shore University Hospital, Northwell Health, Manhasset, NY, USA

Zachary Bloomgarden Department of Medicine, Division of Endocrinology, Diabetes and Bone Disease, Icahn School of Medicine at Mount Sinai, New York, NY, USA

Matthew T. Crow Department of Medicine, Johns Hopkins Bayview Medical Center, Johns Hopkins University School of Medicine, Baltimore, MD, USA

César Fernández-de-las-Peñas Department of Physical Therapy, Occupational Therapy, Physical Medicine and Rehabilitation, Universidad Rey Juan Carlos (URJC), Madrid, Spain

Patricia Garnica Department of Medicine, Division of Endocrinology, North Shore University Hospital, Northwell Health, Manhasset, NY, USA

Kane Genser Comprehensive Wound Healing and Hyperbaric Center, Northwell Health, Lake Success, NY, USA

Junaid Habibullah Division of Pulmonary, Critical Care and Sleep Medicine, Donald and Barbara Zucker School of Medicine at Hofstra/Northwell, New Hyde Park, NY, USA

Ghaleb Halaseh Department of Medicine, Division of Infectious Diseases, Montefiore Albert Einstein, Bronx, NY, USA

Ann Marie Hasse Northwell Health, New Hyde Park, NY, USA

Allyson Hernandez SUNY Downstate College of Medicine, Brooklyn, NY, USA

Erica N. Johnson Department of Medicine, Division of Infectious Diseases, Johns Hopkins University School of Medicine, Baltimore, MD, USA

Hanna J. Lee Department of Medicine, The Fleischer Institute for Diabetes and Metabolism, Albert Einstein College of Medicine, New York, NY, USA

Cecilia C. Low Wang Glucose Management Team, University of Colorado Hospital, Aurora, CO, USA

CPC Clinical Research, Aurora, CO, USA

Department of Medicine, Division of Endocrinology, Metabolism and Diabetes, University of Colorado Anschutz Medical Campus School of Medicine, Aurora, CO, USA

Celia Lu St. John's University College of Pharmacy and Health Sciences, Queens, NY, USA

Department of Medicine, Division of General Internal Medicine, Northwell Health, New Hyde Park, NY, USA

Donald and Barbara Zucker School of Medicine at Hofstra/Northwell, Hempstead, NY, USA

Lyndonna Marrast Department of Medicine, Division of General Internal Medicine, Northwell Health, New Hyde Park, NY, USA

Donald and Barbara Zucker School of Medicine at Hofstra/Northwell, Hempstead, NY, USA

Justin Mathew Department of Medicine, The Fleischer Institute for Diabetes and Metabolism, Albert Einstein College of Medicine, New York, NY, USA

Boonyanuth Maturostrakul Donald and Barbara Zucker School of Medicine at Hofstra/Northwell, Hempstead, NY, USA

Michael T. McDermott Division of Endocrinology, Metabolism and Diabetes, Department of Medicine, University of Colorado Anschutz Medical Campus School of Medicine, Aurora, CO, USA

Endocrinology and Diabetes Practice, University of Colorado Hospital, Aurora, CO, USA

Anoop Misra Fortis-C-DOC Centre of Excellence for Diabetes, Metabolic Diseases and Endocrinology, Diabetes Foundation (India), National Diabetes Obesity and Cholesterol Foundation (NDOC), New Delhi, India

Jaime E. Mogollon Department of Medicine, Division of Infectious Diseases, Montefiore Albert Einstein, Bronx, NY, USA

Alyson K. Myers Donald and Barbar Zucker School of Medicine at Hofstra/ Northwell, Hempstead, NY, USA

Division of Endocrinology, Department of Medicine, North Shore University Hospital, Northwell Health, Manhasset, NY, USA

Albert Einstein College of Medicine, Bronx, NY, USA

Vinay Nair Donald and Barbara Zucker School of Medicine at Hofstra/Northwell, Hempstead, NY, USA

Mahmoud Nassar Department of Medicine, Icahn School of Medicine at Mount Sinai/NYC Health + Hospitals, Queens, NY, USA

Alisha Oropallo Donald and Barbara Zucker School of Medicine at Hofstra/ Northwell, Hempstead, NY, USA

Comprehensive Wound Healing and Hyperbaric Center, Northwell Health, Lake Success, NY, USA

Amit Rao Comprehensive Wound Healing and Hyperbaric Center, Northwell Health, Lake Success, NY, USA

Tirissa J. Reid Department of Medicine, Division of Endocrinology, Diabetes, and Metabolism, Vagelos College of Physicians and Surgeons, Columbia University Irving Medical Center, New York, NY, USA

Jane E. B. Reusch Division of Endocrinology, Metabolism and Diabetes, University of Colorado-Anschutz Medical Campus, Aurora, CO, USA

Center for Women's Health Research, University of Colorado-Anschutz Medical Campus, Aurora, CO, USA

University of Colorado NIH Diabetes Research Center, University of Colorado-Anschutz Medical Campus, Aurora, CO, USA

Departments of Medicine, Integrative Physiology, and Bioengineering, University of Colorado-Anschutz Medical Campus, Aurora, CO, USA

Rocky Mountain Regional VAMC, Aurora, CO, USA

Stacey A. Seggelke Department of Medicine, Division of Endocrinology, Metabolism and Diabetes, University of Colorado Anschutz Medical Campus School of Medicine, Aurora, CO, USA

University of Colorado College of Nursing, University of Colorado Anschutz Medical Campus, Aurora, CO, USA

Neeraja Swaminathan Department of Medicine, Division of Infectious Diseases, Montefiore Albert Einstein, Bronx, NY, USA

Emily D. Szmuilowicz Department of Medicine, Division of Endocrinology, Metabolism and Molecular Medicine, Northwestern University Feinberg School of Medicine, Chicago, IL, USA

Juan Torres-Macho Department of Internal Medicine, Hospital Universitario Infanta Leonor-Virgen de la Torre, Madrid, Spain

Department of Medicine, School of Medicine, Universidad Complutense de Madrid, Madrid, Spain

Jimmy L. N. Vo Department of Medicine, Division of Endocrinology, Diabetes, and Metabolism, Vagelos College of Physicians and Surgeons, Columbia University Irving Medical Center, New York, NY, USA

Janice Wang Division of Pulmonary, Critical Care and Sleep Medicine, Donald and Barbara Zucker School of Medicine at Hofstra/Northwell, New Hyde Park, NY, USA

Justin Jihoon Yoon Advocate Aurora Health, Inc, Milwaukee, WI, USA

Part I
Pathophysiology

Chapter 1
COVID-19: Epidemiology, Etiology, Clinical Manifestations, Diagnosis, Therapeutic Options, and Prevention

Jaime E. Mogollon, Ghaleb Halaseh, and Neeraja Swaminathan

Etiology

The severe acute respiratory syndrome coronavirus 2 (SARS-CoV-2) is the causative agent of COVID-19 and an enveloped ribonucleic acid (RNA) virus. It is called a coronavirus (CoV) because of the crown of spike proteins on its surface. It originated in Wuhan, China, in December 2019 but rapidly spiraled into a global pandemic. The source of the virus is thought to be a novel coronavirus in bats as it has been noted to have significant structural similarity with prior CoV obtained from bats [1]. SARS-CoV-2 infects humans by binding to the angiotensin-converting enzyme 2 (ACE2) receptors of respiratory epithelial cells via the surface S spike glycoprotein. The evolution of new variants globally is a matter of concern as it has significant public health implications. The SARS-CoV-2 interagency group (SIG) divides these variants into subtypes. These include variants of concern (VOC), variants of interest (VUI), variants under monitoring (VUM), and variants of high consequences (VOHC). The important variants thus far described include Alpha, Beta, Gamma, Delta, and Omicron including the sub-lineages BA1 and BA2 [2]. By September 2022, Omicron was the most prevalent circulating variant. It was first identified in Botswana in November 2021. Omicron causes milder infection as compared to Delta, although this may be secondary to higher rates of vaccination globally [3]. The accumulated evidence suggests that most transmission is respiratory, with the virus suspended either on droplets or, less commonly, on aerosols. There is currently no conclusive evidence for fecal-oral, fomite, or direct contact transmission of SARS-CoV-2 in humans [4].

J. E. Mogollon (✉) · G. Halaseh · N. Swaminathan
Department of Medicine, Division of Infectious Diseases, Montefiore Albert Einstein, Bronx, NY, USA
e-mail: jmogollo@montefiore.org; ghalaseh@montefiore.org; nswaminath@montefiore.org

A. K. Myers (ed.), *Diabetes and COVID-19*, Contemporary Endocrinology, https://doi.org/10.1007/978-3-031-28536-3_1

Factors that impact morbidity and mortality include elderly age, premorbid conditions, and immunocompromised status [5]. Diabetes, hypertension, obesity, and smoking have contributed to a third of COVID-19-related deaths [6]. It is especially concerning because diabetes has a high prevalence and a rising incidence globally. As per the International Diabetes Federation, the global burden of diabetes mellitus is as high as 500 million adults as of 2019 and is expected to be over 600 million by the year 2035 [7]. The prevalence of diabetes in COVID-19 is estimated to be anywhere from 5% to 36% in various cohorts in and outside the United States [8]. Patients with diabetes are more likely to have adverse outcomes such as intensive care unit (ICU) admission, need for invasive ventilation, and death [9, 10]. A systematic review and meta-analysis that looked at 25,000 patients with COVID-19 identified that diabetes-associated mortality was as high as 22% [6, 11]. Plasma glucose levels have emerged as an independent risk factor for mortality (see more details in Chap. 8) [11]. In fact, one meta-analysis showed that diabetes was the biggest predictor for poor outcomes in COVID-19, more than even the presence of underlying lung disease like chronic obstructive pulmonary disease (COPD) and this was independent of age or gender [12].

The reasons for this are multifactorial and include the following (see Fig. 1.1):

1. Impaired immune function.
2. Upregulation of enzymes that mediate viral entry and decreased viral clearance.

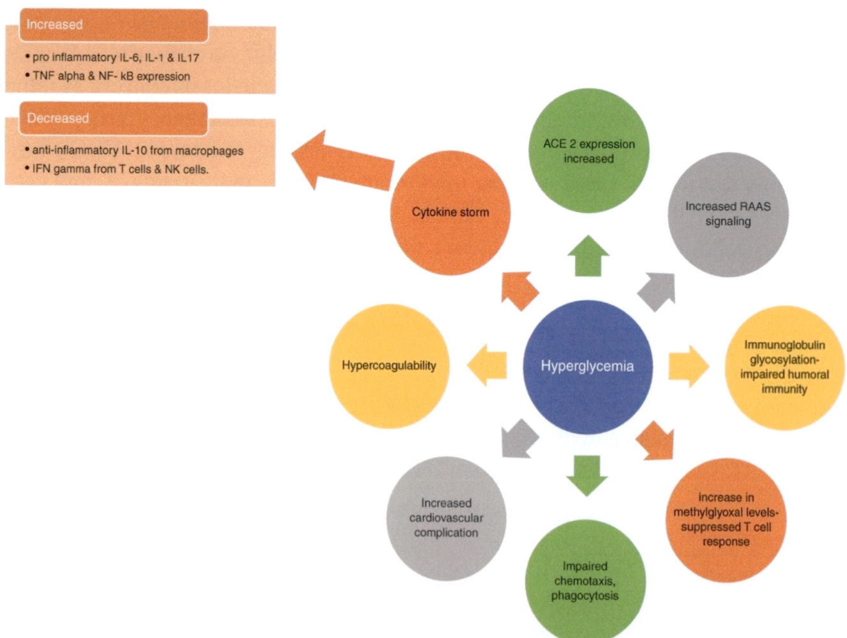

Fig. 1.1 The multiple mechanisms that increase the risk for more severe COVID-19 in persons with diabetes

3. Underlying chronic inflammatory state leading to increased risk of a cytokine storm.
4. Hypercoagulability.
5. Other comorbidities like cardiovascular disease, obesity, chronic kidney disease, etc. [7, 9, 10].

Viral entry into the cell is mediated by various protease enzymes, which cleave the S1 and S2 domains of the viral spike protein and cleave the C-terminal segment of the ACE-2 receptor. Expression of both ACE-2 and protease enzymes such as transmembrane serine protease 2 is increased in persons with diabetes [10].

Diabetes increases the predisposition for hypercoagulability as well, which is associated with COVID-19-related complications. Moreover, COVID-19 infection worsens hyperglycemia in persons with diabetes [10]. Apart from therapy like steroids which also results in hyperglycemia, the impact of the infection on the renin-angiotensin system causes increased insulin resistance, reduced blood supply to pancreatic islet cells, reduced insulin secretion, and a higher chance of diabetic ketoacidosis [7].

One of the mechanisms to explain the impact of diabetes on immunity is the increase in methylglyoxal levels which acts as a suppressor of myeloid and T cells. There is also immunoglobulin glycosylation, which impairs humoral immunity and complement activation. In diabetes, there is a decrease in IL-10 (anti-inflammatory cytokine) production from macrophages and reduced interferon gamma from T cells and NK cells. Hyperglycemia also inhibits neutrophil chemotaxis and phagocytosis. It has been shown that advanced glycation end products (AGEs) can lead to increased basal cytokine release which can be amplified in the setting of getting infected with COVID-19 [7]. Pro-inflammatory cytokines like IL-6, IL-1, and IL17 which in turn regulate the expression of TNF alpha and NF- kB have been noted to be more elevated in COVID-19 patients with concurrent diabetes. In patients with COVID-19 and diabetes, there has also been an elevation of inflammatory markers at admission like lactate dehydrogenase (LDH), C-Reactive protein (CRP), ferritin, D-dimer, and lymphopenia [13].

Clinical Manifestations

Once an individual is exposed to SARS-CoV-2, the incubation period is estimated to be anywhere from 2 to 14 days, although the median is 5 days. The median incubation period for the SARS-CoV-2 Omicron variant appears to be shorter with symptoms appearing within a median of 3 days [14]. The majority of patients with COVID-19 present common symptoms that include fever, shortness of breath, cough (either with or without sputum), sore throat, nasal congestion, dizziness, chills, muscle ache, arthralgia, weakness, fatigue or myalgia, chest tightness, excessive mucus production with expectoration, hemoptysis, and dyspnea [15].

Table 1.1 The National Institute of Health staging for the severity of COVID-19 [16]

Severity	Characteristics
Asymptomatic	Positive test, but no symptoms of COVID-19
Mild	Fever, cough, malaise, headache, myalgia, but no dyspnea and normal chest imaging
Moderate	Evidence of lower respiratory illness clinically or radiographically and oxygen saturation > 94% on room air at sea level
Severe	Oxygen saturation < 94% on room air at sea level and ratio of partial pressure of oxygen to fraction of inspired oxygen <300 mm Hg, tachypnea with respiratory rate > 30/min, or chest imaging with >50% lung infiltrates
Critical	Respiratory failure, septic shock, and/or multi-organ dysfunction

Based on the symptoms at presentation, the National Institute of Health (NIH) has proposed a classification of COVID as mild, moderate, severe, and critical as seen in Table 1.1. This is helpful in order to risk stratify the patients who are at the highest risk of decompensation and death and also have treatment implications.

While the commonest presentation of COVID-19 is a self-limiting viral illness like the flu or common cold, it can have a wide spectrum of systemic disease manifestations. These can be divided as follows:

1. Respiratory: Hypoxic respiratory failure secondary to acute respiratory distress syndrome (ARDS) is the most severe form of respiratory illness caused by COVID-19. However, it more often presents as pneumonia or an acute exacerbation of underlying reactive airway disease like asthma or COPD [17].

2. Cardiovascular: Cardiac manifestations of COVID-19 can be secondary to direct myocardial injury causing heart failure, myocarditis, arrhythmias, and acute coronary syndrome. An elevation of troponin levels is rather observed in a severe course of COVID-19, compared to mild or moderate courses. Increased levels of creatine kinase myocardial band (CK-MB), myohemoglobin, cardiac troponin I, and N-terminal pro-brain natriuretic peptide are associated with the severity of COVID-19 [15]. COVID-19 has been described to cause an acute viral myopericarditis like syndrome, pericardial effusion, or cardiac tamponade [18].

3. Gastrointestinal: The most common digestive symptoms in COVID-19 patients include nausea and/or vomiting, diarrhea, anorexia, or loss of appetite. SARS-CoV-2 infection might involve liver impairments of a wide spectrum of a severity degree. COVID-19 patients show increased levels of alanine transaminase (ALT) and aspartate aminotransferase (AST). Furthermore, serum bilirubin and gamma-glutamyl transferase (GGT) might also be elevated during the course of the disease [15].

4. Renal: Renal manifestations include acute kidney injury (AKI), proteinuria, and hematuria [19] (see Chap. 5 for more details).

5. Hematologic: Hematological complications predominantly include a hypercoagulable state which can lead to venous and arterial thrombosis [20].

6. Neurologic: Neurological manifestations are thought to occur due to viral invasion of the central and peripheral nervous systems through one or more of several portals of entries such as the olfactory pathway, blood-brain barrier and gut-brain axis. The symptoms are due to direct viral invasion, immune-mediated side effects, and hypercoagulability. Symptoms may be central or peripheral and include headache, fatigue, dizziness, confusion/delirium, cognitive changes, seizures, myoclonus, ataxia, neuropathy, vertigo, stroke with hemiplegia, or hemiparesis. Smell and taste disorders such as anosmia and dysgeusia have commonly been reported. Examples of other neurological presentations of COVID-19 include meningoencephalitis, Guillain-Barre Syndrome including the Miller-Fisher variant, and acute necrotizing encephalopathy [15].
7. Psychiatric: Symptoms described include paranoia, hallucinations, anxiety, and depression [21].
8. Dermatologic: Different dermatologic manifestations have been described including maculopapular, morbilliform, vesicular, livedo reticularis, and urticarial eruptions. Digital erythematous – purple nodular lesions known as "COVID toes" are also reported in patients with mild disease [22].
9. Ophthalmologic: SARS-CoV-2 presents its ability of ocular transmission, which might result in ocular manifestations; however, the prevalence of such incidents is extremely low. Ocular manifestations primarily include the onset of conjunctivitis, keratoconjunctivitis, or ocular irritation symptoms [15].

COVID-19 is also associated with an increased risk of secondary bacterial or fungal super-infections. In a study of close to 50,000 hospitalized COVID-19 patients in the UK, it was shown that close to one-fifth of them had positive blood or respiratory cultures that were clinically significant. Of this, the majority were due to *Staphylococcus aureus, Haemophilus influenzae*, and *Enterobacteriae* like *Escherichia coli* [23]. Invasive fungal infections include COVID-19-associated candidiasis, COVID-19-associated pulmonary aspergillosis, and COVID-19-associated mucormycosis (CAM). CAM is a condition for which diabetes is an independent risk factor, and it is especially important to recognize because of the extremely high risk of mortality. Most of the CAM is rhinocerebral and a small percentage is pulmonary. These superinfections are attributed to the immunomodulatory effects of COVID-19 as well as COVID-19 therapy which includes steroids and agents like tocilizumab, baricitinib, etc. [24].

Post-COVID-19 syndrome refers to clinical symptoms that persist for more than 4 weeks after the onset of initial symptoms and diagnosis. These include long COVID-19 or persistent post-COVID-19 symptoms and the effects of COVID-19 treatment and hospitalization. The most common persistent clinical manifestations post-COVID include: fatigue, dyspnea, alopecia, insomnia, hyperhidrosis, and arthralgia. Post-COVID-19 neuropsychiatric manifestations have also been described [25] (see Chap. 14 for further details).

Diagnosis

Diagnostics have proven to be fundamental to the COVID-19 pandemic response. Ideally, all symptomatic individuals or those who are either known or suspected of having been exposed to COVID-19 should be tested. Also testing should be done in asymptomatic individuals with no known contact with COVID-19 who are being hospitalized in areas with a high or low prevalence of COVID-19 in the community.

An exceptional number of diagnostic tests have been developed for COVID-19 using the latest available technologies. Three types of diagnostic tests are relevant to patient management and pandemic control: molecular or nucleic acid amplification tests [e.g., Polymerase Chain Reaction (PCR) tests] that detect SARS-CoV-2 RNA; antigen tests that detect viral proteins (e.g., nucleocapsid or spike proteins); and serology tests that detect host antibodies in response to infection, immunization, or both [26]. Molecular tests such as PCR are highly sensitive and specific at detecting viral RNA and are recommended by the WHO for confirming the diagnosis in individuals who are symptomatic and for activating public health surveillance. Antigen rapid detection tests also called home tests detect viral proteins and have the advantages of being easier to do, giving a faster time to result, a lower cost, and the ability to detect infection in those who are most likely to be at risk of transmitting the virus to others. Antigen tests have a sensitivity of 70% with 99% specificity [27]. Antigen rapid detection tests can be used as a public health tool for screening individuals at enhanced risk of infection, to protect people who are clinically vulnerable, to ensure safe travel and the resumption of schooling and social activities, as well to enable economic recovery strategies. One strategy is to target people attending workplaces in which prolonged daily indoor contact occurs. Another is to target people attending large gatherings in indoor spaces (eg, nightclubs, bars, and karaoke lounges) and indoor or outdoor mass gatherings for religious, sports, music, or other purposes. Antibodies serum levels, which detect the host response to infection or vaccination, can be useful as surveillance tools to advise public policy but should not be used to provide proof of immunity, as the correlates of protection remain unclear [28].

Management

Over the course of the pandemic, periods of time characterized by significant surges in the rates of individuals infected with SARS-CoV-2 severely tested the supply of essential medical items, including, but not limited to, personal protective equipment, and in later surges, the supply of newly developed or repurposed therapeutics [29]. In response to this, a strategy to triage those who are at the highest risk of developing severe illness, and therefore most likely to benefit from therapy such as monoclonal antibodies or antiviral therapy, was developed. The four key elements were: age, vaccination status, immune status, and clinical risk factors. Unvaccinated, immunocompromised, and older individuals with risk factors for developing severe COVID-19 were prioritized [16, 30].

Depending on risk factors, patients with confirmed or suspected COVID-19 should be categorized as higher risk, suggestive of higher risk, and mixed evidence. The higher risk conditions include, but are not limited to, asthma; chronic lung, liver, or heart disease; diabetes mellitus type 1 or 2; human immunodeficiency virus infection; obesity; and pregnancy. Overweight status and substance use disorders are grouped in the suggestive of higher risk category, and conditions such as hypertension and hepatitis B or C are included in the mixed evidence group [31].

Outpatient Management

In the absence of severe shortages in medical supplies necessitating the triage of hospital beds and therapeutics, all individuals with any high-risk condition should be offered treatment. This includes individuals aged 65 and older, those who are unvaccinated, and immunocompromised individuals.

In the face of an evolving pandemic and emerging variants, the data informing the clinical decision of managing patients on an outpatient or inpatient basis are under constant review. However, the principles remain the same: In general, the majority of patients with COVID-19 are appropriate for outpatient management (see Chap. 10). In the absence of clear indications for hospitalization, such as severe dyspnea, hypoxemia, or hemodynamic instability, an individualized risk stratification strategy is appropriate. Several tools have been developed to aid in the decision-making process across medical centers, including patient self-assessment tools, phone triage, and telehealth visits [32]. The overall aim of the tools is to measure the patient's current necessary level of medical care, and/or their risk for disease progression. Based on the above four key elements, an informed clinical decision can be taken in conjunction with the patient. As with many other medical conditions managed on the outpatient side, an assessment of a patient's capability to recognize red flag signs and symptoms, as well as their social support system, is vital. In addition, knowledge of the clinical course of COVID-19 is essential. While many patients might not meet strict criteria for inpatient admission at the time of assessment, the trajectory of their symptoms (i.e., mild dyspnea that is worsening over several days) might herald the development of severe illness, and many of these patients may require in-person evaluation at a minimum.

Therapeutics

Listed on the next page are (Table 1.2) available treatments for the management of high-risk patients with COVID-19 in the ambulatory setting. While the Infectious Disease Society of America (IDSA) does not explicitly list its preferred therapy, the

Table 1.2 Therapeutic options for the management of COVID-19 in the ambulatory setting [33]

Drug name	Mechanism of action	Dosing	Side effects	Contraindications	Notes
Remdesivir	Inhibition of the SARS-CoV-2 RNA polymerase which is central to its replication	*200 mg IV loading dose on day 1, followed by 100 mg IV daily on days 2 and 3.*	Acute kidney injury Elevated liver function tests Gastrointestinal upset	Hypersensitivity Use with caution in eGFR <30 mL/min, toxicity unlikely with 3–5 day course	*Remdesivir is expected to maintain efficacy against all Omicron subvariants, although clinical data is lacking.* *Window of therapy: Within 7 days*
Monoclonal antibodies	Laboratory-made antibody molecules that target the spike protein portion of the SARS-CoV-2 virus	*Bebtelovimab IV 175 mg once*	Infusion reactions	Hypersensitivity	*Bebtelovimab demonstrated* in vitro *activity against all circulating Omicron subvariants, but clinical data is lacking.* *Window of therapy: Within 7 days*
Nirmaltrevir-Ritonavir	Nirmaltrevir is a SARS-CoV-2-3CL protease inhibitor, which is vital for viral replication. Ritonavir is used to slow down the metabolism of Nirmaltrevir	*Nirmaltrelvir 300 mg and Ritonavir 100 mg every 12 h for 5 days*	Rebound phenomenon Hepatic dysfunction Metallic taste in mouth	Hypersensitivity	*Significant drug-drug interactions exist and must be checked prior to prescribing* *Window of therapy:* *Within 5 days*
Molnupiravir	Nucleoside analog that inhibits viral replication	*Molnupiravir 800 mg every 12 h for 5 days*	Dermatologic: Skin rash, etc.	Hypersensitivity	*Window of therapy:* *Within 5 days*
High-titer convalescent plasma	Passive immunotherapy	Optimal dosing has not been defined, commonly administered as 1–2 units (200–250 mL per unit) once	Transfusion reactions (ex. transfusion-associated circulatory overload, transfusion-related acute lung injury, etc.)	Hypersensitivity	*FDA EUA only authorizes use in patients with immunosuppressive disease or receiving immunosuppressive treatment* *Window of therapy: Within 8 days of symptom onset, although maximum benefit is seen within 3 days* [34–36]

National Institute of Health (NIH's) order of preference is: Nirmatrelvir-ritonavir, followed by Remdesivir, monoclonal antibodies (MAbs), Molnupiravir and finally, high-titer antibody convalescent plasma [29]. This takes into account the ease of administration (i.e., whether intravenous access and/or an infusion center is required), efficacy in the context of emerging variants, and potential side effects.

Inpatient Management

The management of patients admitted with COVID-19 depends on the severity of illness. It is now known that COVID-19's clinical course is broadly divided into an early viremic phase and a later inflammatory phase. The viremic phase is driven by viral replication and is characterized by upper respiratory symptoms, and if progression ensues to involve the lower respiratory tract, it leads to the development of dyspnea and hypoxemia. The latter phase is characterized by what was earlier likened to a "cytokine storm syndrome" or macrophage activation syndrome, characterized by profound hypoxemia, ARDS, hemodynamic instability, and eventual progression to multi-organ failure.

In general, therapies are targeted toward reducing viral replication and progression of illness, or toward dampening the hyper-inflammatory immune response to the virus using immunomodulators.

The general issues surrounding management are:

- Coexistence of bacterial pneumonia: The incidence of concomitant bacterial pneumonia from the community is very low, with one meta-analysis estimating it at 3.5% [37]. Empiric antibiotic therapy in patients with COVID-19 is not indicated, unless there is a reasonable degree of suspicion for bacterial co-infection (i.e., leukocytosis, focal or lobar infiltrate, positive cultures) [38, 39].
- Supportive management: including but not limited to antipyretics and oxygen supplementation.
- Thromboprophylaxis: Unless a contraindication is present, all hospitalized patients with COVID-19 should receive thromboprophylaxis. Prophylactic doses of low-molecular weight or unfractionated heparin are preferred, given heparin's short half-life and ability to be reversed if required. For non-critically ill patients on low-flow oxygen, therapeutic doses of heparin are recommended. This recommendation is based on multiple trials (REMAP-CAP, ACTIV-4a, and ATTACC) that showed that those with moderate disease (see Table 1.3) treated with a therapeutic dose of anticoagulation had improved survival rates and required less organ support after 21 days compared to those who had care as usual [16].
- Immunomodulators: Corticosteroids, IL-6, and JAK inhibitors are the most widely studied immunomodulators with demonstrated efficacy in patients who have theoretically progressed to the hyper-inflammatory phase. In addition to their immunomodulatory effects, JAK inhibitors are thought to interfere with viral entry [16].

Table 1.3 Management of COVID-19 inpatients as per NIH guidelines [16]

Severity of illness	Therapeutics	Thromboprophylaxis	Notes
Hospitalized but does not require supplemental oxygen	Recommendation against the use of Dexamethasone. Insufficient evidence for use of Remdesivir, use may be appropriate in high-risk patients	Prophylactic dose of heparin	There is a lack of data regarding the safety and efficacy of corticosteroids in patients who do not require supplemental oxygen, and a theoretical risk of dampening the host's immune response to the virus at an early stage, possibly accelerating viral replication resulting in worse outcomes.
Hospitalized and requires supplemental oxygen through nasal cannula	Dexamethasone and Remdesivir. Consider adding Baricitinib or Tocilizumab if rapidly escalating oxygen requirements.	Prophylactic dose of heparin. Non-pregnant patients with elevated D-dimer: therapeutic dose of heparin.	Based on the RECOVERY trial in the UK, a significant mortality benefit was seen with the use of Dexamethasone in hospitalized patients requiring supplemental oxygen. The addition of IL-6 or JAK inhibitors is based on the potential benefit in select patients on low-flow oxygen seen in subgroup analyses of the RECOVERY trial. However, there is no consensus on which patients would benefit from them.
Hospitalized and requires supplemental oxygen through high-flow nasal cannula or non-invasive ventilation	Dexamethasone and Remdesivir. Consider adding Baricitinib or Tocilizumb if rapidly escalating oxygen requirements.	Prophylactic dose of heparin.	Data from the REMAP-CAP and RECOVERY trials demonstrated a mortality benefit for the addition of IL-6 inhibitors to corticosteroids in patients who rapidly progress to require high-flow oxygen or non-invasive ventilation.
Hospitalized and requires mechanical ventilation or extracorporeal membrane oxygenation	Dexamethasone and Tocilizumab.	Prophylactic dose of heparin.	The use of remdesivir is unlikely to be beneficial during the hyper-inflammatory phase (i.e., in patients on MV/ECMO) as viral replication has already taken place.

– *Note: The use of immunomodulators may place patients at an increased risk of acquiring infections or reactivation of latent infections. It is reasonable to empirically treat for Strongyloidiasis, for example, in patients from endemic regions prior to the availability of test results.*

There are several methods of categorizing the severity of illness; however, as consistent with the NIH's published COVID-19 guidelines, we use the patient's oxygen requirement as a guide.

Prevention

Throughout the COVID-19 pandemic, several community and health-care-based measures have been implemented to slow and prevent viral transmission. However, the general principles remain the same: preventative measures target the virus' main methods of transmission, via large droplets and aerosols [4, 40]. The CDC recommends that all individuals over the age of 2 years old wear well-fitting masks, especially in areas of high community transmission [41]. High-quality data have demonstrated the efficacy of wearing masks at both an individual and community level, particularly when higher quality masks such as the N95 masks are properly fitted and utilized [42]. In addition, the CDC also recommends social distancing, avoiding crowds and poorly ventilated areas when possible, as well as frequent hand washing among other general hygiene measures [41].

1. Vaccination

   There are currently four COVID-19 vaccines that have been either granted emergency use authorization (EUA) or full FDA approval in the United States, with several high-quality trials demonstrating excellent efficacy data and safety profiles [43–51]. Due to waning protection and the emergence of varying degrees of immune escape associated with the Omicron subvariants 30–33, the CDC recommends additional booster shots. The FDA granted emergency use authorization to Moderna and Pfizer-BioNTech's Omicron-specific boosters in late August 2022 [52].

2. Testing

   Especially recommended when displaying symptoms of COVID-19.

   (See "Diagnosis" for more detailed information regarding testing.)

3. Pre-exposure prophylaxis.

   Indicated for certain groups, such as those that have immunosuppressive conditions or are on immunosuppressive medications which will prevent them to mount an adequate immune response to the vaccines. Those individuals that experienced severe adverse events to COVID-19 vaccines are also included. In this cases the FDA recommends a monoclonal antibody cocktail of tixagevimab-cilgavimab which is administered as two separate intravenous injections, with a significant degree of protection expected for up to 6 months. The doses utilized are two times greater than the dose approved, which is due to in vitro studies demonstrating reduced neutralizing activity against the Omicron variants [53, 54].

4. Masking

Mask wearing has been shown to be effective in reducing the risk of infection for individuals and reducing community transmission in areas where government mask mandates were in place [55, 56]. Based on COVID-19 transmission levels in the community, the CDC now categorizes community levels as low (green), medium (yellow), and high (orange). Based on these categories, the CDC recommends a set of preventive actions individuals can take to protect themselves [57]. In situations where masks are recommended, masks with the highest filtration efficacy (i.e., N95 or surgical masks) should be worn reliably over the mouth and nose [58].

5. Social distancing

Close contact with infected individuals is one of the primary risks of exposure. The rationale behind social distancing is to reduce that exposure risk. Despite the appropriate distance not being clearly defined, a minimum distance of 6 feet was widely used during the pandemic. In one meta-analysis examining distance and infection risk with regards to coronaviruses including SARS-CoV-2, proximity and risk of infection were closely associated [59].

Conclusions

In this chapter we have summarized the etiology, clinical manifestations, therapeutic options, and preventive measures regarding the ongoing COVID-19 pandemic. Both type 1 and type 2 diabetes mellitus are major risk factors to develop complications from COVID-19. Symptoms and signs of COVID-19 are broad, from asymptomatic individuals to a vast majority of patients with mild symptoms up to severe complications such as ARDS or multi-organ failure. In addition we have reviewed diagnostic tools, therapeutic options, and preventive measures, vaccines being one of the most important instruments, all of which have allowed the control of the pandemic and the return to a certain level of normal activities across the globe.

References

1. Domingo JL. What we know and what we need to know about the origin of SARS-CoV-2. Environ Res. 2022). Epub 20220826; https://doi.org/10.1016/j.envres.2022.114131.
2. Zella D, Giovanetti M, Benedetti F, Unali F, Spoto S, Guarino M, Angeletti S, Ciccozzi M. The variants question: what is the problem? J Med Virol. 2021;93(12):6479–85. https://doi.org/10.1002/jmv.27196. Epub 2021 Jul 28. PMID: 34255352; PMCID: PMC8426965

3. Ortega M, García-Montero C, Fraile-Martinez O, Colet P, Baizhaxynova A, Mukhtarova K, Alvarez-Mon M, Kanatova K, Asúnsolo A, Sarría-Santamera A. Recapping the features of SARS-CoV-2 and its Main variants: status and future paths. J Pers Med. 2022;12(6):995.
4. Meyerowitz EA, Richterman A, Gandhi RT, Sax PE. (2020) Transmission of SARS-CoV-2: a review of viral, host, and environmental factors. Ann Intern Med. 2021;174(1):69. Epub 2020 Sep 17
5. Nguyen H, Medina A, Golovko G, Evangelista L. Racial and ethnic differences in fatality risk from COVID-19. SAGE Open Nurs. 2022; https://doi.org/10.1177/23779608221107591. PMID: 35769608; PMCID: PMC9234924
6. Mahamat-Saleh Y, Fiolet T, Rebeaud ME, Mulot M, Guihur A, El Fatouhi D, Laouali N, Peiffer-Smadja N, Aune D, Severi G. Diabetes, hypertension, body mass index, smoking and COVID-19-related mortality: a systematic review and meta-analysis of observational studies. BMJ Open. 2021;11(10):e052777. https://doi.org/10.1136/bmjopen-2021-052777. PMID: 34697120; PMCID: PMC8557249
7. Yin Y, Rohli KE, Shen P, et al. The epidemiology, pathophysiological mechanisms, and management toward COVID-19 patients with type 2 diabetes: a systematic review. Prim Care Diabetes. 2021;15(6):899–909. https://doi.org/10.1016/j.pcd.2021.08.014. PMID: 34600859; PMCID: PMC8418914
8. Singh AK, Gupta R, Ghosh A, Misra A. Diabetes in COVID-19: prevalence, pathophysiology, prognosis and practical considerations. Diabetes Metab Syndr. 2020;14(4):303–10. https://doi.org/10.1016/j.dsx.2020.04.004. Epub 2020 Apr 9. PMID: 32298981; PMCID: PMC7195120
9. Vidhya Rekha U, Anita M, Bhuminathan S, Sadhana K. Known data on CoVid-19 infection linked to type-2 diabetes. Bioinformation. 2021;17(8):772–5. https://doi.org/10.6026/97320630017772. PMID: 35540698; PMCID: PMC9049093
10. Gupta P, Gupta M, KAtoch N, Garg K, Garg B. A systematic review and meta-analysis of diabetes associated mortality in patients with COVID-19. Int J Endocrinol Metab. 2021;19(4):e113220. https://doi.org/10.5812/ijem.113220. PMID: 35069750; PMCID: PMC8762284
11. Schlesinger S, Neuenschwander M, Lang A, Pafili K, Kuss O, Herder C, Roden M. Risk phenotypes of diabetes and association with COVID-19 severity and death: a living systematic review and meta-analysis. Diabetologia. 2021;64(7):1480–91. https://doi.org/10.1007/s00125-021-05458-8. Epub 2021 Apr 28. PMID: 33907860; PMCID: PMC8079163
12. Corona G, Pizzocaro A, Vena W, Rastrelli G, Semeraro F, Isidori AM, Pivonello R, Salonia A, Sforza A, Maggi M. Diabetes is most important cause for mortality in COVID-19 hospitalized patients: systematic review and meta-analysis. Rev Endocr Metab Disord. 2021;22(2):275–96. https://doi.org/10.1007/s11154-021-09630-8. Epub 2021 Feb 22. PMID: 33616801; PMCID: PMC7899074
13. Srivastava A, Rockman-Greenberg C, Sareen N, Lionetti V, Dhingra S. An insight into the mechanisms of COVID-19, SARS-CoV2 infection severity concerning β-cell survival and cardiovascular conditions in diabetic patients. Mol Cell Biochem. 2022;477(6):1681–95. https://doi.org/10.1007/s11010-022-04396-2. Epub 2022 Mar 2. PMID: 35235124; PMCID: PMC8889522
14. Jansen L, Tegomoh B, Lange K, Showalter K, Figliomeni J, Abdalhamid B, Iwen PC, Fauver J, Buss B, Donahue M. Investigation of a SARS-CoV-2 B.1.1.529 (omicron) variant cluster—Nebraska, November-December 2021. MMWR Morb Mortal Wkly Rep. 2021;70(5152):1782–4. https://doi.org/10.15585/mmwr.mm705152e3. PMID: 34968376; PMCID: PMC8736273
15. Baj J, Karakuła-Juchnowicz H, Teresiński G, Buszewicz G, Ciesielka M, Sitarz R, Forma A, Karakuła K, Flieger W, Portincasa P, Maciejewski R. COVID-19: specific and non-specific clinical manifestations and symptoms: the current state of knowledge. J Clin Med. 2020;9(6):1753. https://doi.org/10.3390/jcm9061753. PMID: 32516940; PMCID: PMC7356953
16. COVID-19 Treatment Guidelines Panel. Coronavirus disease 2019 (COVID-19) treatment guidelines. National Institutes of Health; 2022. https://www.covid19treatmentguidelines.nih.gov/

17. Li K, Wu J, Wu F, Guo D, Chen L, Fang Z, Li C. The clinical and chest CT features associated with severe and critical COVID-19 pneumonia. Investig Radiol. 2020;55(6):327–31. https://doi.org/10.1097/RLI.0000000000000672. PMID: 32118615; PMCID: PMC7147273

18. Cushion S, Arboleda V, Hasanain Y, Demory Beckler M, Hardigan P, Kesselman MM. Comorbidities and symptomatology of SARS-CoV-2 (severe acute respiratory syndrome coronavirus 2)-related myocarditis and SARS-CoV-2 vaccine-related myocarditis: a review. Cureus. 2022;14(4):e24084. https://doi.org/10.7759/cureus.24084. PMID: 35573496; PMCID: PMC9099161

19. Menez S, Parikh CR. Overview of acute kidney manifestations and management of patients with COVID-19. Am J Physiol Ren Physiol. 2021;321:F403–10.

20. Len P, Iskakova G, Sautbayeva Z, Kussanova A, Tauekelova AT, Sugralimova MM, Dautbaeva AS, Abdieva MM, Ponomarev ED, Tikhonov A, Bekbossynova MS, Barteneva NS. Meta-analysis and systematic review of coagulation disbalances in COVID-19: 41 studies and 17,601 patients. Front Cardiovasc Med. 2022;9:794092. https://doi.org/10.3389/fcvm.2022.794092. PMID: 35360017; PMCID: PMC8962835

21. Varatharaj A, Thomas N, Ellul MA, Davies NWS, Pollak TA, Tenorio EL, Sultan M, Easton A, Breen G, Zandi M, Coles JP, Manji H, Al-Shahi Salman R, Menon DK, Nicholson TR, Benjamin LA, Carson A, Smith C, Turner MR, Solomon T, Kneen R, Pett SL, Galea I, Thomas RH, Michael BD, CoroNerve Study Group. Neurological and neuropsychiatric complications of COVID-19 in 153 patients: a UK-wide surveillance study. Lancet Psychiatry. 2020;7(10):875. Epub 2020 Jun 25

22. Galván Casas C, Català A, Carretero Hernández G, Rodríguez-Jiménez P, Fernández-Nieto D, Rodríguez-Villa Lario A, Navarro Fernández I, Ruiz-Villaverde R, Falkenhain-López D, Llamas Velasco M, García-Gavín J, Baniandrés O, González-Cruz C, Morillas-Lahuerta V, Cubiró X, Figueras Nart I, Selda-Enriquez G, Romaní J, Fustà-Novell X, Melian-Olivera A, Roncero Riesco M, Burgos-Blasco P, Sola Ortigosa J, Feito Rodriguez M, García-Doval I. Classification of the cutaneous manifestations of COVID-19: a rapid prospective nationwide consensus study in Spain with 375 cases. Br J Dermatol. 2020;183(1):71–7. https://doi.org/10.1111/bjd.19163. Epub 2020 Jun 10. PMID: 32348545; PMCID: PMC7267236

23. Russell CD, Fairfield CJ, Drake TM, Turtle L, Seaton RA, Wootton DG, Sigfrid L, Harrison EM, Docherty AB, de Silva TI, Egan C, Pius R, Hardwick HE, Merson L, Girvan M, Dunning J, Nguyen-Van-Tam JS, PJM O, Baillie JK, Semple MG, Ho A, ISARIC4C investigators. Co-infections, secondary infections, and antimicrobial use in patients hospitalised with COVID-19 during the first pandemic wave from the ISARIC WHO CCP-UK study: a multicentre, prospective cohort study. Lancet Microbe. 2021;2(8):e354–65. https://doi.org/10.1016/S2666-5247(21)00090-2. Epub 2021 Jun 2. PMID: 34100002; PMCID: PMC8172149

24. Watanabe A, So M, Mitaka H, Ishisaka Y, Takagi H, Inokuchi R, Iwagami M, Kuno T. Clinical features and mortality of COVID-19-associated mucormycosis: a systematic review and meta-analysis. Mycopathologia. 2022;187(2–3):271–89. https://doi.org/10.1007/s11046-022-00627-8. Epub 2022 Mar 21. PMID: 35312945; PMCID: PMC8935886

25. Almas T, Malik J, Alsubai AK, Jawad Zaidi SM, Iqbal R, Khan K, Ali M, Ishaq U, Alsufyani M, Hadeed S, Alsufyani R, Ahmed R, Thakur T, Antony M, Antony I, Bhullar A, Kotait F, Al-Ani L. Post-acute COVID-19 syndrome and its prolonged effects: an updated systematic review. Ann Med Surg (Lond). 2022; https://doi.org/10.1016/j.amsu.2022.103995. Epub ahead of print. PMID: 35721785; PMCID: PMC9197790

26. Centers for Disease Control and Prevention. Overview of testing for SARS-CoV-2. 2022. https://www.cdc.gov/coronavirus/2019-ncov/hcp/testing-overview.html

27. Infectious Diseases Society of America Guidelines on the Diagnosis of COVID-19 (2021). https://www.idsociety.org/practice-guideline/covid-19-guideline-diagnostics/

28. Peeling R, Heymann D, Teo Y-Y, Garcia P. Diagnostics for COVID-19: moving from pandemic response to control. Lancet. 2021;399 https://doi.org/10.1016/S0140-6736(21)02346-1.

29. National Institute of Health (NIH) COVID-19 Treatment Guidelines (2022). https://www.covid19treatmentguidelines.nih.gov/overview/clinical-spectrum/.

30. Infectious Diseases Society of America. COVID-19 Guideline, Part 1: Treatment and Management. 2022. https://www.idsociety.org/practice-guideline/covid-19-guideline-treatment-and-management/.
31. Centers for Disease Control and Prevention. Covid-19 treatments and medications. In: Centers for Disease Control and Prevention 2022. https://www.cdc.gov/coronavirus/2019-ncov/your-health/treatments-for-severe-illness.html
32. Mehring WM, Poksay A, Kriege J, Prasannappa R, Wang MD, Hendel C, Hochman M. Initial experience with a COVID-19 web-based patient self-assessment tool. J Gen Intern Med. 2020;35(9):2821–2. https://doi.org/10.1007/s11606-020-05893-0. Epub 2020 Jun 15. PMID: 32542495; PMCID: PMC7294986
33. COVID-19 Treatment Guidelines Panel. Coronavirus disease 2019 (COVID-19) therapeutic management of nonhospitalized adults with COVID-19 National Institutes of Health 2022. https://www.covid19treatmentguidelines.nih.gov/management/clinical-management-of-adults/nonhospitalized-adults%2D%2Dtherapeutic-management/.
34. Piechotta V, Iannizzi C, Chai KL, et al. Convalescent plasma or hyperimmune immunoglobulin for people with COVID-19: a living systematic review. Cochrane Database Syst Rev. 2021; https://doi.org/10.1002/14651858.cd013600.pub4.
35. Ortigoza MB, Yoon H, Goldfeld KS, et al. Efficacy and safety of COVID-19 convalescent plasma in hospitalized patients. JAMA Intern Med. 2022;182:115.
36. U.S. Food and Drug Administration. Convalescent Plasma Eua Fact Sheet for healthcare providers. In: Recommendations for Investigational COVID-19 Convalescent Plasma. 2021. https://www.fda.gov/media/141478/download. Accessed 14 Jul 2022.
37. Langford BJ, So M, Raybardhan S, Leung V, Westwood D, MacFadden DR, Soucy JR, Daneman N. Bacterial co-infection and secondary infection in patients with COVID-19: a living rapid review and meta-analysis. Clin Microbiol Infect. 2020;26(12):1622–9. https://doi.org/10.1016/j.cmi.2020.07.016. Epub 2020 Jul 22. PMID: 32711058; PMCID: PMC7832079
38. Kubin CJ, McConville TH, Dietz D, et al. Characterization of bacterial and fungal infections in hospitalized patients with coronavirus disease 2019 and factors associated with health care-associated infections. Open Forum Infect Dis. 2021; https://doi.org/10.1093/ofid/ofab201.
39. Kim D, Quinn J, Pinsky B, Shah NH, Brown I. Rates of co-infection between SARS-COV-2 and other respiratory pathogens. JAMA. 2020;323:2085.
40. Duval D, Palmer JC, Tudge I, Pearce-Smith N, O'Connell E, Bennett A, Clark R. Long distance airborne transmission of SARS-COV-2: rapid systematic review. BMJ. 2022; https://doi.org/10.1136/bmj-2021-068743.
41. Centers for Disease Control and Prevention How to protect yourself & others. In: Centers for Disease Control and Prevention. 2022. https://www.cdc.gov/coronavirus/2019-ncov/prevent-getting-sick/prevention.html
42. Andrejko KL, Pry JM, Myers JF, et al. Effectiveness of facemask or respirator use in indoor public settings for prevention of SARS-COV-2 infection—California, February–December 2021. MMWR Morb Mortal Wkly Rep. 2022;71:212–6.
43. Polack FP, Thomas SJ, Kitchin N, et al. Safety and efficacy of the BNT162B2 mRNA covid-19 vaccine. N Engl J Med. 2020;383:2603–15.
44. Baden LR, El Sahly HM, Essink B, et al. Efficacy and safety of the mrna-1273 SARS-COV-2 vaccine. N Engl J Med. 2021;384:403–16.
45. Sadoff J, Gray G, Vandebosch A, et al. Safety and efficacy of single-dose Ad26.COV2.S vaccine against covid-19. N Engl J Med. 2021;384:2187–201.
46. Dunkle LM, Kotloff KL, Gay CL, et al. Efficacy and safety of NVX-cov2373 in adults in the United States and Mexico. N Engl J Med. 2022;386:531–43.
47. Baden LR, El Sahly HM, Essink B, et al. Phase 3 trial of mRNA-1273 during the delta-variant surge. N Engl J Med. 2021;385:2485–7.
48. Israel A, Merzon E, Schäffer AA, Shenhar Y, Green I, Golan-Cohen A, Ruppin E, Magen E, Vinker S. Elapsed time since BNT162b2 vaccine and risk of SARS-COV-2 infection: test negative design study. BMJ. 2021; https://doi.org/10.1136/bmj-2021-067873.

49. Nordström P, Ballin M, Nordström A. Risk of infection, hospitalization, and death up to 9 months after a second dose of COVID-19 vaccine: a retrospective, total population cohort study in Sweden. Lancet. 2022;399:814–23.
50. Bar-On YM, Goldberg Y, Mandel M, Bodenheimer O, Freedman L, Alroy-Preis S, Ash N, Huppert A, Milo R. Protection against covid-19 by BNT162B2 booster across age groups. N Engl J Med. 2021;385:2421–30.
51. Moreira ED, Kitchin N, Xu X, et al. Safety and efficacy of a third dose of BNT162B2 covid-19 vaccine. N Engl J Med. 2022;386:1910–21.
52. https://www.cdc.gov/media/releases/2022/s0901-covid-19-booster.html
53. Takashita E, Kinoshita N, Yamayoshi S, et al. Efficacy of antibodies and antiviral drugs against covid-19 omicron variant. N Engl J Med. 2022;386:995–8.
54. Bruel T, Hadjadj J, Maes P, et al. Serum neutralization of SARS-COV-2 omicron sublineages BA.1 and BA.2 in patients receiving monoclonal antibodies. Nat Med. 2022;28:1297–302.
55. Rader B, White LF, Burns MR, Chen J, Brilliant J, Cohen J, Shaman J, Brilliant L, Kraemer MUG, Hawkins JB, Scarpino SV, Astley CM, Brownstein JS. Mask wearing and control of SARS-CoV-2 transmission in the United States. medRxiv [Preprint]. 2020 Sep 1:2020.08.23.20078964. doi: 10.1101/2020.08.23.20078964. Update in: Lancet Digit Health. 2021 Mar;3(3):e148-e157. PMID: 32869039; PMCID: PMC7457618.
56. Van Dyke ME, Rogers TM, Pevzner E, et al. Trends in county-level COVID-19 incidence in counties with and without a mask mandate — Kansas, June 1–august 23, 2020. MMWR Morb Mortal Wkly Rep. 2020;69:1777–81. https://doi.org/10.15585/mmwr.mm6947e2externalicon.
57. Centers for Disease Control and Prevention Covid-19 by County. In: Centers for Disease Control and Prevention 2022. https://www.cdc.gov/coronavirus/2019-ncov/your-health/covid-by-county.html.
58. https://www.cdc.gov/coronavirus/2019-ncov/prevent-getting-sick/types-of-masks.html
59. Chu DK, Akl EA, Duda S, Solo K, Yaacoub S, Schünemann HJ. COVID-19 Systematic Urgent Review Group Effort (SURGE) study authors. Physical distancing, face masks, and eye protection to prevent person-to-person transmission of SARS-CoV-2 and COVID-19: a systematic review and meta-analysis. Lancet. 2020;395(10242):1973–87. https://doi.org/10.1016/S0140-6736(20)31142-9. Epub 2020 Jun 1. PMID: 32497510; PMCID: PMC7263814

Chapter 2
Pathophysiology: How COVID-19 Impacts the Pancreas and Peripheral Insulin Resistance

Cecilia C. Low Wang, Stacey A. Seggelke, Michael T. McDermott, and Jane E. B. Reusch

C. C. Low Wang (✉)
Glucose Management Team, University of Colorado Hospital, Aurora, CO, USA

CPC Clinical Research, Aurora, CO, USA

Department of Medicine, Division of Endocrinology, Metabolism and Diabetes, University of Colorado Anschutz Medical Campus School of Medicine, Aurora, CO, USA
e-mail: cecilia.lowwang@cuanschutz.edu

S. A. Seggelke
University of Colorado College of Nursing, University of Colorado Anschutz Medical Campus, Aurora, CO, USA

Department of Medicine, Division of Endocrinology, Metabolism and Diabetes, University of Colorado Anschutz Medical Campus School of Medicine, Aurora, CO, USA
e-mail: Stacey.Seggelke@cuanschutz.edu

M. T. McDermott
Division of Endocrinology, Metabolism and Diabetes, Department of Medicine, University of Colorado Anschutz Medical Campus School of Medicine, Aurora, CO, USA

Endocrinology and Diabetes Practice, University of Colorado Hospital, Aurora, CO, USA
e-mail: Michael.McDermott@cuanschutz.edu

J. E. B. Reusch
Division of Endocrinology, Metabolism and Diabetes, University of Colorado-Anschutz Medical Campus, Aurora, CO, USA

Center for Women's Health Research, University of Colorado-Anschutz Medical Campus, Aurora, CO, USA

University of Colorado NIH Diabetes Research Center, University of Colorado-Anschutz Medical Campus, Aurora, CO, USA

Departments of Medicine, Integrative Physiology, and Bioengineering, University of Colorado-Anschutz Medical Campus, Aurora, CO, USA

Rocky Mountain Regional VAMC, Aurora, CO, USA
e-mail: Jane.Reusch@cuanschutz.edu

A. K. Myers (ed.), *Diabetes and COVID-19*, Contemporary Endocrinology,
https://doi.org/10.1007/978-3-031-28536-3_2

19

Background

As the novel coronavirus SARS-CoV-2 swept through communities and populations globally during the COVID-19 pandemic, astute clinical observations drove basic investigation and vice versa, while knowledge about COVID-19 infection has continued to evolve. One of these clinical observations is the propensity for more severe COVID-19 illness in individuals with diabetes and/or obesity [1, 2]; another was the new-onset of diabetes in individuals with COVID-19 infection [3–12]. These observations have prompted intensive investigations into how SARS-CoV-2 causes infection in the pancreas and in the periphery. This chapter will discuss evidence for COVID-19 infection in the pancreas and mechanisms of peripheral insulin resistance.

COVID-19 Infection and the Pancreas

Disseminating information as quickly as possible was of the highest priority early on during the COVID-19 pandemic, with the goal of informing clinicians and scientists around the world working to learn and understand the clinical manifestations of SARS-CoV-2 infection, and to optimally manage illness resulting from COVID-19 infection. This was also true of manuscripts published about COVID-19 and the pancreas. However, the epidemiologic literature from this period includes studies that were not well-controlled—biased toward hospitalized individuals without rigorous knowledge of the infection rate in the population due to testing and reporting limitations. An important commentary on this literature states that fast-tracking of COVID-19 publications led to a proliferation of literature of variable quality and studies lacking epidemiologic rigor [13]. The authors comment that studies, including those published in major medical journals, reflected hurried approaches and lacked careful epidemiologic design, conduct, and analysis, making it difficult to understand the true contribution of diabetes and other underlying comorbidities to COVID-19 prognosis [13]. It was critical at that moment in history to disseminate as much information as possible. We now need to address specific problems in the literature including: (1) so-called "retrospective cohort studies" that may actually be large case series, (2) conclusions limited by study populations that included only hospitalized and not mild cases, (3) a majority of studies using retrospectively obtained data from electronic health records, (4) studies of comorbidities that included insufficient multivariable adjustment for baseline characteristics, (5) small studies with few clinical events leading to highly imprecise statistical estimates, (6) publication bias, and (7) reporting of results from the same patients in different articles or even duplicate publications, making future meta-analyses problematic [13] and potentially hampering genuine understanding of COVID-19 infection.

Initially, SARS-CoV-2 was thought to mainly affect the pulmonary system leading to severe respiratory symptoms, but evidence accumulated for COVID-19 infection with a variety of clinical manifestations in the hematologic, cardiac, renal, neurologic, dermatologic, gastrointestinal, and endocrine systems [14, 15]. SARS-CoV-2 must bind to a cell surface receptor such as angiotensin-converting enzyme-2 (ACE2), and gain entry with priming of its spike protein by proteases such as transmembrane protease serine 2 (TMPRSS2). Both ACE2 and TMPRSS2 must be co-expressed on the cell surface for entry of SARS-CoV-2, and therefore many studies focus on the degree and location of expression of these proteins in the pancreas, as outlined below.

Studies regarding whether COVID-19 infects the pancreas and causes pancreatic dysfunction are described in this section. An exhaustive list of references is not included; instead, studies were selected based on a higher level of experimental detail and/or because they are representative of similar studies.

Autopsy Evidence for Pancreatic Involvement

Since diabetes and hyperglycemia are associated with an increased risk of severe COVID-19 infection, and new-onset hyperglycemia, ketoacidosis, and diabetes have been observed in those infected with SARS-CoV-2, the question of whether COVID-19 infection can cause new-onset diabetes or accelerate pre-existing pre-diabetes or diabetes has been the subject of intensive investigation. Initial observations suggested that pancreatic beta-cells do not express ACE2 receptors, so a detailed analysis of autopsy samples of pancreatic tissue from 11 obese or overweight patients (age range 40–75 years, 55% male) who died of COVID-19 infection was performed [16]. One patient was previously diagnosed with type 2 diabetes. Immunofluorescence staining for SARS-CoV-2 nucleocapsid protein revealed viral antigen in the lung tissues, the endocrine and exocrine pancreas of all the COVID-19-positive patients but not in the pancreas of negative controls, suggesting that viral infection is systemic and not limited only to beta-cells [16]. The islets were also infiltrated with immune cells (CD-45 positive cells, lymphocytes) and associated with necroptotic cell death. The high protein turnover of the insulin-producing islet cells makes them a susceptible target for viruses. ACE2 is an important route for the entry of SARS-CoV-2 into the cell, but the expression of ACE2 in beta-cells has not been demonstrated consistently. In this small autopsy study, while 70% of the patients were found to express ACE2 in the vasculature, only 30% had expression in beta-cells; thus, the mechanism of viral entry was unclear from this set of studies. The authors noted that the patients died 3 weeks after contracting COVID-19 which could have also impacted the results.

Additional evidence for pancreatic involvement of SARS-CoV-2 comes from examining the expression of ACE2 and TMPRSS2 in postmortem studies of four individuals who died from COVID-19 [17]. The investigators determined that there was persistent SARS-CoV-2 infection of both endocrine and exocrine compartments [17]. Furthermore, endocrine cells infected by SARS-CoV-2 exhibited subcellular changes suggestive of endoplasmic reticular stress and had reduced glucose-sensitive insulin secretion [17]. Islets treated with remdesivir did not display viral replication, thus patients treated with remdesivir may not exhibit beta-cell damage. In cells not treated with remdesivir, investigators demonstrated the permissiveness of pancreatic beta-cells to SARS-CoV-2 infection [17]. However, these studies were limited by small sample size and autolytic necrosis resulting in suboptimal tissue quality, and limited clinical data were available for correlation.

Angiotensin-Converting Enzyme 2 and Transmembrane Protease Serine 2 Expression in the Pancreas

Severe COVID-19 infection in individuals with diabetes and the detection of new-onset diabetes in those with COVID-19 infection suggests that SARS-CoV-2 might be directly toxic to beta-cells of pancreatic islets. Coronaviruses (CoV) enter the body through the respiratory system and bind to specific receptors on the surface of host cells via a surface envelope spike glycoprotein (S-protein) (Fig. 2.1). The S-protein is cleaved by a host cell protease, exposing the receptor binding domain which allows the virus to enter the host cell and replicate [18]. ACE2, the enzyme responsible for cleaving Angiotensin I into Angiotensin II, also serves as the entry point of SARS-CoV-2 into the host cell [19]. S-protein-ACE2 binding is a key factor in the entry of SARS-CoV-2 into the body, its replication, and the pathogenesis of COVID-19 infection (Fig. 2.1), while TMPRSS2 is the transmembrane serine protease responsible for proteolytic cleavage of the S-protein (Fig. 2.1). It is also required for SARS-CoV-2 infectivity, which is higher than that of SARS-CoV due to the stronger affinity of SARS-CoV-2 for the ACE2 receptor [20, 21].

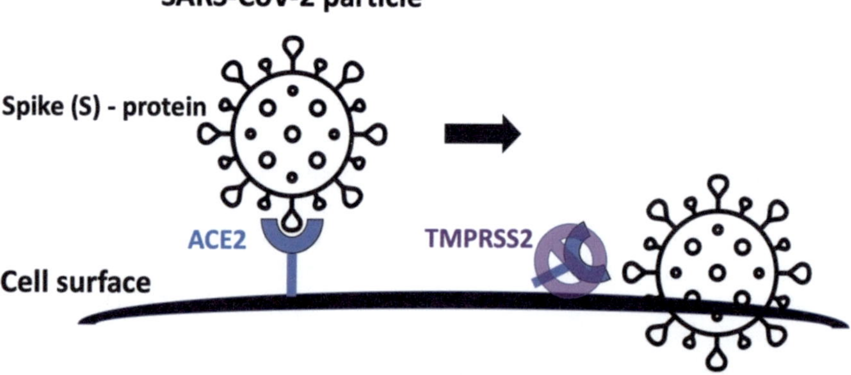

Fig. 2.1 SARS-CoV-2 binds via the viral surface spike (S) – protein to the cell surface angiotensin converting enzyme 2 (ACE2) receptor. The transmembrane protease serine 2 (TMPRSS2) cleaves the ACE2 receptor, allowing the viral particle to enter the cell

Intensive investigations of ACE2 and TMPRSS2 have been performed to understand how each protein is expressed in endocrine and non-endocrine cell types, in individuals with and without diabetes, and in those with and without COVID-19 infection. Some investigators have found significant ACE2 expression in pancreatic microvasculature and ductal cells, but not in pancreatic endocrine cells [22, 23]. In one study, only a very low percentage (<2%) of pancreatic islet cells were found to express the gene for ACE2 while 4–8% of pancreatic acinar or ductal cells were found to express ACE2 in persons without as well as with diabetes [22]. TMPRSS2 was expressed in only ~5% of beta-cells but to a much higher degree in alpha-cells (expressed in ~17% of α-cells in donors without diabetes and 32% of those with diabetes). On the other hand, TMPRSS2 was detectable in a very high proportion of acinar and ductal cells (more than 50% of cells, in donors with or without diabetes) [22]. These findings of high expression in exocrine and vascular but not endocrine compartments of the pancreas are similar to the results of another set of experiments [23]. Investigators analyzed mRNA from primary human islets of persons with and without diabetes, and found minimal expression of *ACE2* and *TMPRSS2* mRNA. Furthermore, ACE2 protein was not found in beta- or alpha-cells, but was found in islet and exocrine tissue microvasculature, and a subset of pancreatic ducts. TMPRSS2 protein was expressed only in pancreatic ductal cells, and not found to be expressed with ACE2, making it less likely that SARS-CoV-2 directly infects beta-cells via ACE2 and TMPRSS2 [23].

In contrast, ACE2 and TMPRSS2 expression has been found in fresh-frozen human pancreatic tissue containing both exocrine and endocrine cell types [17]. Studies of five histologically healthy human pancreata revealed significant co-staining for ACE2 and TMPRSS2 in beta-cells. When human pancreatic islets isolated from four patients were exposed to SARS-CoV-2 ex vivo, both the viral S- and N- (nucleocapsid) proteins were robustly expressed at days 3 and 5 post-infection. Along with subcellular changes in the infected cells, the number of insulin-containing granules decreased by 2.2-fold on day 3 and 2.4-fold on day 5 post-infection [17].

In a separate set of studies, ACE2 expression was evaluated in human pancreata from adult organ donors without pre-existing diabetes, and also in vitro using a human beta-cell line (EndoC-βH1) [24]. ACE2 was found to be expressed in a subset of endothelial cells or pericytes in the exocrine pancreas, scattered ductal cells, and a subset of cells within the islet parenchyma [24]. Within pancreatic islets, ACE2 was preferentially expressed in beta-cells, with a lower degree of expression found in alpha-cells [24]. The ACE2 protein was found to be located mostly in the cytoplasmic/granular compartment, and partially overlapping with insulin granules. The investigators also found ACE2 located close to the plasma membrane, leading them to postulate that ACE2 isoforms may exist in multiple compartments within beta-cells [24]. This is an active area of investigation with inconsistencies in the published literature. Our understanding of ACE2 and TMPRSS2 expression under various conditions will expand as more evidence emerges.

Neuropilin 1 and Transferrin Receptor

SARS-CoV-2 entry into host cells is thought to be mediated not just by ACE2 and TMPRSS2, but also by neuropilin 1 (NRP1) and transferrin receptor (TFRC), with evidence for NRP1 and TFRC facilitation of ACE2-mediated entry of SARS-CoV-2 [25, 26]. The mRNA transcripts and protein for NRP1 and TFRC have been found to be abundantly expressed in pancreatic islets [27]. Ex vivo studies of human islets isolated from healthy donors show that human beta-cells are particularly susceptible to infection with SARS-CoV-2, which may be due to the upregulation of NRP1 expression and resultant increased tropism of SARS-CoV-2 for beta-cells [27]. However, more studies are needed to establish this as a mechanism for the increased susceptibility of beta-cells. Lastly, insulin content is decreased, and glucose-stimulated insulin secretion is reduced in infected islets, an effect that can be reversed partially with an NRP1 antagonist [27]. The latter supports a central role for NRP1 in the suppression of insulin secretion in SARS-CoV-2 infection.

SARS-CoV-2 and β-Cell Transdifferentiation

Most endocrine cell types in the pancreas are susceptible to infection by SARS-CoV-2 [28]. Infection by SARS-CoV-2 results in higher expression of multiple chemokines and cytokines associated with inflammation, including C-X-C motif chemokine ligand 2 (CXCL2), interleukin-1 receptor antagonist (IL1RN), and interleukin-1 β (IL1B). Analysis of the genes enriched in infected human islets reveals upregulation of pathways associated with the cellular stress response, proinflammatory cytokines and bacterial invasion (the eukaryotic translation initiation factor 2 (eIF2) signaling pathway), cellular response to viral infection (interferon pathway), and a vital signaling pathway that mediates inflammation (Janus tyrosine kinase [JAK]-Signal transducer and activator of transcription [STAT] signaling). Further studies demonstrate that upon infection by SARS-CoV-2, beta-cells transdifferentiate. The phenomenon of transdifferentiation occurs when an adult cell undergoes phenotypic switch to another cell type without obvious dedifferentiation. In the setting of SARS-CoV-2 infection, beta-cells have been shown to undergo transdifferentiation to an alpha-cell-type with lower insulin gene expression and greater production of glucagon (GCG), and an acinar (exocrine) cell type with trypsin-1 production [28]. These findings have been confirmed in autopsy samples from COVID-19-infected subjects [28].

Pancreatitis

Individuals with diabetes are at higher risk for developing pancreatitis, and a number of observational studies have been performed to assess the prevalence of acute pancreatitis in COVID-19 infection since SARS-CoV-2 preferentially binds to

ACE2 receptors. Overall, the incidence appears to range from 0.9–2% [29–32]. COVID-19 infection may worsen outcomes in patients with acute pancreatitis [33]. In a large prospective international multicenter cohort study, 1777 patients admitted with acute pancreatitis between March 1 and July 23, 2020, were examined, and 149 (8.3%) had concomitant COVID-19 infection [33]. These patients tended to be older, male, and were more likely to develop severe acute pancreatitis and acute respiratory distress syndrome (ARDS) ($p < 0.001$). In those with concomitant SARS-CoV-2 infection, the adjusted odds ratio was increased for longer length of stay (OR 1.32, $p < 0.001$), higher likelihood of persistent organ failure (OR 2.77, $p < 0.003$), and higher 30-day mortality (OR 2.41, $p < 0.04$) [33]. In a study of patients presenting early in the pandemic in Wuhan, China, 55 critically-ill patients who had undergone transabdominal ultrasound were evaluated for the presence of pancreatitis as defined by the revised Atlanta Classification, if two of the following three criteria were met: (1) abdominal pain; (2) serum lipase and/or amylase higher than three times the upper limit of normal (ULN); and (3) imaging findings characteristic of pancreatitis on contrast-enhanced computed tomography, transabdominal ultrasound, or magnetic resonance imaging [34]. Three of 55 patients were determined to have pancreatitis, with the enzyme peak occurring between hospital days 11–17, and two of the three died of multiorgan failure during the hospitalization [35].

Summary

Existing data suggest that there is a multifaceted insult to the pancreas in the context of COVID-19. Whether the vasculature or the beta-cell is the primary target of injury remains to be defined. Differences in experimental findings regarding ACE2 and TMPRSS2 expression in the pancreas can likely be explained by diverse experimental methods, conditions, and the tissues and cells studied. Variability in the same technique including the specific reagents (e.g., antibodies) used may account for further differences. An additional investigations need to be performed to further elucidate these mechanisms including alternative routes for viral entry into beta-cells, and indirect mechanisms of beta-cell toxicity such as through systemic inflammation and vascular insult plus evaluation of peripheral insulin resistance, which may explain the severity of COVID-19 infection in individuals with diabetes. Additional information is greatly needed on the functional consequences in terms of changes in insulin secretion and/or glucose sensing in individuals at the time of or in the aftermath of SARS-CoV-2 infection.

COVID-19 and Peripheral Insulin Resistance

Insulin resistance is the term used to describe a physical state in which physiologic levels of the hormone insulin do not result in a physiologic insulin response [36]. The cellular and molecular mechanisms of insulin resistance have been elucidated through the intensive investigation and dedication of numerous scientists around the world, and are the subject of excellent reviews over the years [37–42]; these will not be detailed here. This section of the chapter will focus is on what has been discovered regarding COVID-19 and peripheral insulin resistance.

Increased glucose concentration contributes to worsening clinical outcomes in patients with COVID-19 infection [43, 44]. Insulin is the preferred treatment for dysglycemia in the hospital setting and has been used to treat the hyperglycemia complicated by severe insulin resistance found in patients with COVID-19 (see Chap. 8 for inpatient management of COVID-19). Insulin is the key hormone secreted by pancreatic beta-cells that regulates metabolism and maintains glucose homeostasis. Glucose is the primary substrate for human cell metabolism and enters cells via insulin-dependent cellular uptake in most cases [45].

Glucose-stimulated insulin secretion (GSIS) and insulin-mediated glucose uptake (IMGU) are needed to maintain glucose metabolism. Circulating plasma glucose enters beta-cells via glucose transporter 2 (GLUT2), on the beta-cell surface (Fig. 2.2). Once inside the beta-cell, adenosine triphosphate (ATP) is generated through glycolysis, resulting in an increased ATP/ADP ratio triggering closure of ATP-sensitive potassium channels. This causes a decrease in potassium ion efflux resulting in cell membrane depolarization and opening of voltage-dependent calcium channels, with an influx of intracellular calcium triggering the fusion and release of densely clustered insulin granules (Fig. 2.2). The release of insulin promotes IMGU, allowing glucose uptake in skeletal muscle and adipose tissue while simultaneously suppressing hepatic gluconeogenesis. Extracellularly, insulin molecules bind to the alpha subunit of the insulin receptor (Fig. 2.2), leading to tyrosine

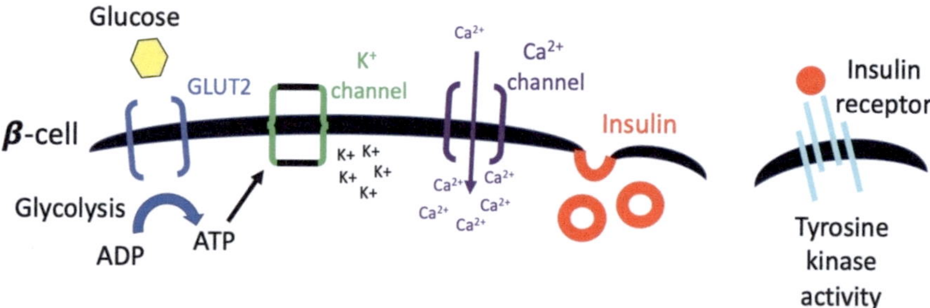

Fig. 2.2 Circulating plasma glucose enters β-cells via glucose transporter 2 (GLUT2) on the β-cell surface. Once inside the β-cell, adenosine triphosphate (ATP) is generated through glycolysis, resulting in an increased ATP/ADP ratio triggering a closure of ATP-sensitive potassium channels. This causes a decrease in potassium ion efflux resulting in cell membrane depolarization and opening of voltage-dependent calcium channels, with an influx of intracellular calcium triggering the fusion and release of densely clustered insulin granules. Extracellularly, insulin molecules bind to the alpha subunit of the insulin receptor, leading to tyrosine kinase phosphorylation of insulin receptor substrates

kinase phosphorylation of insulin receptor substrates and subsequent activation of phosphatidylinositol-3-kinase, resulting in the translocation of the insulin-sensitive glucose transporter 4 (GLUT4) and allowing for glucose entry into cells for metabolism into glycogen [45].

During critical illness, complex interactions between counterregulatory hormones and cytokines can cause excessive production of glucose and insulin resistance, with increased glycogenolysis and gluconeogenesis [46]. Glycogenolysis is triggered by increased catecholamines, whereas gluconeogenesis is triggered by an increase in glucagon and cortisol via a stress response. Additionally, insulin resistance in patients with COVID-19 can occur due to alterations in these pathways. Inflammatory cytokines such as tumor necrosis factor-alpha (TNF-α), interleukin-1 beta (IL-1β), and interleukin-6 (IL-6), which are higher in patients with underlying diabetes and COVID-19, impair insulin signaling and reduce GLUT4 resulting in decreased glucose transport into cells [47].

Adipokines and Insulin Resistance

Adipokines are factors released from adipose tissue with both pro-inflammatory and anti-inflammatory actions [48]. Consequently, dysregulation of adipokine production can cause insulin resistance which contributes to and can be exacerbated by systemic inflammatory responses observed in excess adipose tissue states such as obesity, which correlates with the severity of COVID-19 illness [49].

Leptin, a hormone and pro-inflammatory adipokine, is secreted by adipocytes and also plays a role in insulin resistance. Plasma leptin concentration increases in proportion to body fat mass and regulates food intake and energy expenditure to maintain body fat stores [50]. Leptin is secreted from adipocytes into the circulation and enters the brain through cerebral spinal fluid and across the blood-brain barrier. Leptin acts in the arcuate nucleus of the hypothalamus by inhibiting neuropeptide Y and Agouti-related peptide neurons leading to anorexigenic effects [50]. Leptin also plays a role in peripheral glucose metabolism by decreasing hepatic glucose production, increasing insulin sensitivity, and decreasing glucagon levels. Van der Voort et al. noted higher leptin levels in COVID-19 patients admitted to the ICU as compared with non-COVID-19 ICU patients [51]. Conversely, adiponectin, an anti-inflammatory adipokine and insulin-sensitizing hormone secreted by adipocytes, regulates glucose metabolism and fatty acid oxidation [52]. In patients with COVID-19 and hyperglycemia, Reiterer et al. demonstrated a decrease in adiponectin levels [49]. Di Filippo et al. found that the ratio between adiponectin and leptin levels may predict the severity of COVID-19 illness [52]. Patients with severe COVID-19 had lower adiponectin/leptin ratios (lower adiponectin levels and higher leptin levels with more insulin resistance) [52]. It can therefore be postulated that adipose dysfunction driving hyperglycemia and insulin resistance may be a characteristic of COVID-19 illness.

Prolonged Insulin Resistance

As outlined above, numerous factors lead to the initial insulin resistant and hyperglycemic state seen with COVID-19 infection. However, post-acute illness studies have demonstrated prolonged glycemic alteration even after the remission of COVID-19 infection. The extreme inflammatory state seen in patients with COVID-19 may lead to the worsening of diabetes due to beta-cell exhaustion from glucose toxicity and insulin hypersecretion [53]. Montefusco et al. demonstrated that at six months post-infection, patients without a history of diabetes but with new-onset hyperglycemia during active COVID infection, had elevated fasting plasma glucose levels with increased fasting C-peptide secretion suggesting persistent insulin resistance [53]. Similarly, case studies of adult patients with T2D demonstrate the need for intensification of anti-diabetes therapies for 1–2 months after the resolution of COVID-19 illness [54]. Of note, many epidemiological studies have demonstrated higher rates of incident diabetes after COVID-19 infection [3–12]. It has been suggested that this may be more likely in men than women. There is also a report that incident diabetes post-COVID-19 infection may resolve or undergo remission [55]. Due to the relative newness of SARS-CoV-2, there are limited studies on the prolonged metabolic effects of this disease in the post-acute stage. Investigations are ongoing, and an international group of researchers has established a global registry of patients with new-onset COVID-19–related diabetes called the CoviDIAB Project [9], and many large cohorts have been established to address these questions including the NIH National COVID Cohort Collaborative (N3C) [56]. As with insulin secretion, data specifically measuring insulin sensitivity in individuals with COVID-19 infection are lacking.

Summary

Overwhelming infection with excessive inflammation and cytokines experienced in severe COVID-19 infection is accompanied by extremely high insulin requirements to normalize blood glucose in the hospital, consistent with severe insulin resistance. Persistent post-sepsis inflammatory syndrome is presumed to potentially cause post-infection insulin resistance syndromes. In addition, sarcopenia and decreased functional status could further exacerbate post-infection insulin resistance. How insulin resistance colludes with potential impairments in islet function and insulin secretion and the development of incident diabetes or deterioration of glycemic control post-COVID-19 infection remains to be mechanistically clarified.

Conclusion

Pre-existing diabetes, severe hyperglycemia, and obesity have significantly affected the outcomes of people with COVID-19 infection. In the acute hospital setting, insulin requirements for glucose normalization can be exceptionally high demonstrating profound insulin resistance. Case reports and cohort analysis demonstrate increased incident diabetes potentially more commonly in males. These cases do not suggest that a severe COVID-19 infection is antecedent to the incident diabetes. Smaller analyses suggest deterioration in glycemic control in people with pre-existing diabetes, although this finding has not been consistent in all reports. The contribution of COVID-19-related destruction of beta-cells or islet vasculature is supported by preclinical studies and autopsy studies. Evidence for insulin resistance in the context of SARS-CoV-2 is supported by preclinical studies and case report series. To better understand both incident diabetes and the impact of SARS-CoV-2 infection on long-term glycemic control, formal testing examining insulin secretion and insulin action in individuals with COVID-19 infection is needed. Further, the impact of COVID-19 infection on the long-term consequences of diabetes beyond glycemic control, such as microvascular and macrovascular complications, will require long-term follow-up.

References

1. Kimura T, Namkoong H. Susceptibility of the obese population to COVID-19. Int J Infect Dis. 2020;101:380–1.
2. Gangadharan C, Ahluwalia R, Sigamani A. Diabetes and COVID-19: role of insulin resistance as a risk factor for COVID-19 severity. World J Diabetes. 2021;12(9):1550–62.
3. Khunti K, Del Prato S, Mathieu C, Kahn SE, Gabbay RA, Buse JB. COVID-19, hyperglycemia, and new-onset diabetes. Diabetes Care. 2021;44(12):2645–55.
4. Wander PL, Lowy E, Beste LA, Tulloch-Palomino L, Korpak A, Peterson AC, et al. The incidence of diabetes among 2,777,768 veterans with and without recent SARS-CoV-2 infection. Diabetes Care. 2022;45(4):782–8.
5. Xie Y, Al-Aly Z. Risks and burdens of incident diabetes in long COVID: a cohort study. Lancet Diabetes Endocrinol. 2022;10(5):311–21.
6. Birabaharan M, Kaelber DC, Pettus JH, Smith DM. Risk of new-onset type 2 diabetes in 600 055 people after COVID-19: a cohort study. Diabetes Obes Metab. 2022;24(6):1176–9.
7. Rathmann W, Kuss O, Kostev K. Incidence of newly diagnosed diabetes after Covid-19. Diabetologia. 2022;65(6):949–54.
8. Sathish T, Kapoor N, Cao Y, Tapp RJ, Zimmet P. Proportion of newly diagnosed diabetes in COVID-19 patients: a systematic review and meta-analysis. Diabetes Obes Metab. 2021;23(3):870–4.
9. Rubino F, Amiel SA, Zimmet P, Alberti G, Bornstein S, Eckel RH, et al. New-onset diabetes in Covid-19. N Engl J Med. 2020;383(8):789–90.
10. Shrestha DB, Budhathoki P, Raut S, Adhikari S, Ghimire P, Thapaliya S, et al. New-onset diabetes in COVID-19 and clinical outcomes: a systematic review and meta-analysis. World J Virol. 2021;10(5):275–87.

11. Chen J, Wu C, Wang X, Yu J, Sun Z. The impact of COVID-19 on blood glucose: a systematic review and meta-analysis. Front Endocrinol (Lausanne). 2020;11:574541.
12. Barrett CE, Koyama AK, Alvarez P, Chow W, Lundeen EA, Perrine CG, et al. Risk for newly diagnosed diabetes >30 days after SARS-CoV-2 infection among persons aged <18 years—United States, march 1, 2020-June 28, 2021. MMWR Morb Mortal Wkly Rep. 2022;71(2):59–65.
13. Selvin E, Juraschek SP. Diabetes epidemiology in the COVID-19 pandemic. Diabetes Care. 2020;43(8):1690–4.
14. Gupta A, Madhavan MV, Sehgal K, Nair N, Mahajan S, Sehrawat TS, et al. Extrapulmonary manifestations of COVID-19. Nat Med. 2020;26(7):1017–32.
15. Song E, Zhang C, Israelow B, Lu-Culligan A, Prado AV, Skriabine S, et al. Neuroinvasion of SARS-CoV-2 in human and mouse brain. J Exp Med. 2021;218:3.
16. Steenblock C, Richter S, Berger I, Barovic M, Schmid J, Schubert U, et al. Viral infiltration of pancreatic islets in patients with COVID-19. Nat Commun. 2021;12(1):3534.
17. Muller JA, Gross R, Conzelmann C, Kruger J, Merle U, Steinhart J, et al. SARS-CoV-2 infects and replicates in cells of the human endocrine and exocrine pancreas. Nat Metab. 2021;3(2):149–65.
18. Letko M, Munster V. Functional assessment of cell entry and receptor usage for lineage B beta-coronaviruses, including 2019-nCoV. bioRxiv. 2020;
19. Li W, Moore MJ, Vasilieva N, Sui J, Wong SK, Berne MA, et al. Angiotensin-converting enzyme 2 is a functional receptor for the SARS coronavirus. Nature. 2003;426(6965):450–4.
20. Hoffmann M, Kleine-Weber H, Schroeder S, Kruger N, Herrler T, Erichsen S, et al. SARS-CoV-2 cell entry depends on ACE2 and TMPRSS2 and is blocked by a clinically proven protease inhibitor. Cell. 2020;181(2):271–80 e8.
21. Shang J, Wan Y, Luo C, Ye G, Geng Q, Auerbach A, et al. Cell entry mechanisms of SARS-CoV-2. Proc Natl Acad Sci U S A. 2020;117(21):11727–34.
22. Kusmartseva I, Wu W, Syed F, Van Der Heide V, Jorgensen M, Joseph P, et al. Expression of SARS-CoV-2 entry factors in the pancreas of normal organ donors and individuals with COVID-19. Cell Metab. 2020;32(6):1041–51 e6.
23. Coate KC, Cha J, Shrestha S, Wang W, Goncalves LM, Almaca J, et al. SARS-CoV-2 cell entry factors ACE2 and TMPRSS2 are expressed in the microvasculature and ducts of human pancreas but are not enriched in beta cells. Cell Metab. 2020;32(6):1028–40 e4.
24. Fignani D, Licata G, Brusco N, Nigi L, Grieco GE, Marselli L, et al. SARS-CoV-2 receptor angiotensin I-converting enzyme type 2 (ACE2) is expressed in human pancreatic beta-cells and in the human pancreas microvasculature. Front Endocrinol (Lausanne). 2020;11:596898.
25. Daly JL, Simonetti B, Klein K, Chen KE, Williamson MK, Anton-Plagaro C, et al. Neuropilin-1 is a host factor for SARS-CoV-2 infection. Science. 2020;370(6518):861–5.
26. Cantuti-Castelvetri L, Ojha R, Pedro LD, Djannatian M, Franz J, Kuivanen S, et al. Neuropilin-1 facilitates SARS-CoV-2 cell entry and infectivity. Science. 2020;370(6518):856–60.
27. Wu CT, Lidsky PV, Xiao Y, Lee IT, Cheng R, Nakayama T, et al. SARS-CoV-2 infects human pancreatic beta cells and elicits beta cell impairment. Cell Metab. 2021;33(8):1565–76 e5.
28. Tang X, Uhl S, Zhang T, Xue D, Li B, Vandana JJ, et al. SARS-CoV-2 infection induces beta cell transdifferentiation. Cell Metab. 2021;33(8):1577–91 e7.
29. McNabb-Baltar J, Jin DX, Grover AS, Redd WD, Zhou JC, Hathorn KE, et al. Lipase elevation in patients with COVID-19. Am J Gastroenterol. 2020;115(8):1286–8.
30. Pezzilli R, Centanni S, Mondoni M, Rinaldo RF, Davi M, Stefanelli R, et al. Patients with coronavirus disease 2019 interstitial pneumonia exhibit pancreatic hyperenzymemia and not acute pancreatitis. Pancreas. 2021;50(5):732–5.
31. Troncone E, Salvatori S, Sena G, De Cristofaro E, Alfieri N, Marafini I, et al. Low frequency of acute pancreatitis in hospitalized COVID-19 patients. Pancreas. 2021;50(3):393–8.
32. Bacaksiz F, Ebik B, Ekin N, Kilic J. Pancreatic damage in COVID-19: why? How? Int J Clin Pract. 2021;75(10):e14692.

33. Pandanaboyana S, Moir J, Leeds JS, Oppong K, Kanwar A, Marzouk A, et al. SARS-CoV-2 infection in acute pancreatitis increases disease severity and 30-day mortality: COVID PAN collaborative study. Gut. 2021;70(6):1061–9.
34. Banks PA, Bollen TL, Dervenis C, Gooszen HG, Johnson CD, Sarr MG, et al. Classification of acute pancreatitis—2012: revision of the Atlanta classification and definitions by international consensus. Gut. 2013;62(1):102–11.
35. Ding P, Song B, Liu X, Fang X, Cai H, Zhang D, et al. Elevated pancreatic enzymes in ICU patients with COVID-19 in Wuhan, China: a retrospective study. Front Med (Lausanne). 2021;8:663646.
36. Kahn CR. Insulin resistance, insulin insensitivity, and insulin unresponsiveness: a necessary distinction. Metabolism. 1978;27(12 Suppl 2):1893–902.
37. Yaribeygi H, Farrokhi FR, Butler AE, Sahebkar A. Insulin resistance: review of the underlying molecular mechanisms. J Cell Physiol. 2019;234(6):8152–61.
38. da Silva Rosa SC, Nayak N, Caymo AM, Gordon JW. Mechanisms of muscle insulin resistance and the cross-talk with liver and adipose tissue. Physiol Rep. 2020;8(19):e14607.
39. Petersen MC, Shulman GI. Mechanisms of insulin action and insulin resistance. Physiol Rev. 2018;98(4):2133–223.
40. Romeo GR, Lee J, Shoelson SE. Metabolic syndrome, insulin resistance, and roles of inflammation—mechanisms and therapeutic targets. Arterioscler Thromb Vasc Biol. 2012;32(8):1771–6.
41. Flier JS, Kahn CR, Roth J. Receptors, antireceptor antibodies and mechanisms of insulin resistance. N Engl J Med. 1979;300(8):413–9.
42. Low Wang CC, Draznin B. Chapter 2: insulin resistance: molecular biology and pathophysiology. In: Draznin B, editor. Atypical diabetes: pathophysiology, clinical presentations, and treatment options. Arlington, Virginia: American Diabetes Association, Inc; 2018.
43. Zhu N, Zhang D, Wang W, Li X, Yang B, Song J, et al. A novel coronavirus from patients with pneumonia in China, 2019. N Engl J Med. 2020;382(8):727–33.
44. Wu Z, McGoogan JM. Characteristics of and important lessons from the coronavirus disease 2019 (COVID-19) outbreak in China: summary of a report of 72314 cases from the Chinese Center for Disease Control and Prevention. JAMA. 2020;323(13):1239–42.
45. Roder PV, Wu B, Liu Y, Han W. Pancreatic regulation of glucose homeostasis. Exp Mol Med. 2016;48:e219.
46. Govender N, Khaliq OP, Moodley J, Naicker T. Insulin resistance in COVID-19 and diabetes. Prim Care Diabetes. 2021;15(4):629–34.
47. Santos A, Magro DO, Evangelista-Poderoso R, Saad MJA. Diabetes, obesity, and insulin resistance in COVID-19: molecular interrelationship and therapeutic implications. Diabetol Metab Syndr. 2021;13(1):23.
48. Jaganathan R, Ravindran R, Dhanasekaran S. Emerging role of adipocytokines in type 2 diabetes as mediators of insulin resistance and cardiovascular disease. Can. J Diabetes. 2018;42(4):446–56. e1
49. Reiterer M, Rajan M, Gomez-Banoy N, Lau JD, Gomez-Escobar LG, Ma L, et al. Hyperglycemia in acute COVID-19 is characterized by insulin resistance and adipose tissue infectivity by SARS-CoV-2. Cell Metab. 2021;33(11):2174–88. e5
50. Amitani M, Asakawa A, Amitani H, Inui A. The role of leptin in the control of insulin-glucose axis. Front Neurosci. 2013;7:51.
51. van der Voort PHJ, Moser J, Zandstra DF, Muller Kobold AC, Knoester M, Calkhoven CF, et al. Leptin levels in SARS-CoV-2 infection related respiratory failure: a cross-sectional study and a pathophysiological framework on the role of fat tissue. Heliyon. 2020;6(8):e04696.
52. Di Filippo L, De Lorenzo R, Sciorati C, Capobianco A, Lore NI, Giustina A, et al. Adiponectin to leptin ratio reflects inflammatory burden and survival in COVID-19. Diabetes Metab. 2021;47(6):101268.
53. Montefusco L, Ben Nasr M, D'Addio F, Loretelli C, Rossi A, Pastore I, et al. Acute and long-term disruption of glycometabolic control after SARS-CoV-2 infection. Nat Metab. 2021;3(6):774–85.

54. Downes JM, Foster JA. Prolonged hyperglycemia in three patients with type 2 diabetes after COVID-19 infection: a case series. J Family Med Prim Care. 2021;10(5):2041–3.
55. Laurenzi A, Caretto A, Molinari C, Mercalli A, Melzi R, Nano R, et al. No evidence of long-term disruption of glycometabolic control after SARS-CoV-2 infection. J Clin Endocrinol Metab. 2022;107(3):e1009–e19.
56. Haendel MA, Chute CG, Bennett TD, Eichmann DA, Guinney J, Kibbe WA, et al. The national COVID cohort collaborative (N3C): rationale, design, infrastructure, and deployment. J Am Med Inform Assoc. 2021;28(3):427–43.

Chapter 3
Risk of COVID-19 in Persons with Diabetes

Allyson Hernandez, Ann Marie Hasse, and Justin Jihoon Yoon

Introduction

In late 2019, the entire globe was impacted by the pandemic of the respiratory illness, coronavirus disease 2019 (COVID-19), of which the causative virus was identified to be severe acute respiratory coronavirus 2 (SARS-CoV-2) [1]. As of October 2022, it is estimated that more than 616 million cases of COVID-19 have been detected, and greater than 6.5 million people have died due to the virus [2]. Several medical conditions such as diabetes mellitus (DM), hypertension, coronary artery disease (CAD), and pulmonary diseases have been linked with an increased risk of severity of disease and mortality [1, 3–5]. In this chapter, we will examine the risk of COVID-19 in persons with DM by starting with a brief review of the prevalence of DM, followed by the pathophysiology of COVID-19 in persons with DM, and then complications and mortality related to COVID-19 in patients with different types of DM.

A. Hernandez
SUNY Downstate College of Medicine, Brooklyn, NY, USA

A. M. Hasse
Northwell Health, New Hyde Park, NY, USA
e-mail: AMHaas@northwell.edu

J. J. Yoon (✉)
Advocate Aurora Health, Inc, Milwaukee, WI, USA
e-mail: Justin.Yoon@aah.org

A. K. Myers (ed.), *Diabetes and COVID-19*, Contemporary Endocrinology,
https://doi.org/10.1007/978-3-031-28536-3_3

Prevalence and the Risk of Diabetes in Respiratory Viral Infections

Diabetes mellitus is one of the most widespread medical conditions in the United States and worldwide. The global prevalence of DM in 2019 was estimated to be 9.3% and is expected to rise to 10.2% by 2030 [6, 7]. The United States Centers for Disease Control and Prevention (CDC) estimates that about 11.3% of the US population (37.3 million) has DM, and 38% of the US population aged over 18 years has prediabetes, which comprises 96 million people in the United States [8, 9]. The high prevalence of DM makes it a commonly encountered comorbid disease and a frequent contributor to morbidity among hospitalized patients. The prevalence of DM increases with advanced age, which is associated with an increased risk of DM-related complications [10, 11].

A higher risk of infection has been linked to DM as well [10, 11]. Even prior to the COVID-19 pandemic, patients with DM with good glycemic control (hemoglobin 6–7%) were hospitalized for infections at a 1.4 higher rate relative to the general population, and those with poor glycemic control (HbA1c > 11%) were hospitalized at a rate of 4.7 greater [10]. Persons with DM accounted for a significant proportion of cases during previous pandemics of severe acute respiratory infectious outbreaks including the 2009 influenza A (H1N1) and the Middle East respiratory syndrome coronavirus (MERS-CoV). A systematic review found that the prevalence of DM in MERS-CoV cases was 54.4% compared to 14.6% of DM in H1N1 cases, although those with MERS-CoV were older (mean age: 54.3 ± 7.4 years versus 36.2 ± 6 years) and were associated with comorbid conditions such as CAD or hypertension [12].

Prevalence and Risk of Diabetes and COVID-19

A variable prevalence of DM in patients with COVID-19 has been reported. During the early course of the pandemic, a nationwide study by the Chinese Center for Disease Control (China CDC) showed 5.3% of patients with COVID-19 had DM, and the United States CDC reported a 10.9% prevalence of DM in those with COVID-19 [13, 14]. According to a study done at a major metropolitan New York hospital system (Northwell Health), 33.8% of patients had DM among 5700 patients hospitalized with COVID-19 [15]. A systematic review and meta-analysis of studies conducted in China revealed a prevalence of DM of 11.7% in patients with COVID-19 requiring an ICU level of care, compared to 4% in non-ICU cases [16]. Another Chinese systematic review and meta-analysis of 187 studies involving 77,013 patients revealed an upward trend in the prevalence of DM in accordance with the severity of COVID-19 cases: 7.84%, 8.59%, 17.99%, and 22.68% in mild, moderate, severe, and critical cases, respectively [3].

Over time, retrospective and pooled analyses have shown that 9.8–18% of all patients diagnosed with COVID-19 also carried a diagnosis of DM [17–19]. A pooled analysis of 120 studies (75 studies reported from Asia, 26 from Europe, 16 from the USA, 5 from Latin America, and 1 from South Africa) revealed that DM was present in 14% of COVID-19 patients in Asia, 20% in Europe, 18% in Latin America, and 32% in the USA, respectively [19]. Overall, even though studies have not proven whether DM causes an increase in the risk of contracting SARS-CoV-2, many have demonstrated the positive correlation between DM and a higher risk of more severe COVID-19 and mortality [18, 19].

How the Immunity of Persons with Diabetes Is Impacted by Inflammation of COVID-19

Inflammation plays a pivotal role in the pathogenesis of COVID-19 and many of the complications seen in hospitalized patients with severe disease. Severe COVID-19 is typically defined as the requirement of hospitalization, progressive dyspnea, and the need for oxygenation or ventilatory support, whereas critically ill is defined as the presence of organ damage and the necessity of an ICU level of care [20, 21]. Patients with severe COVID-19, especially those with acute respiratory distress syndrome, often have elevated inflammatory markers such as C-reactive protein (CRP), D-dimer, ferritin, and interleukin 6 (IL-6). Furthermore, the presence of systemic inflammatory infiltrates is a common post-mortem finding in the tissues from deceased COVID-19 patients [22]. The SARS-CoV2 has been shown to trigger a life-threatening "cytokine storm," which is an acute systemic inflammatory syndrome characterized by a prolonged state of elevated levels of circulating cytokines and hyperactivation of the immune system, resulting in widespread end-organ damage and death [22]. The International Study of Inflammation in COVID-19 (ISIC), a multicenter observational study, found that levels of all inflammatory biomarkers including soluble urokinase plasminogen activator (suPAR), IL-6, CRP, D-dimer, ferritin, lactate dehydrogenase, and procalcitonin were associated with an increased likelihood of in-hospital death, need for mechanical ventilation, and need of renal replacement therapy, even after adjustment for demographics and clinical risk factors. In persons with DM, these elevated inflammatory markers were higher than those without DM [23]. Specifically, suPAR was the most reflective of the hyperinflammatory state in persons with DM and COVID-19 in comparison to other inflammatory markers: SuPAR is not an acute-phase reactant, but it is an immune-derived signaling protein that is elevated in the setting of immune activation and inflammation. This protein was found to mediate approximately 80% of DM and COVID-19-related outcomes [23].

Diabetes is characterized by the presence of chronic low-grade inflammation, which is believed to be mediated by glucotoxicity, as well as the widespread oxidative and cellular stress by long-standing hyperglycemia [24]. The low-grade inflammation that drives the pathogenesis of DM perpetuates further insulin resistance and has been associated with many DM-related complications and end-organ damage

[23, 24]. It was initially hypothesized that hyperglycemia and the chronic low-grade inflammation that characterized DM can predispose patients to inflammatory complications that drive the progression to severe COVID-19 and contribute to poor outcomes. However, this was not supported in the ISIC study, which found that among persons with DM hospitalized for COVID-19, hyperglycemia and elevated inflammatory biomarkers (including suPAR) did not correlate with each other. The observed effects between hyperglycemia and poor outcomes were still present after adjustment for suPAR, suggesting the association between hyperglycemia and COVID-19-related outcomes occurs through mechanisms not reflected by inflammatory biomarkers [23]. This suggests that the reason behind the increase in rates of severe COVID-19 and mortality among persons with DM is multifactorial and further research is needed.

Risk of New-Onset Diabetes with COVID-19

It is still unclear whether COVID-19 triggers new-onset DM. Nevertheless, there is a growing body of evidence demonstrating an increase in the number of newly diagnosed DM after COVID-19 infections. In a review of two American databases, new-onset DM was more common in children under 18 within 30 days or more after being diagnosed with COVID-19 [25]. One proposed mechanism for the increase in the trend of new-onset DM with COVID-19 is the impact of government lockdowns, which lead to self-isolation, decreased activity, and dietary indiscretion leading to increased rates of undetected DM prior to admission [26]. This was further exacerbated by a decreased utilization of medical services. According to a survey by the WHO of 163 countries, 49% of countries reported delays in DM and/or DM complications care [27].

It has been proposed that the method of infectivity the SARS-CoV-2 utilizes can contribute to new-onset DM. The uptake of SARS-CoV-2 into cells is mediated through the virus' structural spike S protein that binds primarily to angiotensin-converting enzyme II (ACE2) receptors on the host cell. Early in infection, the virus uses this method to target nasal, bronchial, and alveolar epithelial cells [28]. As viral replication accelerates and the epithelial-endothelial barrier integrity is compromised, the SARS-CoV-2 then starts infecting pulmonary capillary endothelial cells in the later stages of infection [28, 29]. However, the SARS-CoV-2 is shown to directly cause pancreatic beta cell dysfunction and inhibit insulin release when the virus enters pancreatic beta cells via ACE2, transmembrane serine protease 2 (TMPRSS2), neuropilin 1 (NRP1), and transferrin receptor (TFRC), which could increase risk of new-onset DM (see Chap. 2 for more about SARS-CoV-2 in the pancreas) [26, 30]. A multi-institutional research network conducted a retrospective cohort study in 2021 that compared persons diagnosed with COVID-19 with persons diagnosed with influenza. The study revealed an association between COVID-19 infection and an increased risk of new-onset of Type 2 Diabetes (T2D), with higher rates of T2D occurring among persons with moderate-to-severe disease [31]. Although steroid use during the disease course strengthened the association between new-onset T2D and COVID-19, the correlation between new-onset T2D and moderate-to-severe COVID-19 persisted even in the absence of steroid use. Limitations of this study include transient hyperglycemia that may be misdiagnosed as new-onset T2D and incomplete medical health records that miss a known history of pre-existing prediabetes or insulin resistance [31].

Another plausible mechanism of developing new-onset DM in those who are infected with SARS-CoV-2 is insulin resistance resulting in stress hyperglycemia [32]. Even though it is still unclear whether COVID-19 stress hyperglycemia leads to new-onset DM, prior studies of acute and critically ill patients showed that stress hyperglycemia was associated with an increased risk of incidental DM [33, 34]. A recent retrospective review in Boston revealed that among the patients with DM who were admitted at Massachusetts General Hospital for COVID-19 between March and September 2020, 13% had new-onset DM. The study found that patients with new-onset DM had higher inflammatory markers and an increased rate of ICU admission than individuals with pre-existing DM, yet 40.6% of patients with new-onset DM during hospitalization reverted to having either prediabetes or normoglycemia at post-discharge follow-up. Patients with new-onset DM had rapid improvement in glycemic control after discharge, implying that new-onset DM may have been related to stress hyperglycemia [35].

Risk of COVID-19 in Patients with Type 1 Diabetes

A national population-based cohort study from England showed people with type 1 diabetes (T1D) had 3.5 increased odds of in-hospital deaths with COVID-19 compared to people without DM. In comparison, those with T2D had twice the increased odds of in-hospital death with COVID-19 compared to people without DM. These findings were present even after adjustment for age, sex, socioeconomic status, ethnicity, and geography [36]. Another national cohort study from Scotland demonstrated an increased rate of ICU admission and mortality in those with T1D compared to T2D [37].

On the other hand, a recent systematic review and meta-analysis, which included the two studies stated above, revealed no statistical difference between patients with T1D and T2D regarding ICU admission and hospitalization due to COVID-19. Compared to COVID-19 patients with T2D, COVID-19 patients with T1D had a lower mortality rate [adjusted odds ratio 0.83, 95% CI, −0.81 to 0.37]. Nonetheless, this study was limited by high heterogeneity in populations of included studies and an inclusion of unadjusted data for age, gender, and other comorbidities in the quantitative synthesis [38]. Given the contradictory conclusions present in the available literature, more research is warranted to further compare outcomes among different diabetes subtypes.

Risk of COVID-19 in Children with Diabetes

Children under the age of 20 account for 21% of total diagnosed cases of COVID-19 as per data collected from 100 countries [39]. Overall, children with COVID-19 tend to have a milder disease, a more favorable prognosis, and very low death rates [40–42]. There has been no definite evidence that children and adolescents with T1D have an increased risk of more severe disease and mortality associated with COVID-19 compared to children without DM. Most pediatric patients with T1D and COVID-19 did not require hospitalization [43]. For example, a cross-sectional multi-national survey of 303 health-care professionals done by the International Society for Pediatric and Adolescent Diabetes revealed that only 5 out of 86 pediatric diabetes patients with COVID-19 required ICU admission, and no fatality was reported. However, the survey demonstrated that 22% of responders noted a potential delay in diagnosis of new-onset DM in children during the pandemic and 15% of responders noted an increased incidence of diabetic ketoacidosis (DKA) [44].

A retrospective observational study conducted in a medical center in Madrid, Spain, in 2020 found that during the COVID-19 pandemic, the age at presentation of T1DM was younger than in previous years. However, whether this finding was directly influenced by COVID-19 or by other factors such as being under lockdown leading to more contact between children and parents remains unclear [45]. The severity of the presentation during the pandemic also increased, with a greater propensity for presenting with DKA and a high rate of pediatric ICU admission [45]. It was initially postulated that the incidence of pediatric T1D would increase as a result of COVID-19 given that T1D is associated with autoimmunity after viral infections. The traumatic effect of the pandemic and stress associated with the lockdown were also hypothesized to influence the increased incidence. On the other hand, a study in Germany that evaluated over 200 pediatric diabetic centers did not observe a significant deviation from the predicted increase in the incidence of pediatric T1D in the year 2020. The authors noted that the relatively low number of cases of COVID-19 in Germany may have played a role [46]. This finding is in direct contrast to a report published in 2022 by the CDC, which reported a higher incidence of new onset of DM among American patients younger than 18 years old with COVID-19 compared to those without COVID-19 in the same age cohort [25]. The incidence of new-onset DM among COVID-19 patients younger than 18 years of age was higher compared to the pre-pandemic period [25].

Risk of COVID-19 in Patients with Prediabetes

Similar to patients with DM, patients with prediabetes have a poorer clinical course compared with those without. As prediabetes is an enduring state of hyperglycemia preceding the gradual development of T2D, this association is naturally anticipated

[47]. According to a retrospective chart review of 102 patients in India, those with a pre-existing diagnosis of prediabetes had higher inflammatory markers, required more mechanical ventilation, had higher ICU admission rates, and suffered greater mortality [48]. This is exemplified in the single-center consecutive series study done by Smith et al., where there was a 1.3-fold higher prevalence of prediabetes among admitted patients with COVID-19 compared to the general US public; 18.5% of patients with prediabetes required intubation while only 4% of patients without pre-diabetes or diabetes required intubation [49]. These findings were corroborated in a systematic review and meta-analysis that delineated the association of prediabetes with severe COVID-19 outcomes [odds ratio of 2.58 (95%CI, 1.46–4.56)], although this data is limited as the review only included six studies and had a high heterogeneity ($I^2 = 55\%$) [47].

Risk of COVID-19 in Patients with Gestational Diabetes Mellitus

Radan et al. conducted a case-control study that compared pregnant women with and without COVID-19 during the pandemic to historical controls who delivered before the pandemic. Groups were matched by parity, body mass index (BMI), and ethnicity. The study revealed 34.6% of the case group had gestational diabetes mellitus (GDM) compared to 16.1% in the control group. Those who were COVID-19 positive had an increased diagnosis of GDM [50]. Another multicenter retrospective case-control study also depicted a two-fold increase in the incidence of GDM in COVID-19-positive women compared to women who did not have COVID-19 [16/100 (16%) vs. 34/400 (8.5%), $p = 0.03$] [51]. A multinational prospective longitudinal observational study involving 43 institutions from 18 countries named the INTERCOVID study revealed that insulin-using women with GDM were specifically associated with COVID-19 diagnosis regardless of normal, overweight, or obese weight status [overall risk ratio of GDM 1.21; 95% CI 0.99–1.46] [52].

The COVID-19-related Obstetrics and Neonatal Outcome study (CRONOS), a registry-based multicentric prospective observational study conducted in Germany and Austria, delineated that among COVID-19-positive women with pre-existing GDM, BMI $\geq$ 25 was associated with maternal ICU admission, viral pneumonia, and oxygen supplementation requirements (adjusted OR 3.05; 95% CI 1.38–6.73) [53]. Additionally, women with BMI $\geq$ 25 and GDM with higher insulin requirements had higher rates of ICU admission, rapid progression of disease, and a three-fold increased risk of death [53]. However, overall GDM status in the setting of COVID-19 did not seem to worsen fetal and neonatal outcomes; in the multivariable-adjusted model of the CRONOS study, there was no statistically significant difference in adverse outcomes of stillbirth, neonatal ICU stay, and neonatal death less than 7 days after delivery in women with or without GDM (adjusted OR 1.11; 95% CI 0.69–1.79) [53].

Risk of COVID-19 in Patients with Type 2 Diabetes

Most of the data collected on the association between DM and COVID-19 have been centered on T2D given its overwhelming pervasiveness; according to the World Health Organization, more than 95% of people with DM have T2D [6]. Type 2 diabetes is also strongly correlated with other independent risk factors for severe COVID-19 including obesity, older age, hypertension, cardiovascular disease, and chronic kidney disease [4, 36, 54]. Aside from a poor glycemic control, advanced age, male sex, and non-white race when associated with DM are among the strongest independent predictors for COVID-19-related mortality [36, 54–56].

The Risk of Mortality, Severity of Disease, and Glycemic Control and COVID-19

Hyperglycemia has been demonstrated to be an independent poor prognostic marker for severe COVID-19. According to a retrospective study conducted early during the COVID-19 pandemic in Wuhan, China, 47.2% of patients with COVID-19 had hyperglycemia upon admission, but only 13.4% of these patients had a history of DM. In this study, elevated blood glucose at admission and throughout the hospital duration was a predictor of poor outcomes, including increased risk for progression to critical illness and in-hospital mortality in both critical and non-critical cases [57]. Other studies also corroborate these findings, suggesting that fasting or admission hyperglycemia contributes to an increased risk of morbidity and mortality even in the absence of a pre-existing diagnosis of DM [58, 59].

It is uncertain whether HbA1c elevation is a predictor of the severity of COVID-19 disease or mortality due to COVID-19. One multicenter, longitudinal study from Hubei Province, China, retrospectively analyzed 810 patients with T2D hospitalized for COVID-19, where 1:1 propensity score-matched analysis was performed among 500 patients. This study showed that patients with poorly controlled blood glucose, with median glucose of 196 mg/dL and median HbA1c of 8.1%, had worse clinical outcomes compared to patients with better glucose control who had median glucose of 112 mg/dL and median HbA1c of 7.3% [60]. Another population-based cohort study in England based on data from the National Health Services (NHS) showed higher COVID-19-related mortality in patients with T2D with HbA1c $\geq$ 7.6% or T1D with HbA1c $\geq$ 10% when compared to patients with HbA1c between 6.5% and 7% [56].

Nevertheless, this finding was not observed in all studies. The Coronavirus SARS-CoV-2 and Diabetes Outcomes (CORONADO) study (a large French nationwide, multicenter study conducted in 2020) and two additional studies done in New York found that there was no association between HbA1C levels at the time of hospital admission and the risk of dying from COVID-19-related mortality [61–63]. Particularly, Myers et al. demonstrated elevated admitting serum or point-of-care glucose levels, rather than HbA1c, were associated with greater in-hospital mortality due to COVID-19 [62].

Conclusion

As we have explored, there is consistent data suggesting that DM is one of the major risk factors for COVID-19. Epidemiological data have delineated the overall high prevalence of patients with DM among SARS-CoV-19-infected individuals. Although no clear evidence implies an increased risk of COVID-19 infection in persons with DM, it has been demonstrated that DM increases the severity of COVID-19 infection and mortality. Therefore, in the day and age of the COVID-19 pandemic, health-care professionals shall emphasize the importance of glycemic control of DM to patients and continue to work with patients to improve outcomes related to DM and COVID-19.

References

1. Zheng Z, Peng F, Xu B, Zhao J, Liu H, Peng J, et al. Risk factors of critical & mortal COVID-19 cases: a systematic literature review and meta-analysis. J Infect. 2020;81(2):e16–25.
2. WHO Coronavirus (COVID-19) dashboard [Internet]. Who.int. [cited 2022 Oct 7]. https://covid19.who.int/.
3. Chen Z, Peng Y, Wu X, Pang B, Yang F, Zheng W, et al. Comorbidities and complications of COVID-19 associated with disease severity, progression, and mortality in China with centralized isolation and hospitalization: a systematic review and meta-analysis. Front Public Health. 2022;10:923485.
4. de Almeida-Pititto B, Dualib PM, Zajdenverg L, Dantas JR, de Souza FD, Rodacki M, et al. Severity and mortality of COVID 19 in patients with diabetes, hypertension, and cardiovascular disease: a meta-analysis. Diabetol Metab Syndr. 2020;12(1):75.
5. Izcovich A, Ragusa MA, Tortosa F, Lavena Marzio MA, Agnoletti C, Bengolea A, et al. Prognostic factors for severity and mortality in patients infected with COVID-19: a systematic review. Lazzeri C, editor. PLoS One. 2020;15(11):e0241955.
6. Diabetes [Internet]. World Health Organization. 2021 [cited 2022 Apr 2]. https://www.who.int/news-room/fact-sheets/detail/diabetes.
7. Saeedi P, Petersohn I, Salpea P, Malanda B, Karuranga S, Unwin N, et al. Global and regional diabetes prevalence estimates for 2019 and projections for 2030 and 2045: results from the international diabetes federation diabetes atlas, 9th edition. Diabetes Res Clin Pract. 2019;157:107843.
8. National Diabetes Statistics Report [Internet]. Cdc.gov. 2022 [cited 2022 Oct 7]. https://www.cdc.gov/diabetes/data/statistics-report/index.html.
9. CDC. Prediabetes—your chance to prevent type 2 diabetes [Internet]. Centers for Disease Control and Prevention. 2022 [cited 2022 Oct 7]. https://www.cdc.gov/diabetes/basics/prediabetes.html.
10. Critchley JA, Carey IM, Harris T, DeWilde S, Hosking FJ, Cook DG. Glycemic control and risk of infections among people with type 1 or type 2 diabetes in a large primary care cohort study. Diabetes Care. 2018;41(10):2127–35.
11. Pearson-Stuttard J, Blundell S, Harris T, Cook DG, Critchley J. Diabetes and infection: assessing the association with glycaemic control in population-based studies. Lancet Diabetes Endocrinol. 2016;4(2):148–58.
12. Badawi A, Ryoo SG. Prevalence of diabetes in the 2009 influenza a (H1N1) and the Middle East respiratory syndrome coronavirus: a systematic review and meta-analysis. J Public Health Res. 2016;5(3):jphr.2016.733.

13. Team TNCPERE. The epidemiological characteristics of an outbreak of 2019 novel coronavirus diseases (COVID-19)—China, 2020. China CDC Wkly. 2020;2(8):113–22.

14. CDC COVID-19 Response Team, CDC COVID-19 Response Team, Chow N, Fleming-Dutra K, Gierke R, Hall A, et al. Preliminary estimates of the prevalence of selected underlying health conditions among patients with coronavirus disease 2019 — United States, February 12–March 28, 2020. MMWR Morb Mortal Wkly Rep. 2020;69(13):382–6.

15. Richardson S, Hirsch JS, Narasimhan M, Crawford JM, McGinn T, Davidson KW, et al. Presenting characteristics, comorbidities, and outcomes among 5700 patients hospitalized with COVID-19 in the New York City area. JAMA. 2020;323(20):2052.

16. Li B, Yang J, Zhao F, Zhi L, Wang X, Liu L, et al. Prevalence and impact of cardiovascular metabolic diseases on COVID-19 in China. Clin Res Cardiol. 2020;109(5):531–8.

17. Singh AK, Gillies CL, Singh R, Singh A, Chudasama Y, Coles B, et al. Prevalence of comorbidities and their association with mortality in patients with COVID -19: a systematic review and meta-analysis. Diabetes Obes Metab. 2020;22(10):1915–24.

18. Grasselli G, Zangrillo A, Zanella A, Antonelli M, Cabrini L, Castelli A, et al. Baseline characteristics and outcomes of 1591 patients infected with SARS-CoV-2 admitted to ICUs of the Lombardy Region, Italy. JAMA. 2020;323(16):1574.

19. Thakur B, Dubey P, Benitez J, Torres JP, Reddy S, Shokar N, et al. A systematic review and meta-analysis of geographic differences in comorbidities and associated severity and mortality among individuals with COVID-19. Sci Rep. 2021;11(1):8562.

20. Wu Z, McGoogan JM. Characteristics of and important lessons from the coronavirus disease 2019 (COVID-19) outbreak in China: summary of a report of 72 314 cases from the Chinese Center for Disease Control and Prevention. JAMA. 2020;323(13):1239.

21. National Institute of Health. Clinical spectrum of SARS-CoV-2 infection [Internet]. National Institute of Health—COVID-19 Treatment Guidelines. 2022 [cited 2022 Oct 28]. https://www. covid19treatmentguidelines.nih.gov/overview/clinical-spectrum/.

22. Landstra CP, de Koning EJP. COVID-19 and diabetes: understanding the interrelationship and risks for a severe course. Front Endocrinol. 2021;12:649525.

23. Vasbinder A, Anderson E, Shadid H, Berlin H, Pan M, Azam TU, et al. Inflammation, hyperglycemia, and adverse outcomes in individuals with diabetes mellitus hospitalized for COVID-19. Diabetes Care. 2022;45(3):692–700.

24. Yaribeygi H, Sathyapalan T, Jamialahmadi T, Sahebkar A. The impact of diabetes mellitus in COVID-19: a mechanistic review of molecular interactions. Chiefari E, editor. J Diabetes Res. 2020;2020:1–9.

25. Barrett CE, Koyama AK, Alvarez P, Chow W, Lundeen EA, Perrine CG, et al. Risk for newly diagnosed diabetes >30 days after SARS-CoV-2 infection among persons aged <18 years — United States, March 1, 2020–June 28, 2021. MMWR Morb Mortal Wkly Rep. 2022;71(2):59–65.

26. Khunti K, Del Prato S, Mathieu C, Kahn SE, Gabbay RA, Buse JB. COVID-19, hyperglycemia, and new-onset diabetes. Diabetes Care. 2021;44(12):2645–55.

27. World Health Organization. The impact of the COVID-19 pandemic on noncommunicable disease resources and services: results of a rapid assessment [internet]. Geneva: World Health Organization; 2020. [cited 2022 Oct 7]. https://apps.who.int/iris/handle/10665/334136

28. Wiersinga WJ, Rhodes A, Cheng AC, Peacock SJ, Prescott HC. Pathophysiology, transmission, diagnosis, and treatment of coronavirus disease 2019 (COVID-19): a review. JAMA. 2020;324(8):782.

29. Deinhardt-Emmer S, Böttcher S, Häring C, Giebeler L, Henke A, Zell R, et al. SARS-CoV-2 causes severe epithelial inflammation and barrier dysfunction. Gallagher T, editor. J Virol. 2021;95(10):e00110-21.

30. Wu CT, Lidsky PV, Xiao Y, Lee IT, Cheng R, Nakayama T, et al. SARS-CoV-2 infects human pancreatic β cells and elicits β cell impairment. Cell Metab. 2021;33(8):1565–76.e5

31. Birabaharan M, Kaelber DC, Pettus JH, Smith DM. Risk of new-onset type 2 diabetes in 600 055 people after COVID-19: a cohort study. Diabetes Obes Metab. 2022;24(6):1176–9.

32. Da Porto A, Tascini C, Colussi G, Peghin M, Graziano E, De Carlo C, et al. Relationship between cytokine release and stress hyperglycemia in patients hospitalized with COVID-19 infection. Front Med. 2022;9:988686.
33. Jivanji CJ, Asrani VM, Windsor JA, Petrov MS. New-onset diabetes after acute and critical illness. Mayo Clin Proc. 2017;92(5):762–73.
34. Ali Abdelhamid Y, Kar P, Finnis ME, Phillips LK, Plummer MP, Shaw JE, et al. Stress hyperglycaemia in critically ill patients and the subsequent risk of diabetes: a systematic review and meta-analysis. Crit Care. 2016;20(1):301.
35. Cromer SJ, Colling C, Schatoff D, Leary M, Stamou MI, Selen DJ, et al. Newly diagnosed diabetes vs. pre-existing diabetes upon admission for COVID-19: associated factors, short-term outcomes, and long-term glycemic phenotypes. J Diabetes Complicat. 2022;36(4):108145.
36. Barron E, Bakhai C, Kar P, Weaver A, Bradley D, Ismail H, et al. Associations of type 1 and type 2 diabetes with COVID-19-related mortality in England: a whole-population study. Lancet Diabetes Endocrinol. 2020;8(10):813–22.
37. McGurnaghan SJ, Weir A, Bishop J, Kennedy S, Blackbourn LAK, McAllister DA, et al. Risks of and risk factors for COVID-19 disease in people with diabetes: a cohort study of the total population of Scotland. Lancet Diabetes Endocrinol. 2021;9(2):82–93.
38. Shafiee A, Teymouri Athar MM, Nassar M, Seighali N, Aminzade D, Fattahi P, et al. Comparison of COVID-19 outcomes in patients with type 1 and type 2 diabetes: a systematic review and meta-analysis. Diabetes Metab Syndr Clin Res Rev. 2022;16(6):102512.
39. COVID-19 confirmed cases and deaths [Internet]. Unicef. 2022 [cited 2022 Oct 12]. https://data.unicef.org/resources/covid-19-confirmed-cases-and-deaths-dashboard/.
40. Ludvigsson JF. Systematic review of COVID-19 in children shows milder cases and a better prognosis than adults. Acta Paediatr. 2020;109(6):1088–95.
41. Patel NA. Pediatric COVID-19: systematic review of the literature. Am J Otolaryngol. 2020;41(5):102573.
42. Mehta NS, Mytton OT, Mullins EWS, Fowler TA, Falconer CL, Murphy OB, et al. SARS-CoV-2 (COVID-19): what do we know about children? A systematic review. Clin Infect Dis. 2020;71(9):2469–79.
43. Hartmann-Boyce J, Rees K, Perring JC, Kerneis SA, Morris EM, Goyder C, et al. Risks of and from SARS-CoV-2 infection and COVID-19 in people with diabetes: a systematic review of reviews. Diabetes Care. 2021;44(12):2790–811.
44. Elbarbary NS, Santos TJ, Beaufort C, Agwu JC, Calliari LE, Scaramuzza AE. COVID -19 outbreak and pediatric diabetes: perceptions of health care professionals worldwide. Pediatr Diabetes. 2020;21(7):1083–92.
45. Güemes M, Storch-de-Gracia P, Enriquez SV, Martín-Rivada Á, Brabin AG, Argente J. Severity in pediatric type 1 diabetes mellitus debut during the COVID-19 pandemic. J Pediatr Endocrinol Metab. 2020;33(12):1601–3.
46. Tittel SR, Rosenbauer J, Kamrath C, Ziegler J, Reschke F, Hammersen J, et al. Did the COVID-19 lockdown affect the incidence of Pediatric type 1 diabetes in Germany? Diabetes Care. 2020;43(11):e172–3.
47. Heidarpour M, Abhari AP, Sadeghpour N, Shafie D, Sarokhani D. Prediabetes and COVID-19 severity, an underestimated risk factor: a systematic review and meta-analysis. Diabetes Metab Syndr Clin Res Rev. 2021;15(6):102307.
48. Chandrasekaran ND, Velure Raja Rao MR, Sathish T. Clinical characteristics and outcomes of COVID-19 patients with prediabetes. Diabetes Metab Syndr Clin Res Rev. 2021;15(4):102192.
49. Smith SM, Boppana A, Traupman JA, Unson E, Maddock DA, Chao K, et al. Impaired glucose metabolism in patients with diabetes, prediabetes, and obesity is associated with severe COVID-19. J Med Virol. 2021;93(1):409–15.
50. Radan AP, Fluri MM, Nirgianakis K, Mosimann B, Schlatter B, Raio L, et al. Gestational diabetes is associated with SARS-CoV-2 infection during pregnancy: a case-control study. Diabetes Metab. 2022;48(4):101351.

51. Perreand E, Mangione M, Patel M, Miyamoto M, Cojocaru L, Seung H, et al. Gestational diabetes mellitus: a risk factor for COVID-19. Am J Obstet Gynecol. 2022;226(1):S750–1.
52. Eskenazi B, Rauch S, Iurlaro E, Gunier RB, Rego A, Gravett MG, et al. Diabetes mellitus, maternal adiposity, and insulin-dependent gestational diabetes are associated with COVID-19 in pregnancy: the INTERCOVID study. Am J Obstet Gynecol. 2022;227(1):74. e1–74.e16.
53. Kleinwechter HJ, Weber KS, Mingers N, Ramsauer B, Schaefer-Graf UM, Groten T, et al. Gestational diabetes mellitus and COVID-19: results from the COVID-19–related obstetric and neonatal outcome study (CRONOS). Am J Obstet Gynecol. 2022;S0002937822003726
54. Hussain S, Baxi H, Chand Jamali M, Nisar N, Hussain MS. Burden of diabetes mellitus and its impact on COVID-19 patients: a meta-analysis of real-world evidence. Diabetes Metab Syndr Clin Res Rev. 2020;14(6):1595–602.
55. Shah A, Deak A, Allen S, Silfani E, Koppin C, Zisman-Ilani Y, et al. Some characteristics of hyperglycaemic crisis differ between patients with and without COVID-19 at a safety-net hospital in a cross-sectional study. Ann Med. 2021;53(1):1642–5.
56. Holman N, Knighton P, Kar P, O'Keefe J, Curley M, Weaver A, et al. Risk factors for COVID-19-related mortality in people with type 1 and type 2 diabetes in England: a population-based cohort study. Lancet Diabetes Endocrinol. 2020;8(10):823–33.
57. Wu J, Huang J, Zhu G, Wang Q, Lv Q, Huang Y, et al. Elevation of blood glucose level predicts worse outcomes in hospitalized patients with COVID-19: a retrospective cohort study. BMJ Open Diabetes Res Care. 2020;8(1):e001476.
58. Coppelli A, Giannarelli R, Aragona M, Penno G, Falcone M, Tiseo G, et al. Hyperglycemia at hospital admission is associated with severity of the prognosis in patients hospitalized for COVID-19: the Pisa COVID-19 study. Diabetes Care. 2020;43(10):2345–8.
59. Wang S, Ma P, Zhang S, Song S, Wang Z, Ma Y, et al. Fasting blood glucose at admission is an independent predictor for 28-day mortality in patients with COVID-19 without previous diagnosis of diabetes: a multi-Centre retrospective study. Diabetologia. 2020;63(10):2102–11.
60. Zhu L, She ZG, Cheng X, Qin JJ, Zhang XJ, Cai J, et al. Association of Blood Glucose Control and Outcomes in patients with COVID-19 and pre-existing type 2 diabetes. Cell Metab. 2020;31(6):1068–77.e3
61. Wargny M, Potier L, Gourdy P, Pichelin M, Amadou C, Benhamou PY, et al. Predictors of hospital discharge and mortality in patients with diabetes and COVID-19: updated results from the nationwide CORONADO study. Diabetologia. 2021;64(4):778–94.
62. Myers AK, Kim TS, Zhu X, Liu Y, Qiu M, Pekmezaris R. Predictors of mortality in a multiracial urban cohort of persons with type 2 diabetes and novel coronavirus 19. J Diabetes. 2021;13(5):430–8.
63. Agarwal S, Schechter C, Southern W, Crandall JP, Tomer Y. Preadmission diabetes-specific risk factors for mortality in hospitalized patients with diabetes and coronavirus disease 2019. Diabetes Care. 2020;43(10):2339–44.

Chapter 4
Pathophysiology of Lung Dysfunction in Diabetes

Junaid Habibullah and Janice Wang

Introduction

The global pandemic of coronavirus disease 2019 (COVID-19) highly impacted patients with hypertension, diabetes mellitus (DM), coronary heart disease, and obesity [1–3]. These comorbidities are commonly seen in people with metabolic syndrome and highlight the role of pro-inflammatory states of such comorbidities and COVID-19. The underlying pathophysiology of lung disease and diabetes is complex and not fully understood. In this chapter, we review the current understanding of co-existing DM, lung disease, and COVID-19.

The Association Between Diabetes and Lung Disease

Hyperglycemia and hyperinsulinemia appear to play a role in lung disease mechanisms in DM [4] (Fig. 4.1). The physiologic characteristic of lung deflation, also known as elastic recoil, is affected by the presence of Type 1 diabetes (T1D) and can even be seen in juveniles with T1D. Elastic recoil, used as a surrogate measure of airflow and gas exchange within the lungs, has been shown to be reduced in people with T1D and associated with an obstructive respiratory pattern and poor gas exchange on pulmonary function testing [5]. Studies have shown an accelerated decline in lung function linked to poor glycemic control in both T1D and Type 2 diabetes (T2D) [6]. Forced vital capacity (FVC) and forced expiratory volume in

J. Habibullah (✉) · J. Wang
Division of Pulmonary, Critical Care and Sleep Medicine, Donald and Barbara Zucker School of Medicine at Hofstra/Northwell, New Hyde Park, NY, USA
e-mail: jhabibulla@northwell.edu

A. K. Myers (ed.), *Diabetes and COVID-19*, Contemporary Endocrinology,
https://doi.org/10.1007/978-3-031-28536-3_4

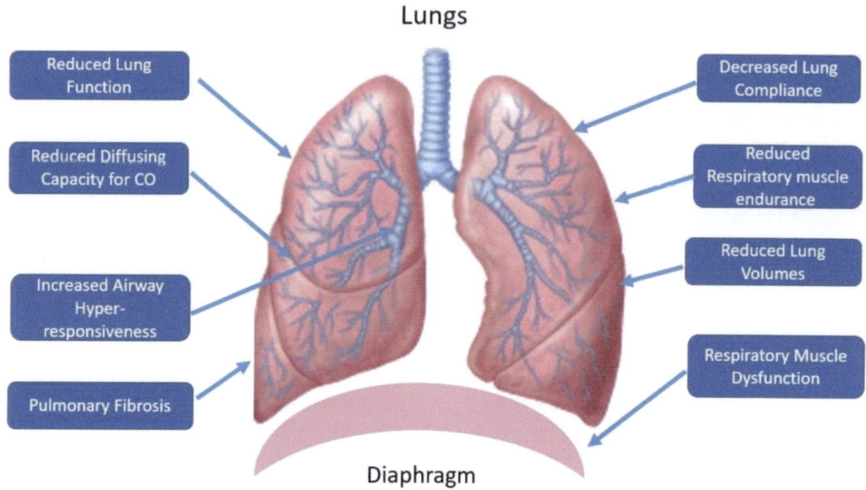

Fig. 4.1 Lung abnormalities associated with diabetes mellitus (DM). People with DM have pulmonary issues, such as reduced lung function and diffusing capacity for carbon monoxide (DLCO) and pulmonary fibrosis resulting from hyperglycemia-induced oxidative stress and activation of fibrotic pathways. Respiratory muscle dysfunction can result from neuropathic damage and increased respiratory muscle rigidity secondary to hyperglycemia

1 second (FEV1) measure the volume of air that can be forcibly blown out after maximum inhalation and in 1 second, respectively. FEV1 declines two to three times faster in diabetic patients compared to nonsmoking patients without diabetes (71 mL/year versus 25 mL/year reduction, respectively) [6]. Cross-sectional analyses also demonstrate that DM is also associated with reduced diffusing capacity for carbon monoxide (DLCO) [7, 8]. This decline in DLCO is likely due to microangiopathy and thickening of the pulmonary capillaries, reduced pulmonary capillary blood volume, nonenzymatic protein glycation in the extracellular matrix, and oxidative stress [7–9]. Reduced DLCO signifies a worsened ability of the lungs to transfer gas from inspired air to the bloodstream [10].

Hyperglycemia can activate multiple pathways of lung damage. Airway hyperresponsiveness may be increased with elevated glucose levels via the Rho/Rock pathway [4]. Rho is part of the Ras superfamily of GTPases and controls several downstream effector proteins. In the GTP-bound state, activated Rho kinase leads to airway inflammation and bronchoconstriction which may contribute to reduced FEV1 and FVC observed in people with DM (PWD) [11]. Hyperglycemia can also accelerate lung fibrosis through the activation of a single transducer and activator of transcription 3 (STAT3), connective tissue growth factor (CTGF), and transforming growth factor beta (TGF- β) [12, 13].

Hyperinsulinemia is commonly seen in T2D in order to overcome the effects of insulin resistance [14]. However, hyperinsulinemia can lead to deleterious effects on the lungs through several mechanisms. Demonstrated in rats through the phosphoinositide-3-kinase pathway, insulin can inhibit the production of surfactant proteins A and D, without which alveoli function can worsen and lead to decreased lung compliance [15, 16]. Immunologically, hyperinsulinemia increases the production of type 2 T helper cells, a key driver of cytokine release, and mast cell survival and degranulation, both seen in disease pathways of asthma [17]. Within the airways, insulin promotes smooth muscle cell proliferation and contraction via Rho kinase and I3K pathways, and lung tissue fibrosis through the deposition of extracellular matrix [18].

Respiratory health is also contributed by lung health and respiratory muscle strength, including the diaphragm and intercostal muscles. Decreased respiratory muscle strength and endurance contributing to decreased lung function have been demonstrated in both T1D and T2D, particularly in association with higher levels of hemoglobin A1C [19, 20].

Lung Pathophysiology of COVID-19 in Diabetes

During the first surge in Wuhan, China moderate to severe acute respiratory distress syndrome (ARDS) was reported to occur in as many as 42% of COVID-19 patients and 52% of them died [21]. PWD are at high risk for COVID-19 and greater illness severity requiring hospital and intensive care unit admission [22]. Major pathways attributing to higher COVID-19 risk seen in PWD are: (1) increased viral entry via angiotensin-converting enzyme 2 (ACE-2) receptors and furin, (2) impaired T-Cell function, (3) increased interleukin-6 (IL-6), and (4) hyperinflammation [22, 23] (see Fig. 4.2).

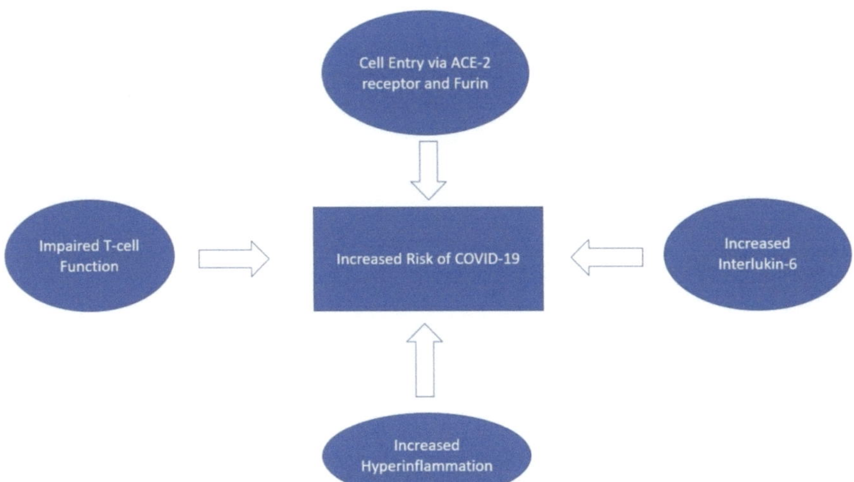

Fig. 4.2 Major pathways attributing to the higher COVID-19 risk in DM: (1) Increased expression of angiotensin-converting enzyme-2 (ACE-2) receptor and furin promote viral cell entry; (2) increased Interleukin-6 accelerates the acute inflammatory process during the infection; (3) impaired T-cell function is seen as a sequela of hyperinsulinemia; and (4) hyperinflammation is due to increased Angiotensin II

The virus responsible for COVID-19, known as severe acute respiratory syndrome coronavirus 2 (SARS-CoV-2), gains host cell entry via ACE-2 which is highly expressed in lung alveolar epithelial cells [24]. ACE-2 is part of renin-angiotensin system (RAS), and converts angiotensin II to angiotensin 1–7. Angiotensin II receptor type 1 regulates increased inflammation, vascular permeability, and vasoconstriction in the lungs, all seen in ARDS [25] (see Fig. 4.3).

Delayed responses from Th1 cell–mediated immunity, as noted previously as a possible effect of hyperinsulinemia, may impair adaptive immunity and be linked to abnormal cytokine release and subsequently a pro-inflammatory state and ARDS. In a study examining Middle Eastern Respiratory Syndrome-Coronavirus (MERS-CoV) infection in a diabetic mouse model, infections were more prolonged and severe in the setting of decreased CD4+ T cell counts and abnormal cytokine release compared to responses in non-diabetic mice. Patients with COVID-19 were found to have decreased CD4+ T cell count [26]. This suggests that a blunted immune response in COVID-19 may indeed be linked to hyperinsulinemia in diabetic patients with insulin resistance.

IL-6 triggers the release of multiple acute phase reactants, which can lead to a hyperinflammatory state and is elevated in airway inflammation and bronchoconstriction. IL-6 is profoundly more elevated in PWD compared to those without diabetes in COVID-19 and has been associated with severe COVID-19 pneumonia [27]. This may contribute to the risk for the progression of COVID-19 severity in PWD.

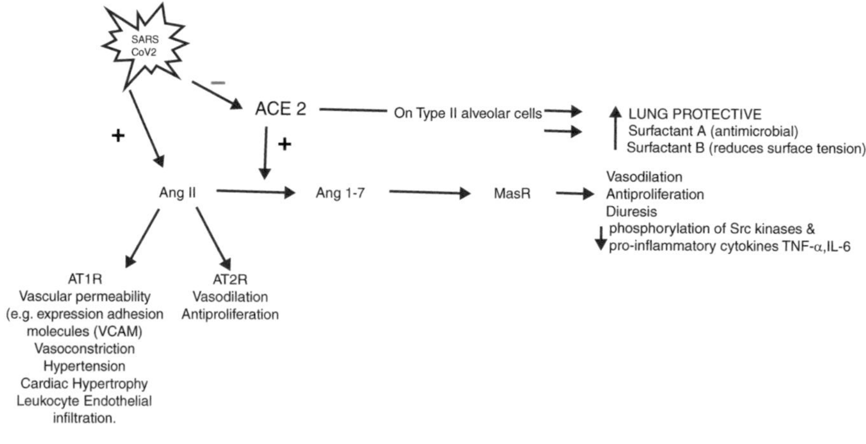

Fig. 4.3 SARS-CoV-2 entry via ACE-2 receptor. This figure illustrates the utilization of ACE-2 receptor by SARS-CoV-2 virus for cellular entry. The binding of ACE-2 receptor also leads to the activation and cleavage of Ang II to Ang 1–7. Ang II leads to increase vascular permeability; release of cytokines (IL-6, TNF-α, IL-1ß); and leukocyte infiltration. Ang 1–7 leads to vasodilation, diuresis, and further cytokine release. ACE-2 = angiotensin converting enzyme-2; Ang II = angiotensin II; Ang 1–7 = angiotensin 1–7; IL-6 = interleukin-6; TNF- α = tumor necrosis factor alpha; IL-1ß = interleukin-1 beta

COVID-19, Diabetes, and Asthma

Immunopathogenic and environmental pathways are known mechanisms of asthma and are observed in people with co-existing diabetes and asthma. Asthma pathways consist of non-Type 2 and Type 2 atopic, or allergic asthma. Non-type 2 asthma is associated with older age, obesity, T2D, and metabolic syndrome; it is characterized by T-helper type 1 cells (Th1) or Th17-dominated inflammation in patients with adult-onset disease [28]. A proposed mechanism linking diabetes and lung disease is the expression of non-enzymatic glycation and oxidation protein products, known as the receptor for advanced glycation end-products (RAGE), which plays a regulatory role in T cell proliferation and differentiation [29]. RAGE products are highly expressed in the lungs and accumulate in hyperglycemia, predisposing patients to chronic airway inflammation [11]. Increased IL-6 in diabetes is associated with more severe asthma, especially in those who are obese, and is also independently elevated in DM, asthma, and COVID-19 [30].

Insulin resistance in T2D is strongly associated with asthma. People with T2D have a two-fold greater risk of developing asthma compared to those without diabetes [31]. Hyperinsulinemia inhibits surfactant A and D production, which are important in preventing alveoli collapse during expiration [15, 16]. Increased insulin levels also shift the production of T cells toward Th2 cells, promote mast cell survival and degranulation, activate inflammatory macrophages, and signal for the proliferation and contraction of airway smooth muscle cells [17, 18, 32, 33].

Asthma prevalence in COVID-19 patients is about 12%; however, there was no difference in intubation frequencies when compared to the patients without asthma [34]. It has been suggested that the use of inhaled steroids by persons with steroids may be the reason for this as it leads to the downregulation of ACE2 [35]. Despite this, there remains an increased risk of severe COVID-19 infection in PWD [36]. There are currently no studies examining the prevalence or severity of COVID-19 in patients with both diabetes and asthma; however, those hospitalized for asthma and who have comorbid diabetes have a longer length of stay, higher cost based on hospital total length of stay and greater risk for 30-day readmission when compared to those without comorbid diabetes [37].

COVID-19, Diabetes, and Chronic Obstructive Pulmonary Disease

In addition to an increased risk of asthma, diabetes also increases the risk of chronic obstructive pulmonary disease (COPD) exacerbation and mortality [38, 39]. Conversely, more advanced COPD is associated with a higher risk for DM, independent of smoking and body mass index (BMI) [39]. Diabetes and COPD share features of chronic inflammation and systemic oxidative stress; however, the underlying mechanism connecting the two comorbidities is not entirely clear. Inflammatory markers of IL-6, tumor necrosis factor alpha (TNF-α) soluble receptor, and C-reactive protein are associated with insulin resistance and are involved in the inflammatory pathways demonstrated in T2DM and impaired lung function as measured by FEV1 in COPD [40].

Hyperglycemia on admission, regardless of diabetes diagnosis, has been associated with an increased need for invasive ventilation for COPD [41]. Metformin treatment in PWD and COPD is associated with reduced emergency room visits and hospitalizations, as well as reduced all-cause mortality [42–44]. Metformin decreases hepatic glucose production and intestinal absorption of glucose, and improves insulin sensitivity thereby attenuating hyperinsulinemia, which may explain the outcome benefits seen in people with COPD [44].

While COPD prevalence has been reported to be low (between 3% and 6.6%) among people with COVID-19, it is linked to high mortality and hospitalizations [45, 46]. Patient outcomes in COVID-19 are influenced by the underlying COPD severity. The pathophysiology of COVID-19 in COPD is similar to asthma. IL-6 levels are elevated in COPD, which can further exacerbate the cytokine storm seen in COVID-19, leading to lung injury [30]. Bronchial epithelium and whole lung tissue from obese COPD patients have increased ACE-2 gene expression when compared to control subjects. COPD patients also have decreased lung function with elevated ACE-2 expression which may contribute to severe COVID-19 infections [47].

COVID-19, Diabetes, and Pulmonary Fibrosis

Idiopathic pulmonary fibrosis (IPF) is a progressive fibrosing interstitial pneumonia of unknown cause. It can present with progressive dyspnea, low lung volumes, and has been shown to have an association with diabetes. PWD and IPF tend to present with a usual interstitial pneumonia pattern on high-resolution computed tomography scan compared to those without DM [48]. In a case-control study of 65 IPF patients, the odds ratio of developing IPF among PWD was found to be 4.06, adjusted for smoking, obesity, hypertension, and hyperlipidemia, [49].

As noted earlier, a proposed mechanism of fibrosis involves hyperglycemia activating STAT3, CTGF, and TGF- β which are signaling pathways in the initiation and progression of pulmonary fibrosis in the diabetic mouse model [12]. In other animal models, hyperglycemia can also lead to oxidative stress, reactive oxygen species, and nitrogen species which are major inducers of pulmonary fibrosis in T1DM [50].

Currently, data is lacking in establishing a direct relationship between DM, IPF, and COVID-19. COVID-19 itself may lead to pulmonary fibrosis which may or may not be reversible (see Fig. 4.4).

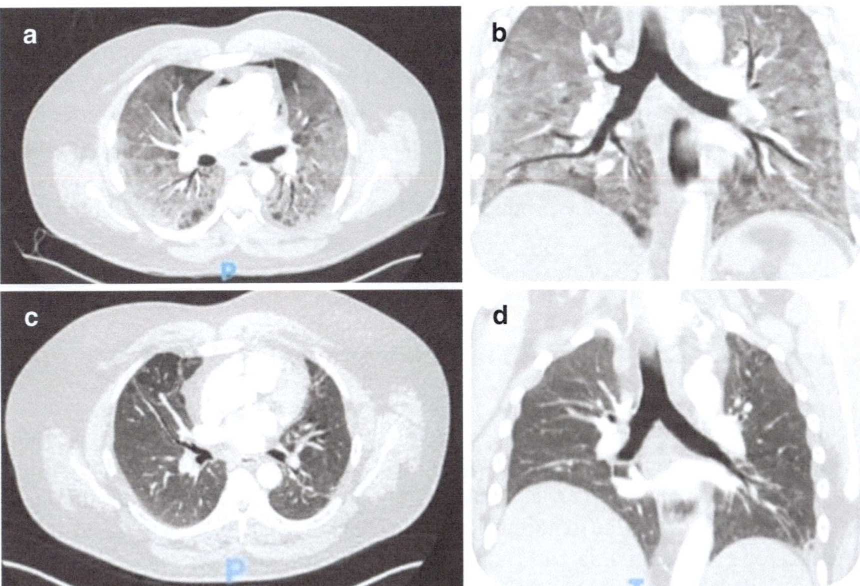

Fig. 4.4 CT chest from a patient with acute COVID-19 infection and one-year follow-up. Images **a** and **b** show acute COVID-19 pneumonia with typical diffuse ground glass opacities. Images **c** and **d** were performed on one-year follow-up, demonstrating resolution of the ground glass opacities and minimal signs of fibrotic changes

COVID-19, Diabetes, and Acute Respiratory Distress Syndrome

Acute respiratory distress syndrome is an acute, diffuse, inflammatory form of lung injury that is associated with a variety of etiologies. It is characterized by bilateral radiographic lung opacities not fully explained by pleural effusions, lung collapse, pulmonary nodules, cardiac failure, or fluid overload. The severity of impaired oxygenation is defined by the ratio of arterial oxygen tension to fraction of inspired oxygen (PaO_2/FiO_2) on ventilator settings delivering positive end expiratory pressure of at least ≥ 5 cm H_2O [51]. According to the Berlin definition, severe ARDS requires a $PaO_2/FiO_2 \leq 100$ mm Hg (normal is greater than 300 mm Hg) [52].

T2D does not appear to affect the progression or mortality of ARDS in those with acute hypoxic respiratory failure [53]. PWD who were obese, older, and had multiple comorbidities were more likely to develop ARDS in a global, multi-center prospective cohort study of 4499 patients in 459 ICUs across 50 countries [53]. The presence of hyperglycemia on admission in those with DM may reduce the development of ARDS in patients with septic shock; however, the mechanism behind this observation is unclear [54]. Intensive insulin therapy has been associated with a shorter duration of mechanical ventilation and decreased mortality and/or morbidity rates among hyperglycemic patients with prolonged ICU stays, regardless of a DM diagnosis [55]. This was then refuted by the NICE-SUGAR study which showed that intensive insulin therapy increased mortality and had no difference on ICU days or ventilator requirement when compared to conventional therapy [56]. Animal models suggest a benefit from insulin therapy in ARDS by negating the effects of endotoxins released during infections, which can cause lung injury [57]. Although this has not been seen in humans, it is known that insulin has anti-inflammatory effects as it can decrease the production of both IL-6 and TNF-α which both contribute to ARDS [58].

COVID-19, Diabetes, and Thromboembolic Disorder

Venous thromboembolism (VTE) presentations range widely from a non-complicated deep venous thrombus (DVT) to small versus life-threatening pulmonary embolism (PE) which carries a risk for long-term morbidities such as pulmonary hypertension and right heart failure (see Fig. 4.5). VTE may be provoked in the presence of a known risk factor(s) or unprovoked. Commonly recognized risks for VTE include but are not limited to immobilization as seen in hospitalized patients, surgery, cancers, obesity, pregnancy, and prior history of VTE. Alarmingly, up to 45% of VTE cases were unprovoked as there were no obvious identifiable risk factors at the time of diagnosis [59]. A population-based study of hospitalized patients demonstrated that people with T2D were 40% more likely to have a PE and 15% more likely to have in-hospital mortality compared to persons without diabetes hospitalized with PE [60]. In turn, patients with VTE have an increased risk for cardiovascular disease, raising the hypothesis of increased risk with metabolic syndrome. Prospective studies and meta-analysis of case-control cohort studies have demonstrated that it is primarily abdominal obesity seen in metabolic syndrome that is an independent risk factor for VTE [59, 61]. Abdominal adiposity is characterized by chronic inflammation and insulin resistance and is associated with increased levels of fibrinogen, tissue factor, and factor VII which can activate the coagulation

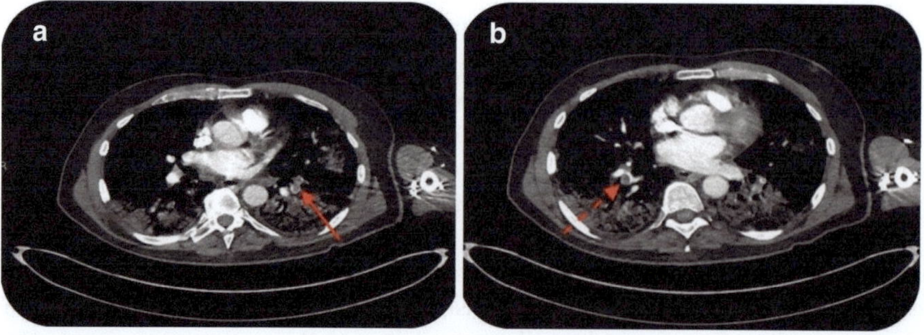

Fig. 4.5 Pulmonary embolus in COVID-19. Images **a** and **b** show the presence of pulmonary embolus (solid and dashed red arrows) in acute COVID-19

cascade. Low fibrinolysis is also seen in obesity because of increased levels of plasminogen activator inhibitor-1 and decreased plasma tissue-type plasminogen activator activity [59]. These factors increase the risk for a hypercoagulable state.

COVID-19 is associated with pro-inflammatory activation through cytokines and angiotensin II effects, immunothrombotic activity, endothelial dysfunction, and vasculopathy on a multi-organ level [62, 63]. The incidence of DVT and PE are reportedly ranging from 16% to 23% and mortality is higher in COVID-19 patients with VTE compared to those without VTE [64, 65]. The prothrombotic state is further increased in COVID-19 patients with DM. Calvisi et al. found a higher incidence of VTE in COVID-19 patients with DM compared to patients without DM (47.1% vs 21.2%, $p = 0.001$). VTE risk factors included DM and stress hyperglycemia which are associated with increased inflammation signified by elevated C reactive protein, higher D-dimer levels, and lower antithrombin III activity [66].

COVID-19's Impact on those with Cystic Fibrosis Bronchiectasis and Diabetes

Chronic inflammation and infection in the lungs can lead to airway scarring and thickening known as bronchiectasis. Bronchiectasis may be due to cystic fibrosis (CF), an autosomal recessive genetic disorder in which disease-causing mutations are found in the cystic fibrosis transmembrane conductance regulator (CFTR) gene. CFTR is a transmembrane chloride ion channel found in the apical membrane of epithelial cells of multiple organs. Dysfunctional CFTR in the lungs leads to significant mucus production in the airways, reduced ciliary function, and increased risk for the acquisition of pathogens and respiratory infections. CF is predominantly a respiratory disorder; however, it also affects the pancreas. Exocrine pancreatic insufficiency is mostly diagnosed at an early age and increases the risk for malnutrition, poor growth, and poor immune defenses, resulting in increased pulmonary infections and exacerbations. Pancreatic insufficiency is treated with pancreatic enzyme replacement therapy and is a life-long therapy. By adulthood, endocrine pancreatic dysfunction resulting in CF-related diabetes (CFRD) may be diagnosed in up to 50% of adults [67]. CFRD is a unique entity because there is insulin deficiency without autoantibodies due to pancreatic fibrosis and destruction as well as varying levels of insulin resistance related to pulmonary exacerbations, corticosteroid use, and genetic variants which may predispose patients with increased susceptibility to beta-cell dysfunction [68]. Treatment of choice in CFRD is insulin therapy, which has been shown to improve FEV1 within 3 months of initial treatment and attenuates decline in lung function by improving nutritional status and glycemic control [69].

As mentioned, diabetes is associated with lower lung function in the general population. However, in people with CF, it is even more impactful in a progressive lung disease that does not have a cure. Patients with hyperglycemia have increased glucose levels in the airway surface liquid, promoting bacterial growth such as *Pseudomonas aeruginosa*, which increases chronic inflammation, mucous production, and furthering bronchiectasis [70, 71]. Chronic respiratory pathogens are difficult to eradicate once colonization is established in bronchiectasis. The lung microbiome is linked to the microbiome of the gut, known as the gut-lung axis [72]. Both microbiomes are affected by inflammation and microbial immunomodulatory metabolites such as short-chain fatty acids. An imbalance of the gut microbiome as seen in frequent antibiotic use may increase the risk for pulmonary exacerbations. It is yet to be elucidated how the dynamics of the gut-lung axis are influenced by hyperglycemia or diabetes; however, DM animal models have demonstrated that dysbiosis of this axis activates the nuclear factor kappa-light-chain-enhancer of activated B cells signaling pathways and results in alveolar wall thickening and fibrosis [73].

Significant advancements have been made in CF treatments, the most recent one being CFTR modulator elexacaftor/tezacaftor/ivacaftor (ETI) which corrects and improves the function of the defective CFTR protein leading to improvement and preservation of lung function. Following the approval of CFTR modulator drugs, the average life expectancy in CF is now 46 years of age compared to 29 in the 1990s [74]. Currently, approximately 90% of the United States CF population is eligible for ETI use; however, patients who do not qualify for this life-changing drug remain at risk for progressing to advanced lung disease and requiring lung transplant. CF lung transplant patients with CFRD pre-transplant have a higher mortality than those without CFRD [75]. The prevalence of new-onset diabetes in patients with CF or bronchiectasis following a lung transplant is also significant and has been observed in up to 67% of patients [76]. The pathophysiologic mechanisms of DM following lung transplant include glucocorticoid-induced hyperglycemia, and the use of calcineurin inhibitors (e.g., cyclosporine, tacrolimus) and inhibitors of mammalian target of rapamycin (e.g., sirolimus) which cause insulin resistance and decrease insulin secretion via beta-cell apoptosis [76].

Further studies are needed to examine the role of DM in the CF COVID-19 population. However, it would not be surprising if it remains a risk factor for COVID-19 as it is in the general population. CFRD is associated with more pathogenic mutations which are linked to increased severity of lung disease, both comorbidities being at risk for severe COVID-19. Another extremely vulnerable CF subpopulation to COVID-19 is the immunosuppressed post-transplant patients, including lung- and/or liver-transplanted patients. The European CF registry data found a higher COVID-19 incidence in the lung-transplanted group compared to the non-transplanted group, while also demonstrating that the mortality rate was lower for all people with CF than for the general population [77]. The reported incidence of COVID-19 in people with CF has thankfully been lower than expected, and it is hypothesized that telemedicine, social distancing, and masking as well as CFTR modulator therapy may have played a role in the low incidence [78, 79].

Conclusion

Diabetes mellitus can influence respiratory mechanics via multiple pathways leading to an increased risk of developing lung disease. These pathways occur at the anatomical and molecular level related to hyperglycemia and insulin levels and share similarities with COVID-19 lung infection via cytokine or secondary messenger pathways. As more knowledge is gained from the disease mechanisms of DM, lung disease, and COVID-19, independently and collectively, a better understanding will be gained of the diabetic lung.

References

1. Du Y, Tu L, Zhu P, Mu M, Wang R, Yang P, et al. Clinical features of 85 fatal cases of COVID-19 from Wuhan. A retrospective observational study. Am J Respir Crit Care Med. 2020;201(11):1372–9. https://pubmed.ncbi.nlm.nih.gov/32242738/ [cited 2022 Feb 6] [Internet]
2. Wang D, Hu B, Hu C, Zhu F, Liu X, Zhang J, et al. Clinical characteristics of 138 hospitalized patients with 2019 novel coronavirus-infected pneumonia in Wuhan, China. JAMA. 2020;323(11):1061–9. [cited 2022 Feb 6] [Internet] https://pubmed.ncbi.nlm.nih.gov/32031570/
3. Kassir R. Risk of COVID-19 for patients with obesity. Obes Rev. 2020;21(6):e13034. https://doi.org/10.1111/obr.13034. [Internet] [cited 2022 Feb 6]
4. Kolahian S, Leiss V, Nürnberg B. Diabetic lung disease: fact or fiction? Rev Endocr Metab Disord. 2019;20(3):303–19. [Internet] [cited 2022 Jan 12] https://pubmed.ncbi.nlm.nih.gov/31637580/
5. Schuyler MR, Niewoehner DE, Inkley SR, Kohn R. Abnormal lung elasticity in juvenile diabetes mellitus. Am Rev Respir Dis [Internet]. 1976;113(1):37–41. [cited 2022 Jan 12] https://pubmed.ncbi.nlm.nih.gov/1247213/
6. Lange P, Groth S, Mortensen J, Appleyard M, Nyboe J, Schnohr P, et al. Diabetes mellitus and ventilatory capacity: a five year follow-up study. Eur Respir J. 1990;3:3.
7. Guvener N, Tutuncu NB, Akcay Ş, Eyuboglu F, Gokcel A. Alveolar gas exchange in patients with type 2 diabetes mellitus. Endocr J [Internet]. 2003;50(6):663–7. [cited 2022 Jan 12] https://pubmed.ncbi.nlm.nih.gov/14709835/
8. Klein OL, Kalhan R, Williams MV, Tipping M, Lee J, Peng J, et al. Lung spirometry parameters and diffusion capacity are decreased in patients with type 2 diabetes. Diabet Med. 2012;29(2):212–9. [cited 2022 Jan 12] [Internet] https://pubmed.ncbi.nlm.nih.gov/21790775/
9. Özşahin K, Tuğrul A, Mert S, Yüksel M, Tuğrul G. Evaluation of pulmonary alveolo-capillary permeability in type 2 diabetes mellitus: using technetium 99mTc-DTPA aerosol scintigraphy and carbon monoxide diffusion capacity. J Diabetes Complications [Internet]. 2006;20(4):205–9. [cited 2022 Jan 12] https://pubmed.ncbi.nlm.nih.gov/16798470/
10. Modi P, Cascella M. Diffusing capacity of the lungs for carbon monoxide. StatPearls. 2021; [cited 2022 Feb 6]; [Internet] https://www.ncbi.nlm.nih.gov/books/NBK556149/
11. Zhang Y, Saradna A, Ratan R, Ke X, Tu W, Do DC, et al. RhoA/rho-kinases in asthma: from pathogenesis to therapeutic targets. Clin Transl Immunology. 2020;9:5. [cited 2022 Feb 6]; [Internet] /pmc/articles/PMC7190398/

12. Zheng F, Lu W, Wu F, Li H, Hu X, Zhang F. Recombinant decorin ameliorates the pulmonary structure alterations by down-regulating transforming growth factor-beta1/SMADS signaling in the diabetic rats. Endocr Res. 2010;35(1):35–49. [Internet] [cited 2022 Jan 12] https://pubmed.ncbi.nlm.nih.gov/20136517/

13. Wang CM, Hsu CT, Niu HS, Chang CH, Cheng JT, Shieh JM. Lung damage induced by hyperglycemia in diabetic rats: the role of signal transducer and activator of transcription 3 (STAT3). J Diabetes Complicat. 2016;30(8):1426–33. [Internet]. [cited 2022 Jan 12]; https://pubmed.ncbi.nlm.nih.gov/27481368/

14. Thomas DD, Corkey BE, Istfan NW, Apovian CM. Hyperinsulinemia: an early indicator of metabolic dysfunction. J Endocr Soc. 2019;3(9):1727. [cited 2022 Feb 10] [Internet] /pmc/articles/PMC6735759/

15. Foster DJ, Ravikumar P, Bellotto DJ, Unger RH, Hsia CCW. Fatty diabetic lung: altered alveolar structure and surfactant protein expression. Am J Physiol Lung Cell Mol Physiol. 2010;298:3. [Internet] [cited 2022 Jan 12] https://pubmed.ncbi.nlm.nih.gov/20061442/

16. Treviñeo-Alanís M, Ventura-Juárez J, Hernández-Piñeero J, Nevárez-Garza A, Quintanar-Stephano A, González-Piñea A. Delayed lung maturation of foetus of diabetic mother rats develop with a diminish, but without changes in the proportion of type I and II pneumocytes, and decreased expression of protein D-associated surfactant factor. Anat Histol Embryol. 2009;38(3):169–76. [cited 2022 Jan 12] [Internet] https://pubmed.ncbi.nlm.nih.gov/19245670/

17. Viardot A, Grey ST, Mackay F, Chisholm D. Potential antiinflammatory role of insulin via the preferential polarization of effector T cells toward a T helper 2 phenotype. Endocrinology. 2007;148(1):346–53. [Internet]. [cited 2022 Jan 12] https://pubmed.ncbi.nlm.nih.gov/17008395/

18. Gosens R, Nelemans SA, Hiemstra M, Grootte Bromhaar MM, Meurs H, Zaagsma J. Insulin induces a hypercontractile airway smooth muscle phenotype. Eur J Pharmacol. 2003;481(1):125–31. [cited 2022 Jan 12] [Internet]. https://pubmed.ncbi.nlm.nih.gov/14637184/

19. Fuso L, Pitocco D, Longobardi A, Zaccardi F, Contu C, Pozzuto C, et al. Reduced respiratory muscle strength and endurance in type 2 diabetes mellitus. Diabetes Metab Res Rev. 2012;28(4):370–5. [cited 2022 Jan 13] [Internet]. https://pubmed.ncbi.nlm.nih.gov/22271438/

20. Wanke T, Formanek D, Auinger M, Popp W, Zwick H, Irsigler K. Inspiratory muscle performance and pulmonary function changes in insulin-dependent diabetes mellitus. Am Rev Respir Dis. 1991;143(1):97–100. [Internet]. [cited 2022 Jan 13] https://pubmed.ncbi.nlm.nih.gov/1986691/

21. Yang X, Yu Y, Xu J, Shu H, Xia J, Liu H, et al. Clinical course and outcomes of critically ill patients with SARS-CoV-2 pneumonia in Wuhan, China: a single-centered, retrospective, observational study. Lancet Respir Med. 2020;

22. Singh AK, Gupta R, Ghosh A, Misra A. Diabetes in COVID-19: prevalence, pathophysiology, prognosis and practical considerations. Diabetes Metab Syndr Clin Res Rev. 2020;14(4):303–10.

23. Muniyappa R, Gubbi S. COVID-19 pandemic, coronaviruses, and diabetes mellitus. Am J Physiol Endocrinol Metab. 2020;318(5):E736–41. [Internet]. [cited 2022 Jan 3]. https://doi.org/10.1152/ajpendo.00124.2020.

24. Hoffmann M, Kleine-Weber H, Schroeder S, Krüger N, Herrler T, Erichsen S, et al. SARS-CoV-2 cell entry depends on ACE2 and TMPRSS2 and is blocked by a clinically proven protease inhibitor. Cell. 2020;181(2):271–80.e8. [Internet] https://pubmed.ncbi.nlm.nih.gov/32142651/ [cited 2022 Feb 6]

25. Kuba K, Imai Y, Penninger JM. Angiotensin-converting enzyme 2 in lung diseases. Curr Opin Pharmacol. 2006;6(3):271–6. [Internet] https://pubmed.ncbi.nlm.nih.gov/16581295/ [cited 2022 Feb 6]

26. Xu Z, Shi L, Wang Y, Zhang J, Huang L, Zhang C, et al. Pathological findings of COVID-19 associated with acute respiratory distress syndrome. Lancet Respir Med. 2020;8(4):420–2. [cited 2022 Jan 13] [Internet] https://pubmed.ncbi.nlm.nih.gov/32085846/

27. Maddaloni E, Buzzetti R. Covid-19 and diabetes mellitus: unveiling the interaction of two pandemics. Diabetes Metab Res Rev. 2020;36:7. [cited 2022 Jan 13] [Internet]. https://pubmed.ncbi.nlm.nih.gov/32233018/

28. Skevaki C, Karsonova A, Karaulov A, Xie M, Renz H. Asthma-associated risk for COVID-19 development. J Allergy Clin Immunol. 2020;146(6):1295. [Internet] /pmc/articles/PMC7834224/ [cited 2022 Jan 16]

29. Akirav EM, Henegariu O, Preston-Hurlburt P, Schmidt AM, Clynes R, Herold KC. The receptor for advanced glycation end products (RAGE) affects T cell differentiation in OVA induced asthma. PLoS One [Internet]. 2014;9:4. [cited 2022 Jan 13]; https://pubmed.ncbi.nlm.nih.gov/24759895/

30. Peters MC, McGrath KW, Hawkins GA, Hastie AT, Levy BD, Israel E, et al. Plasma interleukin-6 concentrations, metabolic dysfunction, and asthma severity: a cross-sectional analysis of two cohorts. Lancet Respir Med. 2016;4(7):574–84. [cited 2022 Jan 13] [Internet]. https://pubmed.ncbi.nlm.nih.gov/27283230/

31. Beuther DA, Sutherland ER. Overweight, obesity, and incident asthma: a meta-analysis of prospective epidemiologic studies. Am J Respir Crit Care Med. 2007;175(7):661–6. [cited 2022 Jan 13]; [Internet]. https://pubmed.ncbi.nlm.nih.gov/17234901/

32. Lessmann E, Grochowy G, Weingarten L, Giesemann T, Aktories K, Leitges M, et al. Insulin and insulin-like growth factor-1 promote mast cell survival via activation of the phosphatidylinositol-3-kinase pathway. Exp Hematol. 2006;34(11):1532–41. [Internet]. [cited 2022 Jan 12]; https://pubmed.ncbi.nlm.nih.gov/17046573/

33. Noveral JP, Bhala A, Hintz RL, Grunstein MM, Cohen P. Insulin-like growth factor axis in airway smooth muscle cells. Am J Physiol [Internet]. 1994;267(6 Pt 1) [cited 2022 Jan 12]; https://pubmed.ncbi.nlm.nih.gov/7528983/

34. Asthma Prevalence | Asthma | CDC [Internet]. [cited 2022 Jan 17]. https://www.cdc.gov/asthma/data-visualizations/prevalence.htm

35. Broadhurst R, Peterson R, Wisnivesky JP, Federman A, Zimmer SM, Sharma S, et al. Asthma in COVID-19 hospitalizations: an overestimated risk factor? Ann Am Thorac Soc. 2020;17(12):1645–8. 1 [cited 2022 Jun 21]; [Internet]. www.atsjournals.org

36. Wu C, Chen X, Cai Y, Xia J, Zhou X, Xu S, et al. Risk factors associated with acute respiratory distress syndrome and death in patients with coronavirus disease 2019 pneumonia in Wuhan, China. JAMA Intern Med. 2020;180(7):934–43. [Internet] [cited 2022 Jan 13] https://jamanetwork.com/journals/jamainternalmedicine/fullarticle/2763184

37. Zhang P, Lopez R, Attaway AH, Georas SN, Khatri SB, Abi-Saleh S, et al. Diabetes mellitus is associated with worse outcome in patients hospitalized for asthma. J Allergy Clin Immunol Pract. 2021;9(4):1562. [cited 2022 Dec 5] [Internet]. Available from: /pmc/articles/PMC8043963/

38. Miller J, Edwards LD, Agustí A, Bakke P, Calverley PMA, Celli B, et al. Comorbidity, systemic inflammation and outcomes in the ECLIPSE cohort. Respir Med. 2013;107(9):1376–84. [cited 2022 Jan 13]; [Internet]. https://pubmed.ncbi.nlm.nih.gov/23791463/

39. Mannino DM, Thorn D, Swensen A, Holguin F. Prevalence and outcomes of diabetes, hypertension and cardiovascular disease in COPD. Eur Respir J. 2008;32(4):962–9. [Internet]. [cited 2022 Jan 13] https://pubmed.ncbi.nlm.nih.gov/18579551/

40. Bolton CE, Evans M, Ionescu AA, Edwards SM, Morris RHK, Dunseath G, et al. Insulin resistance and inflammation—a further systemic complication of COPD. COPD. 2007;4(2):121–6. [Internet]. [cited 2022 Jan 13]; https://pubmed.ncbi.nlm.nih.gov/17530505/

41. Chakrabarti B, Angus RM, Agarwal S, Lane S, Calverley PMA. Hyperglycaemia as a predictor of outcome during non-invasive ventilation in decompensated COPD. Thorax. 2009;64(10):857–62. [Internet]. [cited 2022 Jan 14]; https://pubmed.ncbi.nlm.nih.gov/19454410/

42. Bishwakarma R, Zhang W, Li YL, Kuo YF, Cardenas VJ, Sharma G. Metformin use and health care utilization in patients with coexisting chronic obstructive pulmonary disease and diabetes mellitus. Int J Chron Obstruct Pulmon Dis. 2018;13:793–800. [cited 2022 Jan 14]; [Internet]. https://pubmed.ncbi.nlm.nih.gov/29551895/

43. Yen FS, Chen W, Wei JCC, Hsu CC, Hwu CM. Effects of metformin use on total mortality in patients with type 2 diabetes and chronic obstructive pulmonary disease: a matched-subject design. PLoS One. 2018;13:10. [cited 2022 Jan 14]; [Internet]. https://pubmed.ncbi.nlm.nih.gov/30286138/

44. Metformin: Drug information - UpToDate [Internet]. [cited 2022 Jan 14]. https://www.uptodate.com/contents/metformin-drug-information?search=metformin&source=panel_search_result&selectedTitle=1~149&usage_type=panel&kp_tab=drug_general&display_rank=1#F193820

45. Marcello RK, Dolle J, Grami S, Adule R, Li Z, Tatem K, et al. Characteristics and outcomes of COVID-19 patients in New York City's public hospital system. medRxiv. 2020;2020.05.29.20086645. [cited 2022 Jan 17] [Internet] https://www.medrxiv.org/content/10.1101/2020.05.29.20086645v3

46. Alqahtani JS, Oyelade T, Aldhahir AM, Alghamdi SM, Almehmadi M, Alqahtani AS, et al. Prevalence, severity and mortality associated with COPD and smoking in patients with COVID-19: a rapid systematic review and meta-analysis. PLoS One. 2020;15:5. [Internet]. [cited 2022 Jan 17] https://pubmed.ncbi.nlm.nih.gov/32392262/

47. Higham A, Mathioudakis A, Vestbo J, Singh D. COVID-19 and COPD: a narrative review of the basic science and clinical outcomes. Eur Respir Rev. 2020;29(158):1–13. [Internet]. [cited 2022 Jan 17]; Available from: /pmc/articles/PMC7651840/

48. Raghu G, Collard HR, Egan JJ, Martinez FJ, Behr J, Brown KK, et al. An official ATS/ERS/JRS/ALAT statement: idiopathic pulmonary fibrosis: evidence-based guidelines for diagnosis and management. Am J Respir Crit Care Med. 2011;183(6):788–824. [cited 2022 Jan 14] [Internet] https://pubmed.ncbi.nlm.nih.gov/21471066/

49. Enomoto T, Usuki J, Azuma A, Nakagawa T, Kudoh S. Diabetes mellitus may increase risk for idiopathic pulmonary fibrosis. Chest. 2003;123(6):2007–11. [Internet]. [cited 2022 Jan 14]; https://pubmed.ncbi.nlm.nih.gov/12796182/

50. Gumieniczek A, Hopkała H, Wójtowicz Z, Wysocka M. Changes in antioxidant status of lung tissue in experimental diabetes in rabbits. Clin Biochem. 2002;35(2):147–9. [cited 2022 Jan 14] [Internet]. https://pubmed.ncbi.nlm.nih.gov/11983351/

51. Herridge MS, Tansey CM, Matté A, Tomlinson G, Diaz-Granados N, Cooper A, et al. Functional disability 5 years after acute respiratory distress syndrome. N Engl J Med. 2011;364(14):1293–304. [cited 2022 Jan 17]; [Internet]. https://pubmed.ncbi.nlm.nih.gov/21470008/

52. Ranieri VM, Rubenfeld GD, Thompson BT, Ferguson ND, Caldwell E, Fan E, et al. Acute respiratory distress syndrome: the Berlin definition. JAMA. 2012;307(23):2526–33. [Internet]. [cited 2022 Jan 17] https://jamanetwork.com/journals/jama/fullarticle/1160659

53. Boyle AJ, Madotto F, Laffey JG, Bellani G, Pham T, Pesenti A, et al. Identifying associations between diabetes and acute respiratory distress syndrome in patients with acute hypoxemic respiratory failure: an analysis of the LUNG SAFE database. Crit Care [Internet]. 2018;22:1. [cited 2022 Jan 16] /pmc/articles/PMC6203969/

54. Moss M, Guidot DM, Duhon GF, Wolken R, Parsons PE, Steinberg KP, et al. Diabetic patients have a decreased incidence of acute respiratory distress syndrome. Crit Care Med. 2000;28(7):2187–92. [cited 2022 Jan 16] [Internet]. https://pubmed.ncbi.nlm.nih.gov/10921539/

55. Van den Berghe G, Wilmer A, Hermans G, Meersseman W, Wouters PJ, Milants I, et al. Intensive insulin therapy in the medical ICU. N Engl J Med. 2006;354(5):449–61. [cited 2022 Jan 16]; [Internet] https://pubmed.ncbi.nlm.nih.gov/16452557/

56. Griesdale DEG, De Souza Rd RJ, Van Dam RM, Heyland DK, Cook DJ, Malhotra A, et al. Intensive insulin therapy and mortality among critically ill patients: a meta-analysis including NICE-SUGAR study data. C Can Med Assoc J. 2009;180(8):821. [cited 2022 Dec 6]; [Internet] /pmc/articles/PMC2665940/

57. Chen HI, Yeh DY, Liou HL, Kao SJ. Insulin attenuates endotoxin-induced acute lung injury in conscious rats. Crit Care Med. 2006;34(3):758–64. [cited 2022 Jan 16]; [Internet]. https://pubmed.ncbi.nlm.nih.gov/16505662/

58. Nakhleh A, Shehadeh N. Interactions between antihyperglycemic drugs and the renin-angiotensin system: putative roles in COVID-19. A mini-review. Diabetes Metab Syndr. 2020;14(4):509. [cited 2022 Dec 6]; [Internet] /pmc/articles/PMC7198998/

59. Ageno W, Di Minno MND, Ay C, Jang MJ, Hansen JB, Steffen LM, et al. Association between the metabolic syndrome, its individual components, and unprovoked venous thromboembolism: results of a patient-level meta-analysis. Arterioscler Thromb Vasc Biol. 2014;34(11):2478–85. [cited 2022 Feb 6]; [Internet]. https://pubmed.ncbi.nlm.nih.gov/25212233/

60. Jiménez-García R, Albaladejo-Vicente R, Hernandez-Barrera V, Villanueva-Orbaiz R, Carabantes-Alarcon D, De-Miguel-diez J, et al. Type 2 diabetes is a risk factor for suffering and for in-hospital mortality with pulmonary embolism. A population-based study in Spain (2016-2018). Int J Environ Res Public Health. 2020;17(22):1–15. [cited 2022 Feb 6]; [Internet] https://pubmed.ncbi.nlm.nih.gov/33187341/

61. Steffen LM, Cushman M, Peacock JM, Heckbert SR, Jacobs DR, Rosamond WD, et al. Metabolic syndrome and risk of venous thromboembolism: longitudinal investigation of thromboembolism etiology. J Thromb Haemost. 2009;7(5):746–51. [cited 2022 Feb 6]; [Internet] https://pubmed.ncbi.nlm.nih.gov/19175496/

62. Liu PP, Blet A, Smyth D, Li H. The science underlying COVID-19: implications for the cardiovascular system. Circulation. 2020;142:68–78. [cited 2022 Feb 6]; [Internet]. https://www.ahajournals.org/doi/abs/10.1161/CIRCULATIONAHA.120.047549

63. Ackermann M, Verleden SE, Kuehnel M, Haverich A, Welte T, Laenger F, et al. Pulmonary vascular endothelialitis, thrombosis, and angiogenesis in Covid-19. N Engl J Med. 2020;383(2):120–8. [cited 2022 Feb 6] [Internet]. https://pubmed.ncbi.nlm.nih.gov/32437596/

64. Bilaloglu S, Aphinyanaphongs Y, Jones S, Iturrate E, Hochman J, Berger JS. Thrombosis in hospitalized patients with COVID-19 in a New York City Health System. JAMA. 2020;324(8):799–801. [cited 2022 Feb 6]; [Internet]. https://pubmed.ncbi.nlm.nih.gov/32702090/

65. Nopp S, Moik F, Jilma B, Pabinger I, Ay C. Risk of venous thromboembolism in patients with COVID-19: a systematic review and meta-analysis. Res Pract Thromb Haemost. 2020;4(7):1178–91. [cited 2022 Feb 6]; [Internet]. https://pubmed.ncbi.nlm.nih.gov/33043231/

66. Calvisi SL, Ramirez GA, Scavini M, Da Prat V, Di Lucca G, Laurenzi A, et al. Thromboembolism risk among patients with diabetes/stress hyperglycemia and COVID-19. Metabolism. 2021;123. [cited 2022 Feb 6]; [Internet]. https://pubmed.ncbi.nlm.nih.gov/34364927/

67. Gibson-Corley KN, Meyerholz DK, Engelhardt JF. Pancreatic pathophysiology in cystic fibrosis. J Pathol. 2016;238(2):311–20. [cited 2022 Feb 6]; [Internet]. https://pubmed.ncbi.nlm.nih.gov/26365583/

68. Adler AI, Shine BSF, Chamnan P, Haworth CS, Bilton D. Genetic determinants and epidemiology of cystic fibrosis-related diabetes: results from a British cohort of children and adults. Diabetes Care. 2008;31(9):1789–94. [cited 2022 Feb 6]; [Internet]. https://pubmed.ncbi.nlm.nih.gov/18535191/

69. Mohan K, Israel KL, Miller H, Grainger R, Ledson MJ, Walshaw MJ. Long-term effect of insulin treatment in cystic fibrosis-related diabetes. Respiration. 2008;76(2):181–6. [cited 2022 Feb 6]; [Internet]. https://pubmed.ncbi.nlm.nih.gov/17960051/

70. Brennan AL, Gyi KM, Wood DM, Johnson J, Holliman R, Baines DL, et al. Airway glucose concentrations and effect on growth of respiratory pathogens in cystic fibrosis. J Cyst Fibros. 2007;6(2):101–9. [cited 2022 Feb 6]; [Internet]. https://pubmed.ncbi.nlm.nih.gov/16844431/

71. Prentice BJ, Jaffe A, Hameed S, Verge CF, Waters S, Widger J. Cystic fibrosis-related diabetes and lung disease: an update. Eur Respir Rev. 2021;30:159. [cited 2022 Feb 6]; [Internet]. https://pubmed.ncbi.nlm.nih.gov/33597125/

72. Françoise A, Héry-Arnaud G. The microbiome in cystic fibrosis pulmonary disease. Genes (Basel). 2020;11:5. [cited 2022 Feb 6]; [Internet]. https://pubmed.ncbi.nlm.nih.gov/32403302/

73. Wang G, Hu YX, He MY, Xie YH, Su W, Long D, et al. Gut-lung dysbiosis accompanied by diabetes mellitus leads to pulmonary fibrotic change through the NF-κB signaling pathway. Am J Pathol [Internet]. 2021;191(5):838–56. [cited 2022 Feb 6; https://pubmed.ncbi.nlm.nih.gov/33705752/

74. Fibrosis Foundation C 2019 Patient registry annual data report.
75. Belle-van Meerkerk G, van de Graaf EA, Kwakkel-van Erp JM, van Kessel DA, Lammers JWJ, Biesma DH, et al. Diabetes before and after lung transplantation in patients with cystic fibrosis and other lung diseases. Diabet Med. 2012;29:8. [cited 2022 Feb 6]; [Internet]. https://pubmed.ncbi.nlm.nih.gov/22486317/
76. Sidhaye A, Goldswieg B, Kaminski B, Blackman SM, Kelly A. Endocrine complications after solid-organ transplant in cystic fibrosis. J Cyst Fibros. 2019;18(Suppl 2):S111–9. [cited 2022 Feb 6]; [Internet]. https://pubmed.ncbi.nlm.nih.gov/31679722/
77. Naehrlich L, Orenti A, Dunlevy F, Kasmi I, Harutyunyan S, Pfleger A, et al. Incidence of SARS-CoV-2 in people with cystic fibrosis in Europe between February and June 2020. J Cyst Fibros. 2021;20(4):566–77. [cited 2022 Feb 6]; [Internet]. https://pubmed.ncbi.nlm.nih.gov/34016559/
78. Mondejar-Lopez P, Quintana-Gallego E, Giron-Moreno RM, Cortell-Aznar I, Ruiz de Valbuena-Maiz M, Diab-Caceres L, et al. Impact of SARS-CoV-2 infection in patients with cystic fibrosis in Spain: incidence and results of the national CF-COVID19-Spain survey. Respir Med. 2020;170. [cited 2022 Feb 6]; [Internet]. https://pubmed.ncbi.nlm.nih.gov/32843180/
79. Corvol H, de Miranda S, Lemonnier L, Kemgang A, Gaubert MR, Chiron R, et al. First wave of COVID-19 in French patients with cystic fibrosis. J Clin Med. 2020;9(11):1–12. [cited 2022 Feb 6]; [Internet]. https://pubmed.ncbi.nlm.nih.gov/33182847/

Part II
COVID and Diabetes Complications

Chapter 5
Diabetic Kidney Disease and COVID-19

Mersema Abate, Boonyanuth Maturostrakul, and Vinay Nair

Introduction

The presence of underlying comorbidities including diabetes, kidney disease, and kidney transplant status are well-known factors that increase morbidity and mortality from COVID-19. This chapter discusses the effect of COVID-19 infection on the kidney with a focus on patients with diabetic kidney disease (DKD) and kidney transplant recipients.

Pathophysiology of Diabetic Kidney Disease and Effects of COVID-19

Diabetic Kidney Disease

Chronic kidney disease (CKD) encompasses both diabetic (DKD) and non-diabetic kidney disease (NDKD) [1]. Diabetic nephropathy is characterized by glomerular basement membrane thickening, mesangial matrix expansion, nodular

M. Abate · V. Nair (✉)
Donald and Barbara Zucker School of Medicine at Hofstra/ Northwell, Hempstead, NY, USA
e-mail: vnair5@northwell.edu

B. Maturostrakul
Donald and Barbara Zucker School of Medicine at Hofstra/ Northwell, Hempstead, NY, USA

Kidney Medicine, Cleveland Clinic, Ohio, USA

© The Author(s), under exclusive license to Springer Nature Switzerland AG 2023
A. K. Myers (ed.), *Diabetes and COVID-19*, Contemporary Endocrinology,
https://doi.org/10.1007/978-3-031-28536-3_5

glomerulosclerosis, and arteriolar hyalinosis. This pattern is often seen in patients with type 1 diabetes (T1D) whereas biopsies from patients with type 2 diabetes (T2D) frequently include the presence of other pathologic findings, specifically NDKD. DKD encompasses all the different histopathological patterns of kidney injury related to diabetes. It is a heterogenous disease resulting from a variety of insults including the production of advanced glycation end products (AGEs), reactive oxygen species, pro-inflammatory and fibrogenic gene expression, as well as alterations in glomerular hemodynamics [1]. DKD is responsible for up to 50% of all cases of end-stage kidney disease (ESKD) in Western populations and is an important risk factor for cardiovascular mortality.

Several factors play a role in the pathophysiology of DKD by having distinct effects on the nephron, the basic subcomponent of the kidney.

The nephron is comprised of a glomerulus; the tubule (proximal, loop of Henle, distal tubule); and the collecting duct (see Fig. 5.1). Blood enters the glomerulus via the afferent arteriole and then due to changes in hydrostatic pressure, fluid is filtered into Bowman's space while blood is returned to circulation via the efferent arteriole. The fluid entering Bowman's space is the precursor to urine and travels through the renal tubule until it reaches the collecting duct and then the collecting system.

The effect of hyperglycemia begins with an increase in the amount of glucose filtered through the glomerulus [3]. Increased filtration leads to increased uptake of glucose in the proximal tubule which leads to proximal tubule hypertrophy (see Fig. 5.2).

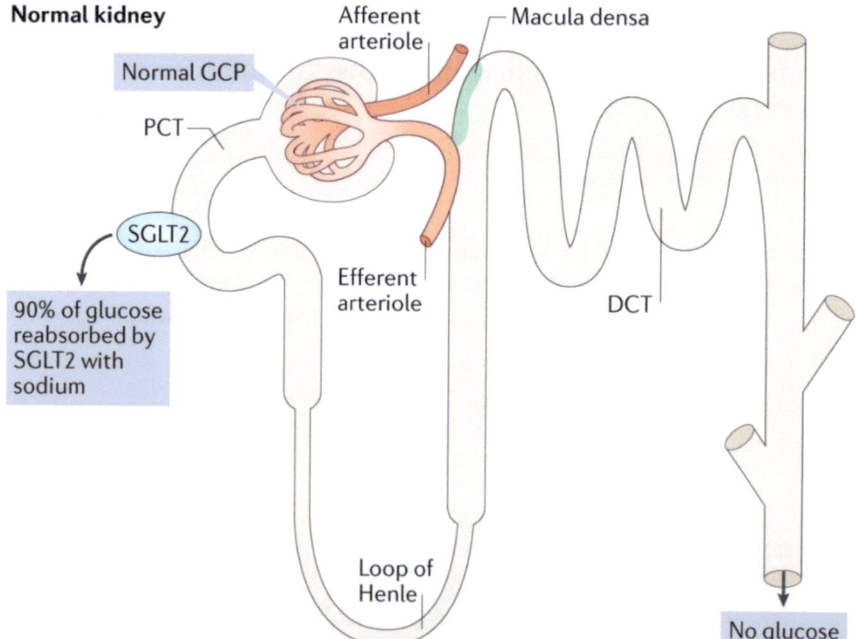

Fig. 5.1 Glucose regulation by the nephron (adapted from DeFronzo et al. [2]). *GCP* glomerular capillary pressure; *PCT* proximal convoluted tubule, *SGLT2* sodium glucose co-transporter 2, *DCT* distal convoluted tubule

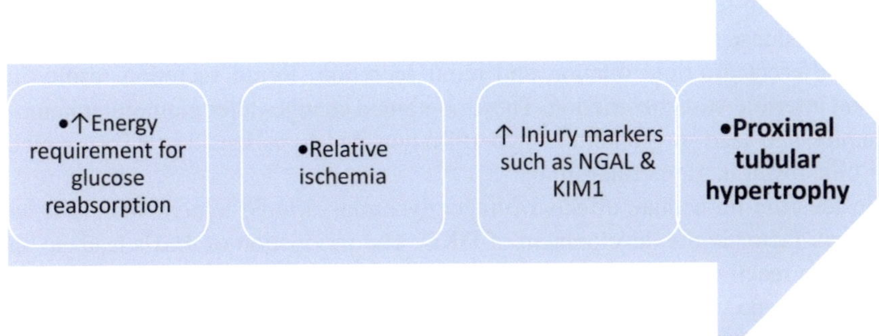

Fig. 5.2 Effect of hyperglycemia on the nephron. *NGAL* neutrophil gelatinase associated lipocalin, *KIM* kidney injury molecule-1

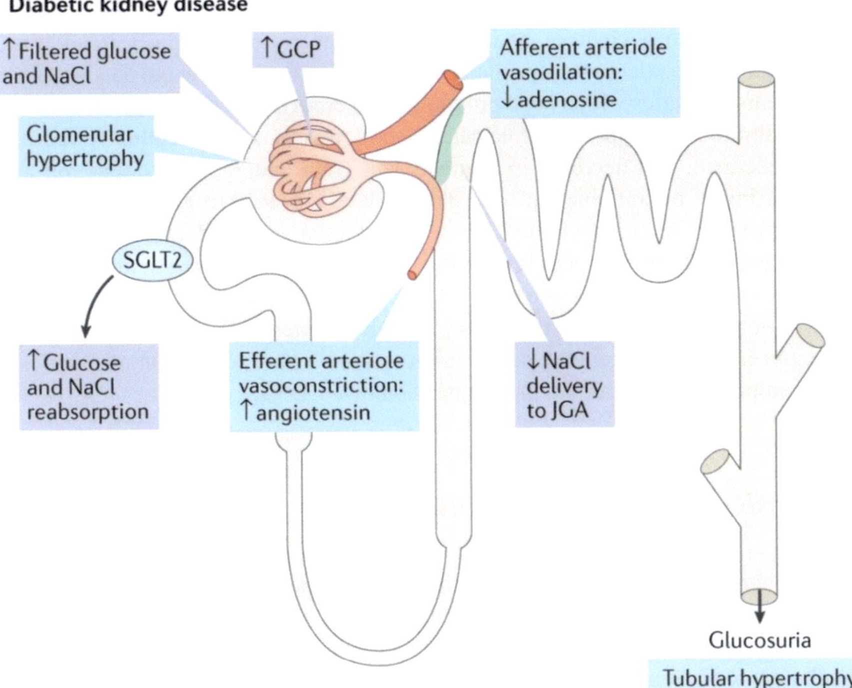

Fig. 5.3 Pathophysiology of diabetic kidney disease (adapted from DeFronzo et al. [2]). *NaCl* sodium chloride, *JGA* juxta glomerular apparatus

The proximal tubule recovers glucose via the sodium-glucose cotransporter-2 (SGLT2) (see Fig. 5.3). By increasing glucose delivery in the proximal tubule, there is an increase in cotransporter activity which increases the recovery of sodium as part of glucose reabsorption, thereby reducing sodium delivery to the distal tubule and the sodium-sensing macula densa. The reduction of distal sodium delivery to the macula densa results in a phenomenon called tubuloglomerular feedback, which causes afferent arteriole dilation and renin secretion. Renin secretion results in efferent arteriole vasoconstriction. These combined changes alter glomerular hemodynamics and lead to glomerular hyperfiltration and hypertension (HTN), which over time result in glomerular injury [3].

Besides the immediate effects of hyperglycemia, chronic hyperglycemia is an important factor in the development of DKD. The production of AGEs leads to an increase in reactive oxygen species. These products result in pro-inflammatory and profibrotic gene expression [4]. Chronic hyperglycemia also results in abnormal activation of transforming growth factor-β (TGFB) which causes renal insufficiency and glomerulosclerosis [5]. It has been demonstrated in mouse models that macrophages accumulate and infiltrate the glomerulus inducing inflammation and tumor necrosis factor - alpha (TNF-a) production, mediating diabetic kidney injury [6].

Additional activation of maladaptive pathways from hyperglycemia results in endothelial dysfunction such as increased permeability from loss of electrostatic charge, inflammatory changes, and dysregulation of vascular tone [7]. In addition, there is damage to podocytes, specialized epithelial cells covering the outside of the glomerular capillaries which keep protein in the serum and prevent it from entering urinary ultrafiltrate. Hyperglycemia causes podocytes to undergo cellular hypertrophy, effacement, and decrease in numbers [8]. Both endothelial dysfunction and podocyte injury in combination with glomerular HTN lead to albuminuria which further propagates kidney injury. These endothelial and podocyte injuries also induce abnormal turnover and remodeling of the glomerular basement membrane (GBM) which contributes to the classic GBM thickening seen in diabetes.

Even if euglycemia is restored, the "metabolic memory" caused by previous hyperglycemia and epigenetic modification results in the progression of microvascular complications furthering the progression of DKD [9].

Diagnosis of Diabetic Kidney Disease

The aforementioned changes in the nephron, and in particular the glomerulus, lead to proteinuria. Proteinuria, particularly albuminuria, remains an important marker used to help define and diagnose diabetic nephropathy. Microalbuminuria is defined as albumin to creatinine ratio of 2.5–25 mg/mmol in males and 3.5–35 mg/mmol in females or urinary albumin excretion rate of 20–200 micrograms per minute. Macroalbuminuria is defined as albumin to creatinine ratio of >25 mg/mmol in males and > 35 mg/mmol in females or urinary albumin excretion rate of >200 micrograms per minute [10]. Several factors affect and increase urinary albumin excretion, including hyperglycemia, HTN, exercise, infection, fever, hematuria, urinary tract infection, menstruation, and pregnancy.

Effect of COVID-19 on the Kidney

Studies have revealed varying degrees of kidney injury in patients with COVID-19 depending on disease severity.

Acute Kidney Injury and COVID-19

Acute kidney injury (AKI) occurs in up to one-third of patients hospitalized with COVID-19 and is as high as 50% in critically ill COVID-19 patients [11–14]. The majority of the observed AKI in the setting of COVID-19 infection is mild, stages I–II (69–85%), 15-31% develop stage III AKI with 12-30% needing renal replacement therapy [11, 12]. Majority of the observed patients (89%) of patients on mechanical ventilation develop AKI which is most likely due to the overall severity of the disease with systemic cardiovascular collapse and multi-organ failure [11]. Observational data suggests that comorbidities associated with AKI in patients hospitalized with COVID-19 include older age, Black race, diabetes, CKD, HTN, and cardiovascular disease [11, 13, 15]. The presence of diabetes mellitus is a significant predictor with a nearly two-fold increased risk of AKI compared to patients without diabetes, as is CKD. Reduced baseline eGFR below 60 ml/min is associated with a 2-to-three-fold increase in the risk of severe AKI [11, 13]. Importantly, during the first COVID-19 surge AKI was a poor prognostic factor associated with a six-fold increase in hospital mortality and of those who lived nearly half had partial or no recovery of kidney function at the time of discharge [13]. In the United States, the rate and severity of AKI declined as the pandemic unfolded with lower rates in July 2020 compared to March 2020 and was lower in places with lower rates of CKD, obesity, diabetes, and hypertension [13]. This may be explained by the differences in COVID-19 variants, a better understanding of the disease process, and better management due to increasing experience.

Interplay of COVID-19 and Diabetic Kidney Disease

COVID-19 and AKI have been shown to be more severe in patients with diabetes and CKD [11, 16]. Whether this risk is cumulative or synergistic is unclear. The similar pro-inflammatory and profibrotic pathways of both COVID-19 and DKD may act in concert to worsen kidney function and recovery from AKI.

Impaired innate immunity and upregulation of ACE2, by hyperglycemia and vasculopathy, may lead to an increase in COVID-19 severity in patients with DKD. Chronic inflammation in diabetic nephropathy may also lead to an exaggerated cytokine storm upon infection by SARS-CoV-2. In addition, patients with diabetes have a high burden of other co-morbid conditions such as cardiac disease, HTN, and obesity, which also impact the severity of COVID-19.

Impact of Diabetic Kidney Disease Therapies on COVID-19

Angiotensin-Converting Enzyme Inhibitors and Angiotensin Receptor Blockers

It is known that the presence of albuminuria increases the risk for diabetic kidney disease progression and kidney failure. ACEi and ARBs are effective agents in reducing albuminuria. The Kidney Disease Improving Global Outcomes (KDIGO) guidelines recommend initiation of ACEi and ARBs as treatment for patients with diabetes, HTN, and proteinuria, and may even be considered in patients with albuminuria and diabetes with normal blood pressure [17]. According to the American Diabetes Association, ACEi or ARBs are recommended for patients with a modestly elevated urine albumin to creatinine ratio (30–299 mg/g creatinine) and are strongly recommended for patients with urine albumin to creatinine ratio of ≥300 mg/g creatinine and/or estimated glomerular filtration rate < 60 mL/min/1.73 m2 [18]. The impact of the continuation of ACEi and ARB therapy in patients hospitalized with COVID-19 is unclear. SARS-CoV-2 binds and uses cell membrane–bound ACE2 to enter the kidney [19]. It is postulated that the use of RAAS inhibitors may increase ACE2 expression, and therefore should be used cautiously in patients with COVID-19 [20]. However, several trials suggest no difference in mortality between patients who are continued on ACEi or ARB therapy compared to those who are not on either medication. This data suggests that the continuation of these therapies does not have an impact on COVID-19 severity [21].

Sodium-Glucose Transport Protein 2 Inhibitors

Sodium-glucose transport protein 2 inhibitors (SGLT2i) have demonstrated a profound effect on the progression of DKD [22]. By blocking this co-transporter, several events take place (Fig. 5.4). Glycosuria and natriuresis occur by reducing sodium reabsorption in the proximal tubule (Fig. 5.4). Natriuresis can improve heart failure outcomes by reducing intravascular volume and blood pressure, which is protective of the kidney. In addition, blocking proximal reabsorption of sodium leads to increased delivery to the macula densa, which normalizes tubuloglomerular feedback (as previously described) (Fig. 5.4). This results in an improvement of glomerular pressure by eliminating vasodilation of the afferent arteriole, preventing glomerular hyperfiltration and hypertension. Other renoprotective mechanisms include reducing oxygen demand, reducing relative ischemia, and reducing cellular edema and apoptosis. These events may also lead to a favorable alteration in pro-inflammatory cytokines seen in diabetic kidney disease [23, 24]. Glycosuria also leads to weight loss and an improvement in blood pressure, reducing hypertensive kidney injury.

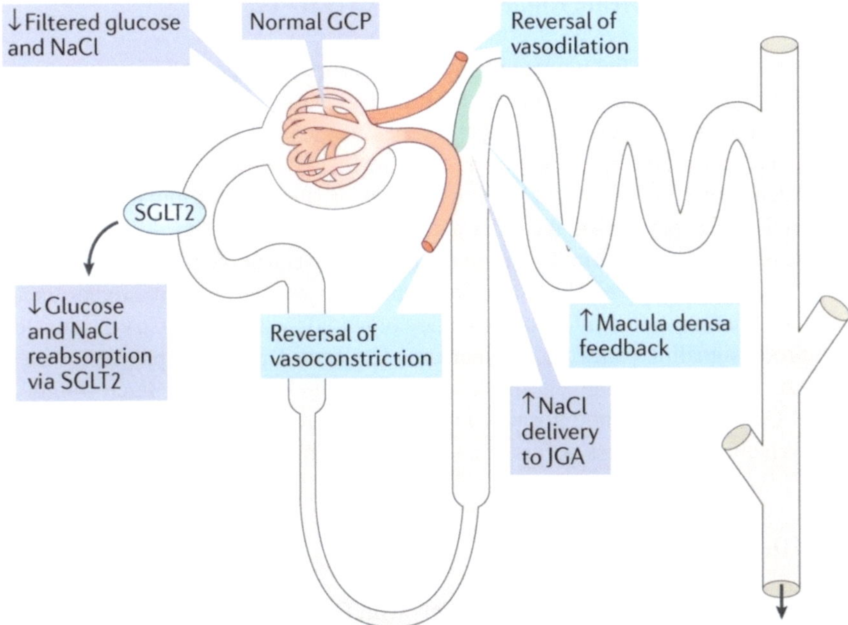

Fig. 5.4 Diabetic kidney disease with SGLT2 inhibitor (adapted from DeFronzo et al. [2]). *NaCl* sodium chloride, *GCP* glomerular capillary pressure, *SGLT2* sodium-glucose cotransport protein 2, *JGA* juxta glomerular apparatus [2]

It is possible that SGLT2i may have a protective effect on DKD during or after COVID-19 [25]. Reducing oxygen demand and improving glycemia may reduce ischemic stress imposed by COVID-19. Improvement in cytokine profile may also be favorable in ameliorating the cytokine storm induced by COVID-19. Finally, improved cardiac function and diuresis may improve tissue homeostasis and oxygenation. However, there are also potential risks when starting or continuing SGLT2i in severely ill patients. It is possible that diuresis or reduction in glomerular pressures could lead to tissue malperfusion and acute tubular necrosis. Severely ill COVID-19 patients may be undergoing peripheral lipolysis from an acute illness which can lead to ketosis. In such a situation, SGLT2i use could precipitate euglycemic or diabetic ketoacidosis. The use of SGLT2i may also lead to ACE2 upregulation which can theoretically increase viral entry into the vascular endothelium of the kidneys. The Dapagliflozin in patients with cardiometabolic risk factors hospitalized with COVID-19 (DARE-19) study was a phase 3 multicenter study evaluating the effect of dapagliflozin in non-critically ill inpatients with COVID-19 and cardiometabolic risk factors [26]. The study found no statistically significant improvement in organ dysfunction or death. However, dapagliflozin was well tolerated, without a significant increase in euglycemic diabetic ketoacidosis, suggesting a neutral effect of SGLT2i in COVID-19.

Pathophysiology of Acute Kidney Injury in COVID-19

Hypotension, endothelial injury, and cytokine storm can induce AKI in any setting. This observation questions whether SARS-CoV-2 itself causes kidney injury or whether it is simply a critical illness. A series of kidney biopsies in patients with severe AKI and COVID-19 revealed a predominance of acute tubular necrosis, with no evidence of viral infection [27]; however, other studies have found evidence of coronavirus-like particles in the kidney [28].

The presence of ACE2 in the vascular endothelium can allow SARS-CoV-2 entry into the kidney, but its mechanism of renal injury is unclear. In vitro studies using stem cells demonstrated infection of kidney organoids with SARS-CoV-2 activates profibrotic signaling pathways and increases Collagen 1 protein expression, which suggests SARS-CoV-2 infects the kidney and promotes fibrosis. Interestingly a SARS-CoV-2 protease inhibitor was able to ameliorate the infection of kidney cells [29]. Whether this process occurs in a similar mechanism in vivo is still unclear.

COVID-19 and Proteinuria

Proteinuria is a common finding in patients with COVID-19 and is present in up to 87% of critically ill patients with COVID-19 [12, 30] . Patients with AKI have a higher incidence of proteinuria compared to those that do not have AKI. The degree of proteinuria among patients with COVID-19-related AKI ranges from 1+ (32%) to 2 + (30%) to 3+ (12%) [11]. Proteinuria subsequently resolves in nearly 70% of patients who recover their kidney function [30]. The high frequency of proteinuria in patients with COVID-19 is similar to patients with other critical illnesses, suggesting that the presence of proteinuria in patients with COVID-19 may nonspecific.

A multi-institutional study that examined kidney tissue from 240 native kidney biopsy specimens from patients actively with COVID-19 showed acute tubular injury was present in 78% of the biopsy specimens but was the sole pathologic finding in only 13% of the cases. Collapsing glomerulopathy (a composition of glomerular capillaries segmental and global collapse, podocytes hyperplasia, and hypertrophy and tubulointerstitial disease) [31] was the predominant finding present in 26% of specimens [32]; diabetic nephropathy was 12% and other findings accounted for 7.5% [32]. A high-risk Apolipoprotein L1 (APOL1) genotype, seen predominately in African American and Hispanic cadavers, was present in most patients (92%) with collapsing glomerulopathy suggesting the pathology of kidney disease in these patients may be related to a "second hit" to APOL1 risk alleles driven by increased circulating interferon generated as an immune response to viral infection.

COVID-19 Outcomes in Chronic Kidney Disease

The "OpenSAFELY" system health analytic platform conducted in England among more than 17,000,000 subjects found that patients with reduced kidney function have increased COVID-19-related mortality compared to the overall population. In patients with a GFR between 30 – 60 ml/min, mortality was 0.3 times higher, while in those with a GFR < 30 ml/min mortality was 2.5 times higher. In patients with ESKD or on dialysis mortality, the risk was 3.7 times higher compared to the overall population [33].

COVID-19 and Kidney Transplantation

The exact incidence of COVID-19 infection in the kidney transplant population is difficult to ascertain due to temporal and geographic differences in viral prevalence, infectivity of the virus variants, and vaccination rates. Based on experience from other respiratory viral infections, kidney transplant recipients are expected to be susceptible to infection with COVID-19. According to one study conducted in Italy, the cumulative incidence of COVID-19 infection in kidney transplant recipients was found to be 1.15% compared to 0.4% in the non-transplant population. The cumulative incidence of COVID-19 infection was three times higher in kidney transplant recipients compared to the general population after adjusting for age and gender differences in the population [34].

The risk of contracting COVID-19 infection is higher in dialysis patients compared to kidney transplant recipients presumably due to difficulty in implementing effective social distancing practices [35–37]. Despite the lower risk in contracting COVID-19 infection, kidney transplant recipients have worse outcomes compared to patients on the kidney transplant waiting list [35–37].

Although kidney transplantation in general offers a survival advantage over dialysis [38], in the presence of COVID-19 infection, kidney transplant recipients exhibit mortality rates 1.3 to 2 times higher compared with age-matched and comorbidity-matched dialysis patients on the transplant waiting list [39, 40].

Mortality rates among kidney transplant recipients hospitalized with COVID-19 range anywhere from 20% to 32% (within 28–90 days of admission) with higher rates reported early during the pandemic [39, 41–45]. Mortality rates declined in late 2020 and onwards, owing to a better understanding of the disease and better management including the routine use of corticosteroids during cytokine storm [44, 45]. While some of the excess mortality may be attributable to existing comorbidities such as diabetes, cardiovascular disease, and chronic kidney disease, there is evidence that the presence of a solid organ transplant is an independent factor for increased morbidity and mortality from COVID-19 [39, 44].

Table 5.1 Clinical symptoms of COVID-19 infection and symptom frequency

Symptom	Frequency
Fever	61–80%
Cough	54–64%
Dyspnea	37–41%
Diarrhea	28–44%
Myalgia or arthralgia	34–40%
Loss of smell or taste	14–24%

Clinical Presentation

Kidney transplant recipients with COVID-19 infection have a heterogenous clinical presentation with varying degrees of severity. About 20% of transplant recipients have mild to no symptoms at diagnosis, while 30–40% have moderate disease and another 30–40% present with severe disease [46, 47]. The onset of symptoms typically ranges from one to three weeks before diagnosis [46, 48]. Approximately one-third of kidney transplant recipients require hospitalization within the first month of diagnosis, although this figure may be an overestimation due to testing bias as asymptomatic and mildly symptomatic patients may not be tested [47].

Common initial presenting clinical symptoms of COVID-19 infection and symptom frequency are shown in Table 5.1 [40–42, 45, 49].

Demographic Characteristics, Baseline Comorbidities, and Immunosuppressant Medications in Transplant Patients Hospitalized with COVID-19 Infection

Nearly two-thirds of kidney transplant recipients hospitalized with COVID-19 infection are male with an average age at presentation of 60 years [39, 44, 49]. Patients can present anywhere from 1 month to >10 years post-transplant, and the average time between presentation and transplantation is 5–7 years [34, 39, 44, 49]. Prevalent comorbidities include HTN 80–90%, diabetes mellitus 30–50%, obesity 30–45%, cardiovascular diseases 30%, and lung disease 10% [39, 40, 45]. Maintenance immunosuppressive medications at the time of COVID-19 diagnosis include calcineurin inhibitors 80–90%, antiproliferative agents 75%, corticosteroids 75–80%, and mTOR inhibitors 12% [34, 39, 40, 44, 45, 49, 50].

Risk Factors for Adverse Outcomes

Advanced age (> 60 years), diabetes mellitus, cardiovascular disease, lower baseline GFR, and chronic lung disease are shown to be predictors of mortality in kidney transplant recipients with COVID-19 infection [33, 39, 45, 51].

Race/ethnicity is an important predictor of COVID-19-related outcomes. The burden of COVID-19 infection and mortality is disproportionately distributed among Black and Hispanic kidney transplant recipients [33, 52]. Although the ethnic/racial disparity became less pronounced over the course of the pandemic, geographic regions with a higher proportion of ethnic/racial minorities demonstrate substantially increased rates of COVID-19-related hospitalization and deaths [53, 54].

The excess COVID-19-related morbidity and mortality in ethnic/racial minority groups is merely a reflection of the long-standing and deep-rooted disparities that existed in health care and were unmasked and amplified during the pandemic [49, 52, 55]. Inequities in COVID-19 infection and outcomes are driven by a higher risk of exposure to the SARS-CoV-2 virus (e.g., occupational exposure in essential workers); higher prevalence of underlying comorbidities (e.g., hypertension, diabetes); and reduced access to health care and health literacy all which are influenced by social determinants of health [54].

The effect of sex and BMI on predicting mortality in kidney transplant recipients is less clear with studies suggesting similar versus slightly increased risk in males and in obese recipients [39, 43, 44]. Obesity is an established risk factor for COVID-19-related mortality in the general population; however, a large meta-analysis failed to demonstrate a significant association between obesity and mortality in kidney transplant recipients with COVID-19 [45].

Transplant recipients experience a high burden of infectious complications in the first year post-transplant when the level of immunosuppression is intense. Although a higher COVID-19-related mortality was reported among recipients within 1 year of transplantation [40], two others (one meta-analysis) demonstrated no difference in the timing of transplantation and COVID-19-related mortality [44, 49].

Similar to the general population, the presence of pneumonia, mechanical ventilation, and AKI in kidney transplant recipients with COVID-19 infection are poor prognostic factors [39, 44, 45, 49]. Among hospitalized kidney transplant recipients with COVID-19, 30–35% require mechanical ventilation [39, 41] and AKI occurs in 40–60% of patients, with 10–20% requiring renal replacement therapy [39, 41, 44]. For most patients, the need for dialysis often coincides with the need for mechanical ventilation which is most likely due to the overall severity of the disease with systemic cardiovascular collapse and multi-organ failure [11].

Vaccination

Vaccination plays a paramount role in the current COVID-19 endemic response. Kidney transplant recipients should preferably receive one of the two currently available mRNA vaccines [BNT162b2 (Pfizer/BioNTech) and mRNA-1273 (Moderna)] ideally prior to transplantation. The mRNA vaccines induce robust titers of anti-spike antibodies that confer >94% protection against severe COVID-19 in the studied population. Unfortunately, nearly half of the transplant recipients do not mount an antibody response after two doses of mRNA vaccine and remain at risk for severe disease [56, 57]. Immunogenicity can be improved by administering a third dose after a minimum of 28 days after the second dose [58, 59]. For patients with moderate to severe immunosuppression including kidney transplant recipients, the current guidelines recommend three primary doses of the mRNA vaccines followed by a fourth dose (booster) administered after a minimum of three months after the third dose. Recently, a bivalent mRNA vaccine has been approved for recent omicron variants by the US FDA [60]. These vaccines are recommended at least 2 months following primary or booster vaccination and contain two mRNA components of the SARS-CoV-2 virus, the original strain of SARS-CoV-2 and the other one in common between the BA.4 and BA.5 lineages of the omicron variant of SARS-CoV-2.

Management

The general management of COVID-19 infection in kidney transplant recipients is similar to that of the non-transplant population. Closer symptom monitoring is needed in kidney transplant recipients due to their immunosuppressed status and risk of rapid clinical deterioration. In addition, the threshold to initiate pre- or post-exposure prophylaxis and treatment is lower. Drugs used in the general population for the treatment of COVID-19 infection such as remdesivir, monoclonal antibodies targeting COVID-19 spike protein, and corticosteroids are used in the treatment of transplant recipients with COVID-19 infection [39, 41, 48]. Interleukin-6 inhibitors (tocilizumab) and JAK inhibitor (Baricitnib or Tofacitinib) should be used with caution due to the risk of profound immunosuppression when used concomitantly with maintenance immunosuppressive medications [61].

Nirmatrelvir-ritonavir significantly reduces the risk of hospitalization or all-cause mortality by 89%; however, its use in transplant recipients is limited by the presence of significant drug interaction with calcineurin inhibitors and mTOR inhibitors [62]. Molnupiravir has a modest effect and reduces COVID-19-related hospitalization or death by 30% and has been safe and effective in transplant recipients without significant adverse effects or drug interactions [63].

Adjustment of Immunosuppression

In patients with mild to moderate COVID-19 infection, complete withdrawal of immunosuppression, especially among recent kidney transplant recipients, is discouraged due to risk of rejection. In general, the immunosuppressive regimen is adjusted based on clinical severity, time post-transplant, and the risk of acute rejection. For mild COVID-19, reduction of antimetabolite by 50% with the continuation of calcineurin inhibitors and corticosteroids is reasonable [64]. Moderate disease can be managed by temporary cessation of antimetabolite or mTOR inhibitors and reduction of calcineurin by 25–50% with the continuation of corticosteroids [48]. In severe disease complicated by ARDS, the need for mechanical ventilation or shock, temporary withdrawal of all maintenance immunosuppressive medication, and the use of intravenous dexamethasone to reduce inflammatory response caused by cytokine storm are the standard treatment. A reinstitution of immunosuppression can be managed case by case depending on the clinical course [41, 43, 48, 65].

Conclusion

COVID-19 is an ongoing pandemic that affects all organ systems including the endocrine system. There is complex clinical and physiological interaction between COVID-19 and diabetes as they pertain to kidney health. Optimal treatments for COVID-19 in patients with diabetic kidney disease are evolving and require further study. Kidney transplant recipients are at a higher risk for severe COVID-19, and immunosuppression should be closely managed. Vaccination against COVID-19 remains the best defense against severe disease, while medical therapy must be used carefully in patients with kidney disease, diabetes, and transplantation.

References

1. Anders HJ, Huber TB, Isermann B, et al. CKD in diabetes: diabetic kidney disease versus nondiabetic kidney disease. Nat Rev Nephrol. 2018;14(6):361–77.
2. DeFronzo RA, Reeves WB, Awad AS. Pathophysiology of diabetic kidney disease: impact of SGLT2 inhibitors. Nat Rev Nephrol. 2021;17(5):319–34.
3. Vallon V. The mechanisms and therapeutic potential of SGLT2 inhibitors in diabetes mellitus. Annu Rev Med. 2015;66:255–70.
4. Pichler R, Afkarian M, Dieter BP, et al. Immunity and inflammation in diabetic kidney disease: translating mechanisms to biomarkers and treatment targets. Am J Physiol Renal Physiol. 2017;312(4):F716–31.
5. Ziyadeh FN, Hoffman BB, Han DC, et al. Long-term prevention of renal insufficiency, excess matrix gene expression, and glomerular mesangial matrix expansion by treatment with monoclonal antitransforming growth factor-beta antibody in db/db diabetic mice. Proc Natl Acad Sci U S A. 2000;97(14):8015–20.
6. Awad AS, You H, Gao T, et al. Macrophage-derived tumor necrosis factor-alpha mediates diabetic renal injury. Kidney Int. 2015;88(4):722–33.
7. Nieuwdorp M, van Haeften TW, Gouverneur MC, et al. Loss of endothelial glycocalyx during acute hyperglycemia coincides with endothelial dysfunction and coagulation activation in vivo. Diabetes. 2006;55(2):480–6.
8. Pagtalunan ME, Miller PL, Jumping-Eagle S, et al. Podocyte loss and progressive glomerular injury in type II diabetes. J Clin Invest. 1997;99(2):342–8.
9. Reddy MA, Zhang E, Natarajan R. Epigenetic mechanisms in diabetic complications and metabolic memory. Diabetologia. 2015;58(3):443–55.

10. Basi S, Fesler P, Mimran A, et al. Microalbuminuria in type 2 diabetes and hypertension: a marker, treatment target, or innocent bystander? Diabetes Care. 2008;31(Suppl 2):S194–201.
11. Hirsch JS, Ng JH, Ross DW, et al. Acute kidney injury in patients hospitalized with COVID-19. Kidney Int. 2020;98(1):209–18.
12. Cummings MJ, Baldwin MR, Abrams D, et al. Epidemiology, clinical course, and outcomes of critically ill adults with COVID-19 in New York City: a prospective cohort study. Lancet. 2020;395(10239):1763–70.
13. Bowe B, Cai M, Xie Y, et al. Acute kidney injury in a National Cohort of Hospitalized US Veterans with COVID-19. Clin J Am Soc Nephrol. 2020;16(1):14–25.
14. Doher MP, Torres de Carvalho FR, Scherer PF, et al. Acute kidney injury and renal replacement therapy in critically ill COVID-19 patients: risk factors and outcomes: a single-Center experience in Brazil. Blood Purif. 2021;50(4-5):520–30.
15. Teoh JY, Yip TC, Lui GC, et al. Risks of AKI and major adverse clinical outcomes in patients with severe acute respiratory syndrome or coronavirus disease 2019. J Am Soc Nephrol. 2021;
16. Richardson S, Hirsch JS, Narasimhan M, et al. Presenting characteristics, comorbidities, and outcomes among 5700 patients hospitalized with COVID-19 in the New York City area. JAMA. 2020;
17. Rossing P, Caramori ML, Chan JCN, et al. Executive summary of the KDIGO 2022 Clinical Practice Guideline for Diabetes Management in Chronic Kidney Disease: an update based on rapidly emerging new evidence. Kidney Int. 2022;102(5):990–9.
18. American Diabetes Association Professional Practice, C, Draznin B, Aroda VR, et al. 11. Chronic kidney disease and risk management: standards of medical care in diabetes-2022. Diabetes Care. 2022;45(Suppl 1):S175–84.
19. Hoffmann M, Kleine-Weber H, Schroeder S, et al. SARS-CoV-2 cell entry depends on ACE2 and TMPRSS2 and is blocked by a clinically proven protease inhibitor. Cell. 2020;181(2):271–80. e8
20. Zheng YY, Ma YT, Zhang JY, et al. COVID-19 and the cardiovascular system. Nat Rev Cardiol. 2020;17(5):259–60.
21. Mehra MR, Desai SS, Kuy S, et al. Cardiovascular disease, drug therapy, and mortality in Covid-19. N Engl J Med. 2020;382(25):e102.
22. Zelniker TA, Wiviott SD, Raz I, et al. SGLT2 inhibitors for primary and secondary prevention of cardiovascular and renal outcomes in type 2 diabetes: a systematic review and meta-analysis of cardiovascular outcome trials. Lancet. 2019;393(10166):31–9.
23. Garvey WT, Van Gaal L, Leiter LA, et al. Effects of canagliflozin versus glimepiride on adipokines and inflammatory biomarkers in type 2 diabetes. Metabolism. 2018;85:32–7.
24. Kaze AD, Zhuo M, Kim SC, et al. Association of SGLT2 inhibitors with cardiovascular, kidney, and safety outcomes among patients with diabetic kidney disease: a meta-analysis. Cardiovasc Diabetol. 2022;21(1):47.
25. Das L, Dutta P. SGLT2 inhibition and COVID-19: the road not taken. Eur J Clin Investig. 2020;50(12):e13339.
26. Kosiborod MN, Esterline R, Furtado RHM, et al. Dapagliflozin in patients with cardiometabolic risk factors hospitalised with COVID-19 (DARE-19): a randomised, double-blind, placebo-controlled, phase 3 trial. Lancet Diabetes Endocrinol. 2021;9(9):586–94.
27. Sharma P, Uppal NN, Wanchoo R, et al. COVID-19-associated kidney injury: a case series of kidney biopsy findings. J Am Soc Nephrol. 2020;31(9):1948–58.
28. Su H, Yang M, Wan C, et al. Renal histopathological analysis of 26 postmortem findings of patients with COVID-19 in China. Kidney Int. 2020;98(1):219–27.
29. Jansen J, Reimer KC, Nagai JS, et al. SARS-CoV-2 infects the human kidney and drives fibrosis in kidney organoids. Cell Stem Cell. 2022;29(2):217–31. e8
30. Pei G, Zhang Z, Peng J, et al. Renal involvement and early prognosis in patients with COVID-19 pneumonia. J Am Soc Nephrol. 2020;31(6):1157–65.
31. Schwimmer JA, Markowitz GS, Valeri A, et al. Collapsing glomerulopathy. Semin Nephrol. 2003;23(2):209–18.

32. May RM, Cassol C, Hannoudi A, et al. A multi-center retrospective cohort study defines the spectrum of kidney pathology in coronavirus 2019 disease (COVID-19). Kidney Int. 2021;100(6):1303–15.
33. Williamson EJ, Walker AJ, Bhaskaran K, et al. Factors associated with COVID-19-related death using OpenSAFELY. Nature. 2020;584(7821):430–6.
34. Trapani S, Masiero L, Puoti F, et al. Incidence and outcome of SARS-CoV-2 infection on solid organ transplantation recipients: a nationwide population-based study. Am J Transplant. 2021;21(7):2509–21.
35. Thaunat O, Legeai C, Anglicheau D, et al. IMPact of the COVID-19 epidemic on the moRTAlity of kidney transplant recipients and candidates in a French Nationwide registry sTudy (IMPORTANT). Kidney Int. 2020;98(6):1568–77.
36. Ravanan R, Callaghan CJ, Mumford L, et al. SARS-CoV-2 infection and early mortality of waitlisted and solid organ transplant recipients in England: a national cohort study. Am J Transplant. 2020;20(11):3008–18.
37. Mohamed IH, Chowdary PB, Shetty S, et al. Outcomes of renal transplant recipients with SARS-CoV-2 infection in the eye of the storm: a comparative study with waitlisted patients. Transplantation. 2021;105(1):115–20.
38. Tonelli M, Wiebe N, Knoll G, et al. Systematic review: kidney transplantation compared with dialysis in clinically relevant outcomes. Am J Transplant. 2011;11(10):2093–109.
39. Nair V, Jandovitz N, Hirsch JS, et al. An early experience on the effect of solid organ transplant status on hospitalized COVID-19 patients. Am J Transplant. 2021;21(7):2522–31.
40. Goffin E, Candellier A, Vart P, et al. COVID-19-related mortality in kidney transplant and haemodialysis patients: a comparative, prospective registry-based study. Nephrol Dial Transplant. 2021;36(11):2094–105.
41. Caillard S, Anglicheau D, Matignon M, et al. An initial report from the French SOT COVID registry suggests high mortality due to COVID-19 in recipients of kidney transplants. Kidney Int. 2020;98(6):1549–58.
42. Requiao-Moura LR, Sandes-Freitas TV, Viana LA, et al. High mortality among kidney transplant recipients diagnosed with coronavirus disease 2019: results from the Brazilian multicenter cohort study. PLoS One. 2021;16(7):e0254822.
43. Kates OS, Haydel BM, Florman SS, et al. Coronavirus disease 2019 in solid organ transplant: a multicenter cohort study. Clin Infect Dis. 2021;73(11):e4090–9.
44. Kremer D, Pieters TT, Verhaar MC, et al. A systematic review and meta-analysis of COVID-19 in kidney transplant recipients: lessons to be learned. Am J Transplant. 2021;21(12):3936–45.
45. Udomkarnjananun S, Kerr SJ, Townamchai N, et al. Mortality risk factors of COVID-19 infection in kidney transplantation recipients: a systematic review and meta-analysis of cohorts and clinical registries. Sci Rep. 2021;11(1):20073.
46. Alfishawy M, Elbendary A, Mohamed M, et al. COVID-19 mortality in transplant recipients. Int J Organ Transplant Med. 2020;11(4):145–62.
47. Hadi YB, Naqvi SFZ, Kupec JT, et al. Outcomes of COVID-19 in solid organ transplant recipients: a propensity-matched analysis of a large research network. Transplantation. 2021;105(6):1365–71.
48. Kataria A, Yakubu I, Winstead R, et al. COVID-19 in kidney transplantation: epidemiology, management considerations, and the impact on kidney transplant practice. Transplant Direct. 2020;6(8):e582.
49. Cravedi P, Mothi SS, Azzi Y, et al. COVID-19 and kidney transplantation: results from the TANGO international transplant consortium. Am J Transplant. 2020;20(11):3140–8.
50. Jager KJ, Kramer A, Chesnaye NC, et al. Results from the ERA-EDTA registry indicate a high mortality due to COVID-19 in dialysis patients and kidney transplant recipients across Europe. Kidney Int. 2020;98(6):1540–8.
51. Oto OA, Ozturk S, Turgutalp K, et al. Predicting the outcome of COVID-19 infection in kidney transplant recipients. BMC Nephrol. 2021;22(1):100.

52. Mohan S, King KL, Husain SA, et al. COVID-19-associated mortality among kidney transplant recipients and candidates in the United States. Clin J Am Soc Nephrol. 2021;16(11):1695–703.
53. Wadhera RK, Wadhera P, Gaba P, et al. Variation in COVID-19 hospitalizations and deaths across New York City boroughs. JAMA. 2020;323(21):2192–5.
54. Romano SD, Blackstock AJ, Taylor EV, et al. Trends in racial and ethnic disparities in COVID-19 hospitalizations, by region—United States, march-December 2020. MMWR Morb Mortal Wkly Rep. 2021;70(15):560–5.
55. Mountantonakis SE, Epstein LM, Coleman K, et al. The association of structural inequities and race with out-of-hospital sudden death during the COVID-19 pandemic. Circ Arrhythm Electrophysiol. 2021;14(5):e009646.
56. Boyarsky BJ, Werbel WA, Avery RK, et al. Antibody response to 2-dose SARS-CoV-2 mRNA vaccine series in solid organ transplant recipients. JAMA. 2021;325(21):2204–6.
57. Caillard S, Chavarot N, Bertrand D, et al. Occurrence of severe COVID-19 in vaccinated transplant patients. Kidney Int. 2021;100(2):477–9.
58. Hall VG, Ferreira VH, Ku T, et al. Randomized trial of a third dose of mRNA-1273 vaccine in transplant recipients. N Engl J Med. 2021;385(13):1244–6.
59. Masset C, Kerleau C, Garandeau C, et al. A third injection of the BNT162b2 mRNA COVID-19 vaccine in kidney transplant recipients improves the humoral immune response. Kidney Int. 2021;100(5):1132–5.
60. Food and Drug Administration. *Coronavirus (COVID-19) update: FDA authorizes Moderna, Pfizer-BioNTech bivalent COVID-19 vaccines for use as a booster dose.* 2022, August 12.; https://www.fda.gov/news-events/press-announcements/coronavirus-covid-19-update-fda-authorizes-moderna-pfizer-biontech-bivalent-covid-19-vaccines-use.
61. Mella A, Mingozzi S, Gallo E, et al. Case series of six kidney transplanted patients with COVID-19 pneumonia treated with tocilizumab. Transpl Infect Dis. 2020;22(6):e13348.
62. Fishbane S, Hirsch JS, Nair V. Special considerations for Paxlovid treatment among transplant recipients with SARS-CoV-2 infection. Am J Kidney Dis. 2022;
63. Poznanski P, Augustyniak-Bartosik H, Magiera-Zak A, et al. Molnupiravir when used alone seems to be safe and effective as outpatient COVID-19 therapy for Hemodialyzed patients and kidney transplant recipients. Viruses. 2022;14:10.
64. Devresse A, De Greef J, Yombi JC, et al. Immunosuppression and SARS-CoV-2 infection in kidney transplant recipients. Transplant Direct. 2022;8(3):e1292.
65. Nair V, Jandovitz N, Hirsch JS, et al. COVID-19 in kidney transplant recipients. Am J Transplant. 2020;20(7):1819–25.

Chapter 6
The Impact of COVID-19 on Diabetic Foot Ulcers

Alisha Oropallo, Kane Genser, Amit Rao, Inthuja Baskaran, and Alyson K. Myers

Diabetic Foot Ulcers

Background and Epidemiology

The number of persons across the world with diabetes mellitus (DM) has surpassed 425 million in 2017 and is projected to reach 629 million by 2045 [1]. In conjunction, chronic wound occurrence is increasing, affecting 1–2 per 100,000 in the United States [2]. While the majority of these wounds are caused by venous disease, neuropathy related to DM trails closely behind [3, 4].

Attributing an exact tally of chronic lower extremity wounds as sequelae of DM is difficult as there is significant overlap between DM and other comorbidities,

A. Oropallo (✉)
Donald and Barbara Zucker School of Medicine at Hofstra/Northwell, Hempstead, NY, USA

Comprehensive Wound Healing and Hyperbaric Center, Northwell Health,
Lake Success, NY, USA
e-mail: Aoropallo@northwell.edu

K. Genser · A. Rao
Comprehensive Wound Healing and Hyperbaric Center, Northwell Health,
Lake Success, NY, USA
e-mail: KGenser@northwell.edu; arao3@northwell.edu

I. Baskaran
Department of Medicine, Center for Health Innovations and Outcomes Research, Northwell
Health, Manhasset, NY, USA

A. K. Myers
Albert Einstein College of Medicine, Bronx, NY, USA

Department of Medicine, Endocrinology Division, Montefiore Medical Center,
Bronx, NY, USA
e-mail: alymyers@montefiore.org

A. K. Myers (ed.), *Diabetes and COVID-19*, Contemporary Endocrinology,
https://doi.org/10.1007/978-3-031-28536-3_6

particularly peripheral arterial disease (PAD). DM is the second most powerful predictor of PAD after tobacco use. There are more than 8.5 million people with PAD in the United States, and approximately one-third of them also have diabetes [5, 6]. The lifetime risk of chronic lower extremity wound in patients with diabetes (PWD) is 34% [7]. Diabetic foot ulcers (DFU) complicated with infections and/or ischemia account for approximately a quarter of all hospital admissions for PWD and at least two-thirds of non-traumatic amputations in the United States [8, 9].

Pathophysiology

Diabetes induces many biochemical and physiologic changes which precipitate lower extremity ulcer formation and impair wound healing (see Fig. 6.1). These changes often work synergistically with concomitant comorbid conditions, more commonly PAD, to cause and then subsequently to negatively affect DFUs. Although a complete analysis of the effects of DM is beyond the scope of this chapter, the major pathophysiological effects are reviewed here.

Neuropathy

Diabetes mellitus is the most common cause of neuropathy in industrialized countries, with approximately half of PWD developing it in their lifetime [10]. Recent studies have greatly expanded the understanding of the biochemical mechanisms of

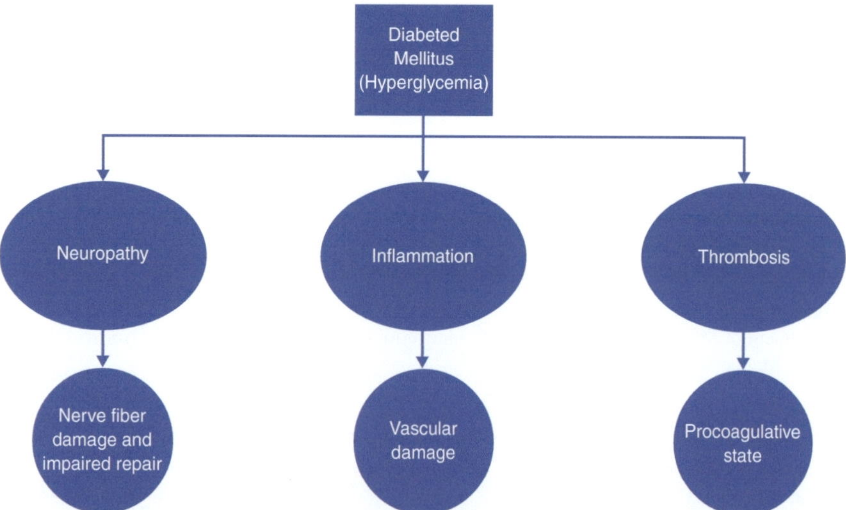

Fig. 6.1 *Diabetes and impaired wound healing.* The disease state affects three aspects that result in a poor healing environment

peripheral nerve damage occurring with DM. The dysregulation of multiple different metabolic pathways is responsible in aggregate for nerve fiber damage and the downregulation of nerve fiber repair [11]. In PWD, the increased production of reactive oxygen species (ROS) and glycated end products leads to protein misfolding, endoplasmic reticulum (ER) malfunction, impaired mitochondrial function, and further production of ROS [12–14]. The excess of ROS causes a pro-inflammatory effect. Misfolded proteins and subsequent loss of function due to glycation have been shown to affect transmission along the dorsal root ganglia [11] and play a role in neuropathy. Studies have shown that ER stress is associated with peripheral nerve damage due to DM [15]. Mitochondrial dysfunction leads to inefficient energy production further reducing nerve signal transmission [16]. Once present, peripheral neuropathy can cause PWD to overlook foot wounds due to a blunted pain response.

Inflammation

Diabetes is known to increase inflammation in the body, as measured by increased circulating levels of C-reactive protein as well as other markers of inflammation. Many of these markers have been implicated in vascular damage and the induction of a procoagulant state [17]. Hyperglycemia activates the protein kinase C (PKC) pathway in mitochondria, resulting in increased cellular permeability, apoptosis, and extracellular matrix expansion [18]. The increased PKC activity caused by hyperglycemia also upregulates the production of endothelin-1 (ET-1) and in turn results in increased vasoconstriction and platelet aggregation. This ET-1 upregulation has been directly observed in patients with Type II DM (T2D). Additionally, increased ET-1 activity also interferes with nitric oxide (NO) signaling leading to vasoconstriction (NO being an important endogenous vasodilator) [19, 20]. Vasoconstriction promotes thrombus formation and ultimately leads to atherosclerosis [21].

Thrombosis

Diabetes mellitus induces a prothrombotic state in several ways. Circulating levels of plasminogen activator inhibitor-1 and fibrinogen are increased in patients with insulin resistance [22]. Persistently elevated insulin levels and hyperglycemia have been shown to increase the expression of tissue factor monocytes [23]. In PWD, glycoproteins Ib and IIb/IIIa are upregulated, which in turn interacts with von Willebrand factor and fibrin, leading to a prothrombotic state [20]. There is also an increase in circulating vesicles – deemed microparticles – which are produced by various types of cells in response to activation and apoptosis. This increase in microparticles has been shown to promote coagulation at sites of endothelial injury and has been linked with thrombosis in both coronary artery disease and PAD [24, 25].

Management

Management of DFUs has evolved to incorporate a multidisciplinary approach that relies heavily on care coordination and close follow-up.

Screening

All patients with DM should have detailed examinations of their feet performed by providers with appropriate experience and training. These examinations should take place at least annually and should incorporate four major components: dermatological, vascular, neurological, and musculoskeletal. From a dermatological standpoint, any ulcer should be evaluated for size and depth as well as the potential for infection (discharge, malodor, etc.). Pedal pulse checks should be performed, at a minimum, with follow-up ultrasound testing for vascular evaluation if needed. Of the various neurological examinations that can be performed during the evaluation, the Semmes-Weinstein monofilament test or Ipswitch Touch Test is most commonly used for pressure and light touch assessment. Finally, muscle strength and range of motion should be evaluated as pedal deformities can lead to further ulceration [26]. Early intervention with proper shoes for PWD may help prevent further recourse.

Assessment of Contributing Factors and Comorbid Conditions

Once DFUs are found, a survey of contributing factors should be undertaken. It is important for the treatment team to explore underlying and adjacent issues that are ultimately responsible for the visible wound. Improving suboptimal glycemic control would benefit the healing of a diabetic wound. However, there are no randomized trials (and little evidence overall) that tight glucose control improves the healing of DFUs in the short term [27]. Despite this, there are numerous studies – the Action to Control Cardiovascular Risk in Diabetes, the United Kingdom Prospective Diabetes Study, and Action in Diabetes and Vascular Disease trials being among the most notable – which clearly demonstrate the benefits of good glycemic control, as defined by Hemoglobin A1c < 7%, on long-term cardiovascular and renal function [28–30]. A review of diet should also include a discussion of dyslipidemia as lipid overload has been shown to damage neurons, especially under the conditions of hyperglycemia, and further exacerbate neuropathy [31].

Compromised vasculature is a known associated risk factor for DFU. Therefore, all patients with DFU should be screened for PAD. The accepted standard for PAD screening remains a good clinical exam and measurement of the ankle/brachial index (ABI). Social history should cover tobacco abuse as smoking has been associated with the early development of microvascular complications [32].

In addition to these medical considerations, a patient's social infrastructure must also be evaluated. Proper care of DFUs, like all chronic wounds, requires frequent office visits and good care at home. The absence of an adequate support system – whether in the form of family, friends, and/or adjunctive health-care services – can seriously impact the efficacy of wound care. Any additional stressors to the ability of patients to seek consistent treatment for their DFUs can result in irreversible damage.

Wound Care

Local wound care is a fundamental aspect of treatment for DFUs. Any necrotic infected tissue should be sharply debrided. While this can often be accomplished in the outpatient setting, progression to abscess, gas formation (crepitus), or any sign of necrotizing soft tissue infection should prompt immediate transfer to an inpatient setting for surgical evaluation. Dressings vary drastically but the following standards should be met: (1) maintain a moist wound bed, (2) control any exudate, and (3) protect the surrounding tissues from maceration.

The optimal frequency of wound care is a matter of debate. In general, more frequent visits seem to result in better outcomes. A large review of the United States Wound Registry conducted in 2017 concluded that patients who visited a clinic at an average of 7.5 weeks times or more during a four-week period healed faster than patients seen at intervals of every two weeks or less [33]. The frequency of these visits had benefits beyond wound debridement, as providers were able to address other issues, such as compliance and adequacy of home care services. Frequent visitation may not be practical in all settings, but patients should be seen no less than once every four weeks.

Treatment of Concomitant Peripheral Arterial Disease

Roughly 50% of PWD presenting with DFU have some degree of arterial insufficiency [34]. Any PAD (ABI < 0.8) in a PWD increases the risk of limb loss by up to 13% [35]. Patients with both DM and PAD have a five-year mortality rate of nearly 50%. If a patient with DM and PAD requires amputation, their two-year mortality rate rises to 50% as well [36]. For these reasons, the American Diabetes Association recommends screening for PAD in all patients with DM by 50 years of age using ABI measurements. The use of ABI with toe pressure measurements or transcutaneous partial pressure of oxygen (T_CP_{O2}) measurements in all DFU patients is necessary to evaluate lower extremity blood supply [7]. Lower values are associated with an increased risk of amputation, particularly ABIs under 0.4 and toe pressures less than 30 mm Hg [37]. Once PAD is identified in a patient with a DFU, revascularization is recommended. Several options are available, involving bypass surgery or other noninvasive interventions individualized to the patient. The optimal approach in any given anatomical and physiological variation of PAD continues to be a matter of debate, but both options have yielded good results in DFU patients. A systematic review conducted in 2012 found that one-year limb salvage rates for PAD treated in DFU patients were a median of 85% following open surgery and 78% following endovascular interventions, and that 60% or more of foot ulcers had healed at one year following either open or endovascular revascularization [38].

Treatment of Infection

Infected DFUs are the leading cause of requiring hospitalization in PWD [39]. Neuropathic, vasculopathic, and diabetic effects on the immune system are the chief underlying risk factors for diabetic foot infections (DFI) [40]. Osteomyelitis, which can significantly complicate the treatment of a DFI and exacerbate patient outcomes, can be present in up to 60% of severely infected DFUs and even up to 20% of mild DFIs [41]. Careful evaluation and treatment of DFI are therefore recommended.

Depending upon the structures involved and the anatomical depth, surgical debridement may be necessary. To evaluate for osteomyelitis, two screening tests are recommended: the probe to bone (PTB) test and serial plain radiographs of the foot. PTB poses minimal risk, carries no additional cost, and offers a high-positive predictive value of 89% [42]. PTB does suffer from poor reproducibility. Serial plain radiographs of the foot are also easy to obtain and relatively low-cost, but only have a sensitivity and specificity of 54% and 68%, respectively [43]. It should be noted that these values have only been measured for single studies – radiographic changes over an interval of at least two weeks were more likely to diagnose osteomyelitis accurately [44]. If there remains uncertainty as to the presence of osteomyelitis, MRI is recommended. As MRI carries a sensitivity of 90% and specificity of 79% for osteomyelitis in DFUs, it is an excellent diagnostic tool (albeit at a greatly increased cost and time commitment).

To guide antimicrobial therapy, culture of the ulcer base should be performed by curettage, *after* debridement is performed. If osteomyelitis is present or highly suspected, a biopsy of the bone is preferred [44]. There are multiple empiric regimens available to treat DFI, and they vary based upon the severity of the infection present. No single regimen appears superior to the others, with clinical cure rates ranging from 48% to 90% [45]. Once culture or biopsy results are available, the antibiotic regimen should be appropriately tailored.

COVID-19 and Diabetic Foot Ulcer Care

Logistical Impact

Coronavirus disease caused by the severe acute respiratory syndrome coronavirus 2 (SARS-CoV-2) has both complicated the care of and worsened the outcomes of patients with DFUs. As has been widely reported across many fields (medical and non-medical), the COVID-19 pandemic has massively diverted resources. Personnel, funding, and physical assets once available for routine *and* emergent care of diabetic wounds have been reallocated to combat the pandemic [46, 47]. In an Italian study from 2020, patients with DFU were more likely to be admitted with wound complication emergencies and there was a more than three-fold increase in the likelihood of amputation due to DFU complications as compared to the previous year [48].

Since the earliest cases were reported in China during the end of 2019, over 500 million cases of COVID-19 infections have been reported worldwide. This enormous number underestimates the true rate of infection, as studies have shown that the incidence of seropositivity outstrips the number of reported cases by roughly ten-fold [49, 50]. The widespread global disruption caused by this pandemic, to everything from global shipping to simple activities of daily life, has been well documented. Due to the short-term necessity of diverting resources and staff to deal with the pandemic, medical fields were severely impacted. Organizing a patient's wound care with a multidisciplinary team results in better outcomes [51]. Outpatient wound centers have become recognized as the most effective implementation of comprehensive wound care strategy [52].

In the wake of the pandemic, many wound clinics were closed temporarily [53]. The centers that were not closed faced many logistical challenges. In-person visits were limited to those patients with severe wounds that were deemed to require urgent care [54, 55]. Centers that offered hyperbaric oxygen therapy decreased their daily operating capacity by a third (from three patients per chamber per day down to two patients per chamber per day) [56]. Caregivers were often prohibited from attending visits to wound care centers during this period [57]. A 2021 study that surveyed data from a wound center company with clinics in 45 US states found that visitation volume dropped 40% within the first 12 weeks of 2020 [58]. The burden of these missed visits shifted to home health-care providers, families, and the patients themselves [59]. There was a marked increase in telehealth visits for patients with wounds, as there was for all patients. In the United States, the Center for Medicare and Medicaid Services (CMS) significantly lowered barriers to the use of telemedicine by granting many waivers for its use [60]. However, the widespread adoption of telehealth was not without its challenges. Many wound care centers had never implemented telehealth and experienced significant difficulties as they transitioned. Even centers which had utilized telehealth prior to the pandemic found their infrastructure overwhelmed by the influx of new patients to the services [61].

The CMS covers three types of virtual services: telehealth visits, virtual check-ins, and e-visits. Telehealth services have been utilized for over 20 years with satisfying results [62]. A 2017 meta-analysis compared 213 patients treated using telehealth services and 301 patients treated in the usual fashion. The system utilized home visitation by nursing services who collected relevant patient information, performed exams, and obtained digital images. These data were then referred to a physician for decision-making. Rates of ulcer healing, healing time, and amputation rates were similar between the two groups [63]. In addition to these objective data regarding outcomes, patients themselves have reported good satisfaction with these systems [64].

Although these data are striking, perhaps the most concerning statistic is that the number of new wounds seen in wound centers in the United States in 2020 fell significantly. By June 2020, the patient volume in the wound centers studied had essentially returned to 2019 levels, and outcomes for these patients who were seen were largely unchanged [65]. However, the number of new wounds seen had fallen 19% as compared to 2019. Taken together, these data can be interpreted to signify that while patients who managed to be seen and followed up in the clinic (even with some delay) fared well, there may be large numbers of untreated wound patients who were never evaluated or treated in wound centers as a direct result of the pandemic [65]. This highlights the need for the clinician to review a patient's social well-being and ensure that they will be able to maintain an adequate level of care in face of external factors that hinder the patient's ability to do so.

There is evidence out of Italy that restrictions to wound care have already resulted in worsened patient outcomes. PWD with DFU admitted to an Italian hospital during the Spring of 2020 were compared to similar patients admitted during the same time of the previous year [62]. As compared to the 2019 cohort, the 2020 patients had significantly worsened outcomes. There were more cases of gangrene (64% vs. 29%, $P = 0.009$) and the need for amputation (60% vs. 18%, $P = 0.001$) [62]. While the study's population is admittedly small, at 63 patients in total, it suggests a concerning trend among patients with DFU.

Pathophysiological Synergy

Many of the same comorbid conditions that place PWD with wounds at risk of complications are similar to those conditions that predispose patients to more severe infection with COVID-19. Cardiovascular disease, smoking, chronic kidney disease, and chronic obstructive pulmonary disease (COPD) were all found in a systematic review to be among the most common comorbid conditions in patients hospitalized with COVID-19 [66].

In addition to the overlap of comorbid conditions, COVID-19 has been associated with hyper-inflammatory and prothrombotic states that may worsen DFUs. Severe cases of COVID-19 result in complement activation and a hypercoagulable state, linked to increased risk for pulmonary embolism and arterial thrombosis [67]. Of note is the clinical finding of "covid foot," which is described as a painful rash on the plantar surfaces of the foot; however, current research is limited to case reports and any link to DFU has yet to be determined.

Triaging Wound Care

In order to continue with good care of the patients, the CMS has promoted the concept of "hospitals without walls." In the early days of the pandemic, this referred to utilizing all facilities with available space, staff, and supplies to be used as makeshift triage units and hospitals. More broadly speaking, it refers to a transition away from the necessity to see every patient in the hospital, or in the office, in person. Keeping patients and their families away from one another was seen to be an effective strategy for limiting the spread of SARS-CoV-2 early in the pandemic, and it remains a useful strategy now.

Table 6.1 Categories of the wound patient

Critical (priority 1)	These are patients with gas gangrene, sepsis, or acute limb-threatening ischemia. They meet the Infectious Disease Society of America (IDSA) severe systemic signs of infection such as temperature > 38 °C, tachycardia, tachypnea, and abnormal white blood cell count. They should be seen urgently in the hospital setting.
Serious (priority 2)	These are patients with osteomyelitis, chronic limb ischemia, dry gangrene, worsening foot ulcers, and active Charcot foot. They exhibit IDSA-defined mild and some moderate infections. They should be seen in outpatient settings – such as wound centers, surgery centers, or podiatric offices – for their care.
Guarded (priority 3)	These are patients with stable or improving foot ulcers or active Charcot foot (not yet placed in stable footwear), who exhibit no signs of active infection. They may be seen in the office, or at home, with oversight of this process provided via telehealth.
Stable (priority 4)	These are patients with uncomplicated venous leg ulcers, healed foot wounds or amputations, and inactive Charcot (in stable footwear). Together, this population represents 94% of all patients with diabetic foot wounds. They can be treated at home or through telehealth.

A model for determining patients' needs, and subsequently meeting them, was developed in 2020. Deemed "Wound Centers Without Walls," it defined a strategy to triage wound patients and effectively care for them during the pandemic (See Table 6.1) [68].

Conclusion

COVID-19 has strained every aspect of the worldwide health-care system. As reviewed here, the pandemic deferred the care of many patients with DFUs. The overlap of many comorbid conditions, as well as the direct pathophysiological effects of the SARS-CoV-2 infection itself, put patients with diabetic wounds at particular risk of poorer outcomes.

These patients require close attention to their wounds, and diligent care by providers. The pandemic may have forever changed the proportion of DFU patients, and chronic wound patients in general, who are routinely seen in person. However, sophisticated systems of triage and telehealth together can mitigate these systemic changes and continue to ensure excellent care for patients with diabetic wounds.

References

1. International Diabetes Federation. IDF diabetes atlas. 8th ed. Brussels: International Diabetes Federation; 2017. http://www.diabetesatlas.org. Accessed 1 Nov 2022
2. Martinengo L, Olsson M, Bajpai R, et al. Prevalence of chronic wounds in the general population: systematic review and meta-analysis of observational studies. Ann Epidemiol. 2019;29:8–15.

3. Hicks CW, Selvarajah S, Mathioudakis N, et al. Burden of infected diabetic foot ulcers on hospital admissions and costs. Ann Vasc Surg. 2016;33:149–58.
4. Körber A, Klode J, Al-Benna S, et al. Etiology of chronic leg ulcers in 31,619 patients in Germany analyzed by an expert survey. JDDG. J Dtsch Dermatol Ges. 2011;9(2):116–21.
5. Barnes JA, Eid MA, Creager MA, Goodney PP. Epidemiology and risk of amputation in patients with diabetes mellitus and peripheral artery disease. Arterioscler Thromb Vasc Biol. 2020;40(8):1808–17. https://doi.org/10.1161/ATVBAHA.120.314595. Epub 2020 Jun 25. PMID: 32580632; PMCID: PMC7377955
6. Olesen KKW, Gyldenkerne C, Thim T, Thomsen RW, Maeng M. Peripheral artery disease, lower limb revascularization, and amputation in diabetes patients with and without coronary artery disease: a cohort study from the Western Denmark heart registry. BMJ Open Diabetes Res Care. 2021;9(1):e001803. https://doi.org/10.1136/bmjdrc-2020-001803. PMID: 33414173; PMCID: PMC7797253
7. Boulton AJ, Armstrong DG, Albert SF, et al. Comprehensive foot examination and risk assessment: a report of the task force of the foot care interest group of the American Diabetes Association, with endorsement by the American Association of Clinical Endocrinologists. Diabetes Care. 2008;31(8):1679–85.
8. Geraghty T, LaPorta G. Current health and economic burden of chronic diabetic osteomyelitis. Expert Rev Pharmacoecon Outcomes Res. 2019;19(3):279–86. https://doi.org/10.108 0/14737167.2019.1567337. Epub 2019 Jan 21
9. American Diabetes Association. 2. Classification and diagnosis of diabetes: standards of medical Care in Diabetes-2020. Diabetes Care. 2020;43(Suppl 1):S14–31. https://doi.org/10.2337/dc20-S002.
10. Anandhanarayanan A, Teh K, Goonoo M, Tesfaye S, Selvarajah D. Diabetic Neuropathies. 2022 Mar 15. In: Feingold KR, Anawalt B, Boyce A, Chrousos G, de Herder WW, Dhatariya K, Dungan K, Hershman JM, Hofland J, Kalra S, Kaltsas G, Koch C, Kopp P, Korbonits M, Kovacs CS, Kuohung W, Laferrère B, Levy M, McGee EA, McLachlan R, Morley JE, New M, Purnell J, Sahay R, Singer F, Sperling MA, Stratakis CA, Trence DL, Wilson DP, editors. Endotext [Internet]. South Dartmouth (MA): MDText.com, Inc.; 2000.
11. Feldman EL, Nave KA, Jensen TS, Bennett DL. New horizons in diabetic neuropathy: mechanisms, bioenergetics, and pain. Neuron. 2017;93(6):1296–313.
12. O'Brien PD, Hinder LM, Sakowski SA, Feldman EL. ER stress in diabetic peripheral neuropathy: a new therapeutic target. Antioxid Redox Signal. 2014;21(4):621–33.
13. Pinti MV, Fink GK, Hathaway QA, et al. Mitochondrial dysfunction in type 2 diabetes mellitus: an organ-based analysis. Am J Physiol Endocrinol Metabol. 2019;316(2):E268–85.
14. Chowdhury SK, Smith DR, Fernyhough P. The role of aberrant mitochondrial bioenergetics in diabetic neuropathy. Neurobiol Dis. 2013;51:56–65.
15. Lupachyk S, Watcho P, Stavniichuk R, Shevalye H, Obrosova IG. Endoplasmic reticulum stress plays a key role in the pathogenesis of diabetic peripheral neuropathy. Diabetes. 2013;62:944–52.
16. Rumora AE, et al. Dyslipidemia impairs mitochondrial trafficking and function in sensory neurons. FASEB J. 2018;32:195–207.
17. Beckman JA, Creager MA. Vascular complications of diabetes. Circ Res. 2016;118(11):1771–85.
18. Geraldes P, King GL. Activation of protein kinase C isoforms and its impact on diabetic complications. Circ Res. 2010;106(8):1319–31.
19. Cardillo C, Campia U, Bryant MB, Panza JA. Increased activity of endogenous endothelin in patients with type II diabetes mellitus. Circulation. 2002;106(14):1783–7.
20. Creager MA, Lüscher TF, Cosentino F, Beckman JA. Diabetes and vascular disease: pathophysiology, clinical consequences, and medical therapy: part I. Circulation. 2003;108(12):1527–32.
21. Kaur R, Kaur M, Singh J. Endothelial dysfunction and platelet hyperactivity in type 2 diabetes mellitus: molecular insights and therapeutic strategies. Cardiovasc Diabetol. 2018;17(1):121. https://doi.org/10.1186/s12933-018-0763-3. PMID: 30170601; PMCID: PMC6117983

22. Cefalu WT, Schneider DJ, Carlson HE, et al. Effect of combination glipizide GITS/metformin on fibrinolytic and metabolic parameters in poorly controlled type 2 diabetic subjects. Diabetes Care. 2002;25(12):2123–8.
23. Boden G, Rao AK. Effects of hyperglycemia and hyperinsulinemia on the tissue factor pathway of blood coagulation. Curr Diab Rep. 2007;7(3):223–7.
24. Sinning JM, Losch J, Walenta K, et al. Circulating CD31+/annexin V+ microparticles correlate with cardiovascular outcomes. Eur Heart J. 2011;32(16):2034–41.
25. Tsimerman G, Roguin A, Bachar A, et al. Involvement of microparticles in diabetic vascular complications. Thromb Haemost. 2011;106(08):310–21.
26. Song K, Chambers AR. Diabetic Foot Care. [Updated 2022 Jul 25]. In: StatPearls [Internet]. Treasure Island (FL): StatPearls Publishing; 2022. Available from: https://www.ncbi.nlm.nih.gov/books/NBK553110/.
27. Fernando ME, Seneviratne RM, Tan YM, et al. Intensive versus conventional glycaemic control for treating diabetic foot ulcers. Cochrane Database Syst Rev. 2016;1:CD010764.
28. Action to Control Cardiovascular Risk in Diabetes Follow-On (ACCORDION) Eye Study Group and the Action to Control Cardiovascular Risk in Diabetes Follow-On (ACCORDION) Study Group. Persistent Effects of Intensive Glycemic Control on Retinopathy in Type 2 Diabetes in the Action to Control Cardiovascular Risk in Diabetes (ACCORD) Follow-On Study. Diabetes Care. 2016;39(7):1089–100. https://doi.org/10.2337/dc16-0024. Epub 2016 Jun 11. PMID: 27289122; PMCID: PMC4915557
29. Adler AI, Stevens RJ, Manley SE, Bilous RW, Cull CA, Holman RR, UKPDS GROUP. Development and progression of nephropathy in type 2 diabetes: the United Kingdom prospective diabetes study (UKPDS 64). Kidney Int. 2003;63(1):225–32. https://doi.org/10.1046/j.1523-1755.2003.00712.x.
30. Patel A, Chalmers J, Poulter N. ADVANCE: action in diabetes and vascular disease. J Hum Hypertens. 2005;19(Suppl 1):S27–32. https://doi.org/10.1038/sj.jhh.1001890.
31. Padilla A, Descorbeth M, Almeyda AL, Payne K, De Leon M. Hyperglycemia magnifies Schwann cell dysfunction and cell death triggered by PA-induced lipotoxicity. Brain Res. 2011;1370:64–79. https://doi.org/10.1016/j.brainres.2010.11.013. Epub 2010 Nov 23. PMID: 21108938; PMCID: PMC3018544
32. Śliwińska-Mossoń M, Milnerowicz H. The impact of smoking on the development of diabetes and its complications. Diabetes Vasc Dis Res. 2017;14(4):265–76. https://doi.org/10.1177/1479164117701876.
33. Carter MJ, Fife CE. Clinic visit frequency in wound care matters: data from the US wound registry. J Wound Care. 2017;26(Sup1):S4–10.
34. Prompers L, Schaper N, Apelqvist J, et al. Prediction of outcome in individuals with diabetic foot ulcers: focus on the differences between individuals with and without peripheral arterial disease. The EURODIALE Study. Diabetologia. 2008;51(5):747–55.
35. Gazzaruso C, Gallotti P, Pujia A, Montalcini T, Giustina A, Coppola A. Predictors of healing, ulcer recurrence and persistence, amputation and mortality in type 2 diabetic patients with diabetic foot: a 10-year retrospective cohort study. Endocrine. 2021;71(1):59–68. https://doi.org/10.1007/s12020-020-02431-0. Epub 2020 Jul 25
36. Armstrong DG, Kanda VA, Lavery LA, et al. Mind the gap: disparity between research funding and costs of care for diabetic foot ulcers. Diabetes Care. 2013;36(7):1815–7.
37. Kalani M, Brismar K, Fagrell B, Ostergren J, Jörneskog G. Transcutaneous oxygen tension and toe blood pressure as predictors for outcome of diabetic foot ulcers. Diabetes Care. 1999;22(1):147–51.
38. Hinchliffe RJ, Andros G, Apelqvist J, Bakker K, Fiedrichs S, Lammer J, Lepantalo M, Mills JL, Reekers J, Shearman CP, Valk G. A systematic review of the effectiveness of revascularization of the ulcerated foot in patients with diabetes and peripheral arterial disease. Diabetes Metab Res Rev. 2012;28:179–217.
39. Palestro CJ, Love CNuclear medicine and diabetic foot infections. Seminars in nuclear medicine 2009 (vol. 39, no. 1, pp. 52–65). WB Saunders.

40. Pecoraro RE, Ahroni JH, Boyko EJ, Stensel VL. Chronology and determinants of tissue repair in diabetic lower-extremity ulcers. Diabetes. 1991;40(10):1305–13.
41. Lipsky BA. Osteomyelitis of the foot in diabetic patients. Clin Infect Dis. 1997;25(6):1318–26.
42. Grayson ML, Gibbons GW, Balogh K, Levin E, Karchmer AW. Probing to bone in infected pedal ulcers: a clinical sign of underlying osteomyelitis in diabetic patients. JAMA. 1995;273(9):721–3.
43. Aragón-Sánchez J, Lipsky BA, Lázaro-Martínez JL. Diagnosing diabetic foot osteomyelitis: is the combination of probe-to-bone test and plain radiography sufficient for high-risk inpatients? Diabet Med. 2011;28(2):191–4.
44. Lipsky BA, Berendt AR, Cornia PB, et al. 2012 Infectious Diseases Society of America clinical practice guideline for the diagnosis and treatment of diabetic foot infections. Clin Infect Dis. 2012;54(12):e132–73.
45. Peters EJ, Lipsky BA, Berendt AR, et al. A systematic review of the effectiveness of interventions in the management of infection in the diabetic foot. Diabetes Metab Res Rev. 2012;28:142–62.
46. Grande R, Fiori G, Russo G, et al. A multistage combined approach to promote diabetic wound healing in COVID-19 era. Int Wound J. 2020;17(6):1863–70.
47. Coronavirus disease (COVID-19) outbreak situation. World Health Organization. Available at: www.who.int/emergencies/diseases/novel-coronavirus-2019.
48. Caruso P, Longo M, Signoriello S, et al. Diabetic foot problems during the COVID-19 pandemic in a tertiary care center: the emergency among the emergencies. Diabetes Care. 2020;43(10):e123–4.
49. Stringhini S, Wisniak A, Piumatti G, et al. Seroprevalence of anti-SARS-CoV-2 IgG antibodies in Geneva, Switzerland (SEROCoV-POP): a population-based study. Lancet. 2020;396(10247):313–9.
50. Havers FP, Reed C, Lim T, et al. Seroprevalence of antibodies to SARS-CoV-2 in 10 sites in the United States, March 23-May 12, 2020. JAMA Intern Med. 2020;180(12):1576–86.
51. Weck M, Slesaczeck T, Paetzold H, et al. Structured health care for subjects with diabetic foot ulcers results in a reduction of major amputation rates. Cardiovasc Diabetol. 2013;12(1):1–9.
52. Kim PJ, Evans KK, Steinberg JS, Pollard ME, Attinger CE. Critical elements to building an effective wound care center. J Vasc Surg. 2013;57(6):1703–9.
53. El Hawa AA, Bekeny JC, Phillips NW, Johnson-Arbor K. Hyperbaric oxygen therapy for paediatric patients: an unintended consequence of the COVID-19 pandemic. J Wound Care. 2021;30(Sup9):S24–8.
54. Shankhdhar K. Diabetic foot amputation prevention during COVID-19. Adv Skin Wound Care. 2021;34(5):1–4.
55. Scalise A, Falcone M, Avruscio G, et al. What COVID-19 taught us: new opportunities and pathways from telemedicine and novel antiseptics in wound healing. Int Wound J. 2021;19(5):987–95.
56. El Hawa AA, Charipova K, Bekeny JC, Johnson-Arbor KK. The evolving use of hyperbaric oxygen therapy during the COVID-19 pandemic. J Wound Care. 2021;30(Sup2):S8–11.
57. Queen D, Harding K. The legacy of the COVID-19 pandemic and potential impact on persons with wounds. Int Wound J. 2021;18(4):417.
58. Cho SK, Mattke S, Sheridan M, Ennis W. Outpatient wound clinics during COVID-19 maintained quality but served fewer patients. J Am Med Dir Assoc. 2021;23(4):660–5.
59. Vowden K, Hill L. What is the impact of COVID-19 on tissue viability services and pressure ulceration? J Wound Care. 2021;30(7):522–31.
60. Centers for Medicare and Medicaid Services (CMS). Medicare telemedicine health care provider fact sheet. Centers for Medicare and Medicaid Services March17, 2020.
61. Scalise A, Torresetti M, Di Benedetto G. Wound healing Center: analysis of preventive measures and new indications in a teaching hospital in Central Italy during the Covid-19 emergency. Int Wound J. 2020;17(5):1538.

62. Kim HS. A randomized controlled trial of a nurse short-message service by cellular phone for people with diabetes. Int J Nurs Stud. 2007;44(5):687–92.
63. Tchero H, Noubou L, Becsangele B, et al. Telemedicine in diabetic foot care: a systematic literature review of interventions and meta-analysis of controlled trials. Int J Low Extrem Wounds. 2017;16(4):274–83.
64. Myra Kim H, Lowery JC, Hamill JB, Wilkins EG. Patient attitudes toward a web-based system for monitoring chronic wounds. Telemed J e-Health. 2004;10(Supplement 2):S-26.
65. Sen CK. Human wound and its burden: updated 2020 compendium of estimates. Adv Wound Care. 2021;10(5):281–92. https://doi.org/10.1089/wound.2021.0026.
66. Emami A, Javanmardi F, Pirbonyeh N, Akbari A. Prevalence of underlying diseases in hospitalized patients with COVID-19: a systematic review and meta-analysis. Arch Acad Emerg Med. 2020;8(1):e35.
67. Zhang Y, Xiao M, Zhang S, et al. Coagulopathy and antiphospholipid antibodies in patients with Covid-19. N Engl J Med. 2020;382(17):e38.
68. Rogers LC, Armstrong DG, Capotorto J, et al. Wound center without walls: the new model of providing care during the COVID-19 pandemic. Wounds A Compendium Clin Res Pract. 2020;32(7):178.

Chapter 7
Comorbid Obesity and Its Impact on Diabetes and COVID-19

Jiali Fang, Jimmy L. N. Vo, and Tirissa J. Reid

Introduction

As severe acute respiratory syndrome coronavirus 2 (SARS-CoV-2) spread through-out the world and reached a pandemic stage, comorbid medical conditions such as diabetes and obesity were reported to be associated with a more severe disease course and increased mortality [1, 2]. Given the close relationship between obesity and type 2 diabetes (T2D), with a diagnosis of obesity increasing the risk for T2D by seven-fold [3], the question naturally arises whether these are dependent or independent risk factors. This chapter will explore the interaction between these disease states in novel coronavirus 2019 (COVID-19) to affect disease severity.

The consistent trend toward increased morbidity and mortality in patients with diabetes infected with COVID-19 falls in line with previous viral outbreaks, including SARS-CoV-1 (2002–2004) and H1N1 (2009), where hyperglycemia or diabetes was found to be an independent predictor for death and morbidity and tripled the risk of hospitalization [4, 5]. While early studies reported both obesity and diabetes mellitus as risk factors for increased morbidity and mortality with COVID-19 [1, 6],

---

Jiali Fang and Jimmy L. N. Vo contributed equally with all other contributors.

J. Fang
Division of Endocrinology, Diabetes, and Metabolism, Department of Medicine, Vagelos College of Physicians and Surgeons, Columbia University Irving Medical Center, New York, NY, USA
e-mail: jf3404@cumc.columbia.edu

J. L. N. Vo · T. J. Reid (✉)
Department of Medicine, Division of Endocrinology, Diabetes, and Metabolism, Vagelos College of Physicians and Surgeons, Columbia University Irving Medical Center, New York, NY, USA
e-mail: jv2765@cumc.columbia.edu; tjr2122@cumc.columbia.edu

© The Author(s), under exclusive license to Springer Nature Switzerland AG 2023
A. K. Myers (ed.), *Diabetes and COVID-19*, Contemporary Endocrinology, https://doi.org/10.1007/978-3-031-28536-3_7

there remained questions as to whether there were unidentified confounders or population-specific differences, making these associations not applicable on a wider scale. More recent studies have confirmed some of these findings in more diverse populations or narrowed the specific circumstances under which an increased risk exists [7–9]. A 2021 study of 1019 patients found that obesity was associated with complications in COVID-19, including intubation, septic shock, and the need for renal replacement therapy in a diverse cohort. The same study also found that mortality was increased, particularly in those with a body mass index (BMI) above 40 kg/m^2, and that both morbidity and mortality increases were independent of comorbid diseases, including a diagnosis of diabetes [8]. Similarly, a prospective cohort study of nearly seven million patients found a linear increase in the risk for hospitalization, ICU admission, and death due to COVID-19 as BMI increased above 23 kg/m^2. Interestingly, the increased risk for hospitalization and ICU admission in those with increasing BMIs was lower in those with a diagnosis of diabetes than in those without. While a diagnosis of T2D attenuated these associations for severe disease, an increased BMI was still found to be an independent risk factor for severe COVID-19, especially in younger patients when compared to older patients, as well as Black patients when compared to White patients. The increased risk of death due to COVID-19 was not altered based on diabetes status in this study [7].

Morbidity has been consistently shown to be increased in patients with both type 1 diabetes (T1D) and T2D and COVID-19 [6, 9]. While mortality was initially reported to be increased in patients with diabetes, this has not been consistently shown to be an independent risk factor when controlling for age and BMI [9]. Several studies which drew this conclusion did not control for all likely confounders such as cardiovascular disease and BMI and were also not able to distinguish between patients with diabetes and those with a normal Hemoglobin A1c (HbA1c) experiencing stress hyperglycemia [6].

Some of the most prominent features of severe COVID-19 disease include a heightened inflammatory state, coagulopathy, and an impaired immune response, all of which have previously been described in patients with diabetes and obesity [10–12]. These abnormalities have long been established as detriments to overall health in patients with diabetes and obesity. There is a distinct possibility that further stress to these already dysfunctional pathways by a SARS-CoV-2 infection sets the stage for a more severe disease course. We will explore in detail the possible pathogenic mechanisms explaining why obesity and diabetes may worsen the prognosis for individuals diagnosed with COVID-19. As there is limited data on COVID-19 outcomes in patients with T1DM, we will focus primarily on patients with T2DM.

Inflammatory Response

Our current understanding of COVID-19 has identified inflammation as a key driver of pathophysiologic disease. SARS-CoV-2 invasion and infection of cells leads to an overproduction of cytokines [Interleukin (IL)-1β, IL-6, IL-8, IL-10, IL-12; Tumor Necrosis Factor-α (TNF-α); Interferon (IFN)-γ; IFN-β; C-X-C motif chemokine ligand-10 (CXCL-10); Monocyte chemoattractant protein-1 (MCP-1);

Macrophage inflammatory protein-1-α (MIP-1-α)] thus leading to cytokine storm [13] (Fig. 7.1). Diabetes, with its dysregulation of glycemic control, results in the uncoupling of inflammatory mediators from their natural feedback mechanisms. The ensuing inflammation and loss of immune cell regulation contribute to a β-cell cytotoxic environment due to the expression of pro-inflammatory cytokines and generation of autoreactive T-cells. Obesity augments inflammation via adipocytes, which secrete a number of inflammatory factors. Hypertrophic adipocytes increase activation of the endoplasmic reticulum and mitochondrial stress response promoting the upregulation of pro-inflammatory molecules, including TNF-α, IL-6,

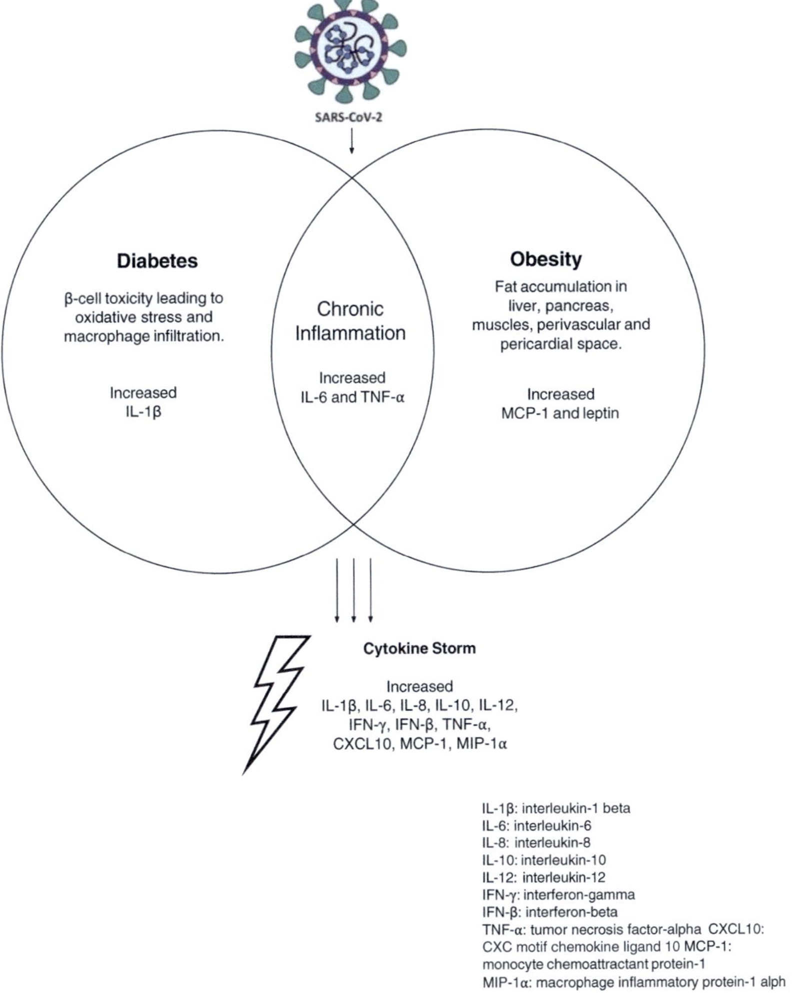

Fig. 7.1 SARS-CoV-2 leads to exacerbation of chronic inflammation in diabetes and obesity. Diabetes and obesity are states of chronic low-grade inflammation with overlapping mechanisms including increased expression of IL-6 and TNF-α. Viral infection with SARS-CoV-2 leads to acute exacerbation of this chronic inflammatory state. Elevated expression of cytokines can lead to worsened outcomes via cytokine storm

MCP-1, and leptin [14]. Decreased blood flow to adipocytes leads to hypoxia, necrosis, and macrophage infiltration with further upregulation of inflammatory markers causing oxidative stress, and endothelial and microvascular dysfunction [14]. The acute inflammation of COVID-19 exacerbates underlying chronic inflammation in patients with obesity and diabetes leading to increased hospitalizations, more severe disease, and worsened outcomes [15] (Fig. 7.1).

Interleukin-6

Interleukin-6 (IL-6) has been identified as one of the key participants of cytokine dysregulation in COVID-19 infection, upregulating angiotensin-converting enzyme-2 (ACE-2) receptors which allow the virus to bind and enter human cells as well as contributing to the severe acute respiratory distress syndrome seen in patients with COVID-19 [16]. IL-6 is a pleiotropic cytokine with both pro-inflammatory and anti-inflammatory functions. With regards to its pro-inflammatory properties, IL-6 is a driver of T helper 17 (Th17) cell differentiation from naive T-cells. Th17 T-cells trigger the production of numerous downstream cytokines, which enhance the antiviral immune response, as well as stimulate anti-apoptotic molecules, which can lead to viral replication. Studies demonstrate that IL-6-deficient mice have increased lung injury following influenza infections as well as an impaired antiviral immune response [17]. In this regard, IL-6 provides a protective advantage, but this benefit is quickly lost when signaling is altered. The balance between the inflammatory and anti-inflammatory effects of IL-6 is critical for a functional immune system.

In diabetes and obesity, IL-6 levels are chronically elevated and contribute to the development of detrimental metabolic effects [18]. In patients with T2D, IL-6 levels have been found to be elevated. Two small studies demonstrated that IL-6 levels are further elevated when there is chronic hyperglycemia in these patients, with IL-6 levels positively correlated to HbA1c values [19, 20]. The exact cause of IL-6 elevation in patients with T2D is unknown. One possibility is the presence of hyperglycemia creating advanced glycosylation end products (AGEs). AGEs activate the transcription factor NF-kappa beta, which in turn induces IL-6 [20, 21]. As much as 35% of IL-6 originates from adipose tissue and levels are proportional to fat mass, so patients with obesity have increased levels at baseline [22]. Elevated IL-6 levels, in turn, result in increased leptin secretion, worsening the anti-inflammatory milieu. Interestingly IL-6 has been found to be an independent predictor of COVID-19 severity and mortality [23]. IL-6 is one of the main effectors of cytokine storm, the aggressive inflammatory response seen in the most severe COVID-19 cases causing pulmonary inflammation, lung damage, and multi-organ failure [24].

Knowledge of IL-6 as a key driver of the inflammatory response in COVID-19 has resulted in therapeutic trials utilizing IL-6 inhibitors (see Chap. 1 for further discussion of the management of COVID-19). These agents include anti-IL-6 receptor monoclonal antibodies (e.g., sarilumab and tocilizumab) and anti-IL-6 monoclonal antibodies (e.g., siltuximab). The results of the Randomized Evaluation of COVID-19 Therapy (RECOVERY) and Randomized Embedded Multifactorial Adaptive Platform for Community-Acquired Pneumonia (REMAP-CAP) trials showed evidence that tocilizumab, when co-administered with corticosteroids, offered only a modest mortality benefit in certain patients with COVID-19 who are severely ill, rapidly deteriorating, have increasing oxygen needs, and who have a significant inflammatory response, defined by elevated levels of C-reactive protein and ferritin [25–27]. While further studies are ongoing, this therapeutic approach seeks to address one of the drivers of inflammation in COVID-19 which is also invariably elevated in patients with diabetes and obesity.

Tumor Necrosis Factor-α

TNF-α has also been identified as a driver of COVID-19-induced inflammation and cytokine storm [27]. Similar to IL-6, TNF-α is also found in adipose tissue and overexpressed in obesity, contributing to the development of peripheral insulin resistance and progression of diabetes by inhibiting the production of anti-inflammatory adiponectin and increasing the circulation of fatty acids (see Chap. 2 for more on insulin resistance) [28]. High levels of TNF-α and IL-6 seen in cytokine storm impair pancreatic β-cell function and inhibit insulin secretion, worsening hyperglycemia and leading to oxidative stress and gluco-lipotoxicity. This stress from hyperglycemia exacerbates the hyper-inflammatory state and perpetuates the destructive process of cytokine storm.

The inflammatory effects of TNF-α and IL-6 have also been shown to cause endothelial dysfunction and levels are elevated in obesity. Increased leptin, secreted in proportion to adipose tissue mass, is a potent stimulator of TNF-α and IL-6. TNF-α stimulates reactive oxygen species and induces mobilization of macrophages and smooth muscle proliferation, creating a pro-inflammatory and prothrombotic environment [29].

Strategies targeted at reducing TNF-α expression have also been offered as a potential therapy for reducing the severity of COVID-19-induced inflammation. Specifically, hydroxychloroquine was initially explored due to its well-established ability to suppress TNF-α and IL-6 levels in in-vitro studies [30]. Unfortunately, improved outcomes have never been established on a consistent basis. One study suggesting a therapeutic benefit required high-dose (600 mg/day) hydroxychloroquine which introduces the potential for multiple side effects including retinopathy, cardiomyopathy, neuromyopathy, and myopathy [31]. Furthermore, combination therapy with azithromycin has also been explored, but unfortunately, data indicates no additional benefit compared to controls as well as increased risk of QT corrected for heart rate (QTc) interval prolongation [31, 32].

Angiotensin Pathway

One proposed pathway through which SARS-COV-2 acts to worsen inflammation is the modulation of the renin-angiotensin pathway via an imbalance of angiotensin-converting enzyme 1 (ACE1) and angiotensin-converting enzyme 2 (ACE2). In the traditional renin-angiotensin pathway, angiotensinogen is converted to angiotensin 1 (AT1) via renin. AT1 is then converted by ACE1 to angiotensin 2 (AT2). AT2 has multiple downstream functions which include the promotion of vasoconstriction and inflammation. One counter-regulatory mechanism to AT2 activity is conversion of AT2 to angiotensin (1–9) [AT(1–9)] and angiotensin (1–7) [AT(1–7)] via ACE2 which results in vasodilation and anti-inflammatory activity. During viral infection, there is viral-induced downregulation of ACE2 [33]. Decreased ACE2 activity leads to the buildup of AT2. This results in a shift toward vasoconstriction, increased vascular permeability, volume overload, cardiac dysfunction, apoptosis of pulmonary endothelial cells, impaired insulin secretion, thrombus formation, and a global inflammatory response [33] (Fig. 7.2).

The imbalance of ACE1/ACE2 is likely more significant in patients with obesity as angiotensinogen, the precursor to angiotensin I and II, is highly expressed in adipose tissue [28]. The increase in angiotensinogen leads to chronically higher levels of AT2 at baseline. AT2 has tissue-dependent activity, but it leads to the development of metabolic syndrome by decreasing insulin sensitivity and insulin

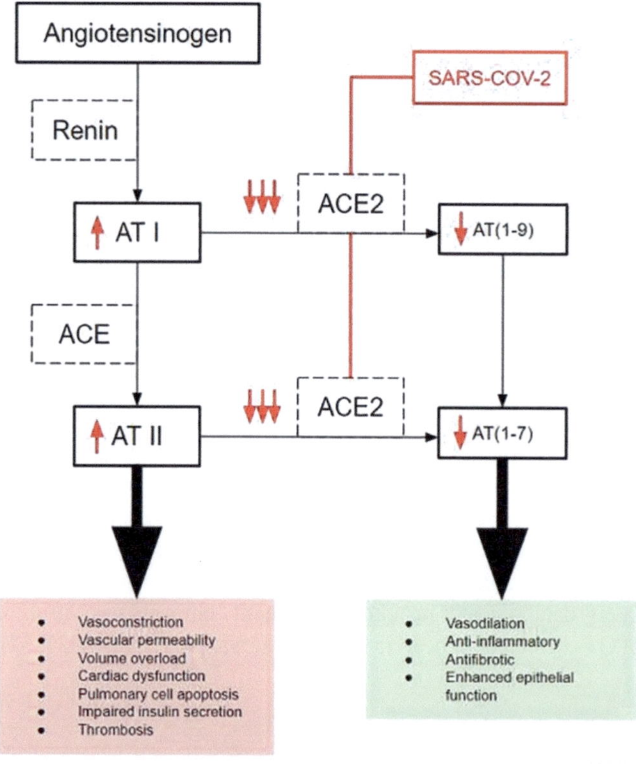

Fig. 7.2 Effect of SARS-CoV-2 on the angiotensin pathway

secretion, increasing white adipose tissue hypertrophy, and increasing vasoconstriction [34]. AT2 also impairs endothelial cell function, as well as promotes monocyte differentiation and chemotaxis [33]. The combination of chronically elevated AT2 levels in subjects with obesity combined with an acute increase of AT2 production from ACE 2 downregulation from SARS-CoV-2 is likely one pathway in which COVID-19 is worsened in patients with obesity.

Additionally, SARS-COV-2 infiltrates cells via binding to ACE2 which is expressed in a variety of locations including alveolar cells, bronchial epithelial cells, myocardial cells, adipose tissue, and pancreatic endocrine cells. Expression on pancreatic cells is of particular interest due to glycemic dysregulation seen in patients with COVID-19 [9]. While increases in glycemic counter-regulatory mechanisms leading to stress-hyperglycemia are routinely seen in severe illness, SARS-CoV-2's unique ability to target pancreatic β-cells further exacerbates this process. In fact, patients without previously diagnosed diabetes are frequently shown to have sustained hyperglycemia suggesting that ACE2-mediated pancreatic inflammation may unveil or even possibly induce diabetes in previously euglycemic patients [35].

Immune Dysfunction

An impaired immune function has also been explored as a mechanism that leads to worsened COVID-19 outcomes in patients with diabetes and obesity [36]. Hyperglycemia alone results in immune dysfunction on the cellular level. Normal physiologic response to infection is also altered leading to impaired priming of the immune system [36]. Abnormalities in immune function noted in patients with obesity include chronic innate immune system activation, adaptive immune system dysregulation, and lymphopenia. Elevated levels of inflammatory monocytes; neutrophils; TH1, TH2, and TH17 helper cells; and pro-inflammatory cytokines all contribute to an altered pro-inflammatory stance for the immune system. The imbalance between pro-inflammatory leptin, increased in patients with obesity, and anti-inflammatory adiponectin, decreased in patients with obesity, also contributes to the pro-inflammatory environment [37]. This results in the overstimulation of immune-regulatory pathways at baseline, which then impairs the immune system response to acute infections like SARS-CoV-2 [38]. Coupled with aberrations seen in obesity such as leptin-mediated dysregulation, an additional diagnosis of diabetes further magnifies the altered immune state of affected patients.

Hyperglycemia

The detrimental effect of poor glycemic control on the immune system has been well documented, and these effects have been extrapolated to explain the relationship between COVID-19 severity and uncontrolled hyperglycemia. Alterations in the number and function of immune cells underscore one mechanism that leads to increased susceptibility to infections and decreased clearance of pathogens. Both innate and adaptive arms of the immune system are susceptible to dysregulation.

Virtually all aspects of the innate immune system are affected by hyperglycemia. Dendritic cells, which function in the recognition and generation of the targeted immune response, are reduced in number due to accelerated maturation and apoptosis in mice models [39]. Macrophages, which act in the direct killing of pathogens and promotion of inflammation, are trafficked to lung tissue and driven toward differentiation to their pro-inflammatory subtype [40]. Neutrophils, which also act in direct killing through the generation of reactive oxygen species, release of antimicrobial peptides, and generation of neutrophil extracellular traps, are more prone to activation and can delay wound healing [41]. This is particularly important in pulmonary tissue. These deficiencies in the frontline defense against pathogens lead to impaired immune function and set the stage for increased COVID-19 infection severity.

The adaptive immune response is driven primarily by B and T-lymphocytes which work in conjunction with the innate immune system to deliver a target-specific response. B-cells produce antigen-directed antibodies as well as signaling molecules that can either promote or suppress further immune function. Patients with T2DM have disease-associated changes in B-cell function that are associated with promoting systemic inflammation, adipose tissue inflammation, and insulin resistance. Additionally, one study has shown that the SARS-CoV-2-directed CD4+ T-cell response is blunted in patients with diabetes [42]. Dipeptidyl peptidase-4 (DPP-4) has also been explored as a means of facilitating immune dysregulation in COVID-19 infection. DPP-4 (formerly known as "T-cell antigen CD26") is widely expressed in immune cells [CD4+ and CD8+ T-cells, B-cells, natural killer (NK) cells, dendritic cells, macrophages] and has been suggested as an entry point for SARS-CoV-2. This has sparked interest in the use of DPP-4 inhibitors, which are commonly used for the treatment of T2DM, as a means of improving COVID-19 outcomes. Unfortunately supporting data is inconsistent and further investigations are underway.

Interferon-γ

IFN-γ has also been identified as an important indicator of COVID-19 severity. In normal human physiology, acute respiratory viral infections lead to increased production of IFN-γ. IFN-γ leads to increased muscle insulin resistance and this in turn allows for more glucose to be available to meet the increased metabolic demands of immune cells. As a result of this hyperglycemia, insulin secretion is increased, and this is believed to benefit the priming of the immune system [43]. CD28, a potent co-stimulatory signal for activation of CD8+ T-cells, like insulin has a phosphoinositide 3-kinase in its signaling cascade. Co-stimulation of the CD28 and insulin receptor on CD8+ T-cells thereby serves to enhance the anti-viral CD8+

response [44]. It is therefore proposed that those with impaired glycemic response are unable to mount a sufficient insulin response, placing them at risk of developing complications from hyperglycemia as well as impaired antiviral immune activity.

Multiple studies have shown that patients with moderate COVID-19 had elevated levels of IFN-γ compared to healthy patients and patients with mild COVID-19 infections. Early on, IFN-γ levels peaked in patients with severe COVID-19 [45] and were associated with earlier death [46]. This overactivation of IFN-γ and other pro-inflammatory cytokines in COVID-19 infection is deleterious and has been shown to synergistically induce cell death [45] as well as impair lung epithelial repair [46]. In patients with obesity, there is an increase in CD4+ Th1 cells expressing IFN-γ [47]. IFN-γ has been shown to stimulate adipose tissue to increase the expression of chemokines and cytokines, contributing to chronic inflammation seen in obesity. Furthermore, sustained activation of IFN-γ has been shown to polarize macrophages (M1 macrophages), which are more responsive to inflammatory stimuli [47]. IFN-γ also suppresses anti-inflammatory factors that promote the resolution of inflammation and return to homeostasis [47]. Stimulation of M1 macrophages leads to an exaggerated inflammatory response, which may contribute to the severity of COVID-19 seen in patients with obesity [47].

Leptin

Adipose tissue is a complex structure involved in inflammation and metabolic signaling. Adipose tissue not only contains a significant number of immune cells but also produces both inflammatory and anti-inflammatory factors including TNF-α, IL-6, and adipokines, such as leptin [48].

Leptin is mainly produced by adipocytes and increases proportionally to adipose mass in order to control satiety through binding of leptin receptors in the hypothalamus [49]. Leptin is also secreted by multiple cells in the lungs and is a mediator of pulmonary immunity [49]. Pulmonary function is further exacerbated by obese patients' decreased lung compliance and diabetic lung disease (see Chap. 4). Although leptin deficiency is associated with immune dysfunction, chronic hyperleptinemia, typically seen in patients with obesity due to increased adipocyte mass, increases leptin resistance and decreases immune function [49]. In mouse influenza models, hyperleptinemia in obesity is associated with increased mortality, viral spread, and pro-inflammatory cytokines in the lungs [50].

Similarly, in humans, higher levels of leptin in patients corresponded with more severe COVID-19 infection and worsened mortality [13]. Specifically, patients with BMI > 24 kg/m^2 had overall higher leptin levels in SARS-CoV-2 infection compared to patients with normal BMI, and patients with severe levels had higher leptin levels than patients with mild disease [13]. Patients with obesity have baseline chronically elevated leptin levels, and further acute elevation leads to more severe COVID-19 disease through increased virus susceptibility, impaired pulmonary immunity, and increased inflammation.

As we now have a COVID-19 vaccine, it will be interesting to see if there are differences in immune response in patients with obesity compared to those without obesity post-vaccination. Studies have shown that leptin resistance can inhibit the production and activation of T-cells, impairing immune response [49]. Patients with obesity who receive the influenza vaccine have a two-fold increased risk of getting the flu compared to non-obese individuals due to blunted CD8+ memory T-cell response, impairing vaccine efficacy [51]. Unlike previous vaccines, the COVID-19 vaccine is an mRNA vaccine so it is unclear if the same phenomenon may occur. Although early data suggests that patients with obesity are more susceptible to vaccine-breakthrough infection, more data is still needed at this time [52].

Coagulopathy

Thromboembolic diseases, such as deep venous thrombosis and pulmonary embolism, are a major cause of mortality in COVID-19 infection [53]. Current data shows that patients with obesity with COVID-19 have an increased risk of venous thromboembolism (VTE) as well as a greater risk for mortality [53].

The increase of prothrombotic factors is thought to arise from the pro-inflammatory state. Patients with obesity also have an increased risk of VTE at baseline likely due to the overproduction of prothrombotic molecules including factor VII, fibrinogen, and vWF [54], as well as inflammatory markers.

Elevated levels of TNF-α and IL-6 are also known to have deleterious effects on the vasculature [55], in patients with obesity and T2D. As previously mentioned, TNF-α induces the production of reactive oxygen species, causing endothelial dysfunction. Likewise, IL-6 induces oxidative stress and endothelial dysfunction via activation of AT1 receptors, ultimately resulting in vasoconstriction [56]. This endothelial dysfunction resulting from TNF-α and IL-6 activity, including impaired vasodilation and enhanced vasoconstriction, contributes to the prothrombotic environment seen in patients with obesity and T2D and appears to be exacerbated with COVID-19 infection.

Clinical Considerations

Respiratory

Early studies of the COVID-19 pandemic demonstrated increased intubation and ICU admission of patients with obesity [30]. Obesity is often associated with negative effects of lung pathophysiology, both due to potential anatomic difficulty with intubation and an increased incidence of obstructive lung disease and complications while ventilated [57]. Proning has been one of the key management strategies for patients with COVID-19 infections and hypoxia. In patients with obesity, proning is thought to have even more benefits compared to non-obese patients and greatly improves functional residual capacity, lung compliance, and oxygenation [58].

Long-Term Sequelae

More than 2 years have passed after COVID-19 was declared a pandemic, but the full scope of the long-term impact of COVID-19 infection remains uncertain (see Chap. 14). Multiple reports of long COVID have been published, but we still cannot predict which patients experience long-term sequelae. It is unknown if obesity worsens the risk for long COVID; however, one study has shown increased hospital readmission after initial infection in patients with BMI > 30 kg/m^2 [59]. Whether obesity is a direct cause of rehospitalization is unclear as there are many confounding factors as patients with obesity tend to have more comorbidities.

Conclusion

The preponderance of evidence currently reveals an increased risk for more severe disease and increased morbidity in patients with obesity or diabetes and COVID-19. There is increased mortality in patients with obesity and COVID-19 and in patients with diabetes and COVID-19 if they experience significant hyperglycemia. A diagnosis of diabetes in and of itself does not increase the risk for mortality with COVID-19. Stress hyperglycemia in those without diabetes is known to cause immune dysfunction and lead to poor clinical outcomes in hospitalized patients, so it is not surprising that severe hyperglycemia likewise contributes to increased mortality in some patients with diabetes and COVID-19. The multiple pathophysiologic pathways described above are likely all contributing to the increased risk for more severe disease in patients with obesity and diabetes. At baseline, patients with obesity and diabetes are known to have a heightened inflammatory response, coagulopathies, and an impaired immune response. Hyperactivation of these already impaired systems in patients with diabetes and obesity once infected with SARS-CoV-2 appears to be the key pathway linking and explaining the increased risk for more severe disease with COVID-19. Further studies are underway to elucidate the relative import of these specific pathways and how they may be utilized for therapeutic benefits in COVID-19.

References

1. Barron E, Bakhai C, Kar P, Weaver A, Bradley D, Ismail H, et al. Associations of type 1 and type 2 diabetes with COVID-19-related mortality in England: a whole-population study. Lancet Diabetes Endocrinol. 2020;8(10):813–22. https://doi.org/10.1016/S2213-8587(20)30272-2.

2. Huang Y, Lu Y, Huang YM, Wang M, Ling W, Sui Y, et al. Obesity in patients with COVID-19: a systematic review and meta-analysis. Metabolism. 2020;113:154378. https://doi.org/10.1016/j.metabol.2020.154378.

3. Abdullah A, Peeters A, de Courten M, Stoelwinder J. The magnitude of association between overweight and obesity and the risk of diabetes: a meta-analysis of prospective cohort studies. Diabetes Res Clin Pract. 2010;89(3):309–19. https://doi.org/10.1016/j.diabres.2010.04.012.

4. Yang JK, Feng Y, Yuan MY, Yuan SY, Fu HJ, Wu BY, et al. Plasma glucose levels and diabetes are independent predictors for mortality and morbidity in patients with SARS. Diabet Med. 2006;23(6):623–8. https://doi.org/10.1111/j.1464-5491.2006.01861.x.

5. Jain S, Kamimoto L, Bramley AM, Schmitz AM, Benoit SR, Louie J, et al. 2009 pandemic influenza a (H1N1) virus hospitalizations investigation team. Hospitalized patients with 2009 H1N1 influenza in the United States, April-June 2009. N Engl J Med. 2009;361(20):1935–44. https://doi.org/10.1056/NEJMoa0906695. Epub 2009 Oct 8

6. Bode B, Garrett V, Messler J, McFarland R, Crowe J, Booth R, et al. Glycemic characteristics and clinical outcomes of COVID-19 patients hospitalized in the United States. J Diabetes Sci Technol. 2020;14(4):813–21. https://doi.org/10.1177/1932296820924469.

7. Gao M, Piernas C, Astbury NM, Hippisley-Cox J, O'Rahilly S, Aveyard P, et al. Associations between body-mass index and COVID-19 severity in 6·9 million people in England: a prospective, community-based, cohort study. Lancet Diabetes Endocrinol. 2021;9(6):350–9. https://doi.org/10.1016/S2213-8587(21)00089-9.

8. Page-Wilson G, Arakawa R, Nemeth S, Bell F, Girvin Z, Tuohy MC, et al. Obesity is independently associated with septic shock, renal complications, and mortality in a multiracial patient cohort hospitalized with COVID-19. PLoS One. 2021;16(8):e0255811. https://doi.org/10.1371/journal.pone.0255811.

9. Stevens JS, Bogun MM, McMahon DJ, Zucker J, Kurlansky P, Mohan S, et al. Diabetic ketoacidosis and mortality in COVID-19 infection. Diabetes Metab. 2021;47(6):101267. https://doi.org/10.1016/j.diabet.2021.101267.

10. Berbudi A, Rahmadika N, Tjahjadi AI, Ruslami R. Type 2 diabetes and its impact on the immune system. Curr Diabetes Rev. 2020;16(5):442–9. https://doi.org/10.2174/1573399815666191024085838[tr1]. PMID: 31657690; PMCID: PMC7475801

11. Paneni F, Beckman JA, Creager MA, Cosentino F. Diabetes and vascular disease: pathophysiology, clinical consequences, and medical therapy: part I. Eur Heart J. 2013;34(31):2436–43. https://doi.org/10.1093/eurheartj/eht149.

12. Samad F, Ruf W. Inflammation, obesity, and thrombosis. Blood. 2013;122(20):3415–22. https://doi.org/10.1182/blood-2013-05-427708.

13. Wang J, Xu Y, Zhang X, Wang S, Peng Z, Guo J, et al. Leptin correlates with monocytes activation and severe condition in COVID-19 patients. J Leukoc Biol. 2021;110(1):9–20. https://doi.org/10.1002/JLB.5HI1020-704R. Epub 2021 Jan 6

14. Zhou Y, Chi J, Lv W, Wang Y. Obesity and diabetes as high-risk factors for severe coronavirus disease 2019 (Covid-19). Diabetes Metab Res Rev. 2021;37(2):e3377. https://doi.org/10.1002/dmrr.3377. Epub 2020 Jul 20. PMID: 32588943; PMCID: PMC7361201

15. Kompaniyets L, Goodman AB, Belay B, Freedman DS, Sucosky MS, Lange SJ, et al. Body mass index and risk for COVID-19–related hospitalization, intensive care unit admission, invasive mechanical ventilation, and death — United States, march–December 2020. MMWR Morb Mortal Wkly Rep. 2021;70:355–61. https://doi.org/10.15585/mmwr.mm7010e4.

16. Gubernatorova EO, Gorshkova EA, Polinova AI, Drutskaya MS. IL-6: relevance for immunopathology of SARS-CoV-2. Cytokine Growth Factor Rev. 2020;53:13–24. https://doi.org/10.1016/j.cytogfr.2020.05.009.

17. Yang ML, Wang CT, Yang SJ, Leu CH, Chen SH, Wu CL. IL-6 ameliorates acute lung injury in influenza virus infection. Sci Rep. 2017;7:43829.

18. Han MS, White A, Perry RJ, Camporez J-P, Hidalgo J, Shulman GI, et al. Regulation of adipose tissue inflammation by interleukin 6. Proc Natl Acad Sci. 2020;117:2751.

19. Mirza S, Hossain M, Mathews C, Martinez P, Pino P, Gay JL, Rentfro A, McCormick JB, Fisher-Hoch SP. Type 2-diabetes is associated with elevated levels of TNF-alpha, IL-6 and adiponectin and low levels of leptin in a population of Mexican Americans: a cross-sectional study. Cytokine. 2012;57(1):136–42. https://doi.org/10.1016/j.cyto.2011.09.029. Epub 2011 Oct 28. PMID: 22035595; PMCID: PMC3270578

20. Kado S, Nagase T, Nagata N. Circulating levels of interleukin-6, its soluble receptor and interleukin-6/interleukin-6 receptor complexes in patients with type 2 diabetes mellitus. Acta Diabetol. 1999;36(1–2):67–72. https://doi.org/10.1007/s005920050147.

21. Yan SD, Schmidt AM, Anderson GM, Zhang J, Brett J, Zou YS, Pinsky D, Stern D. Enhanced cellular oxidant stress by the interaction of advanced glycation end products with their receptors/binding protein. J Biol Chem. 1994;269:9889–97.

22. Mohamed-Ali V, Goodrick S, Rawesh A, Katz DR, Miles JM, Yudkin JS, et al. Subcutaneous adipose tissue releases interleukin-6, but not tumor necrosis factor-alpha, in vivo. J Clin Endocrinol Metab. 1997;82(12):4196–200. https://doi.org/10.1210/jcem.82.12.4450.

23. Henry BM, de Oliveira MHS, Benoit S, Plebani M, Lippi G. Hematologic, biochemical and immune biomarker abnormalities associated with severe illness and mortality in coronavirus disease 2019 (COVID-19): a meta-analysis. Clin Chem Lab Med. 2020;58(7):1021–8. https://doi.org/10.1515/cclm-2020-0369.

24. Tang L, Yin Z, Hu Y, Mei H. Controlling cytokine storm is vital in COVID-19. Front Immunol. 2020;11:570993. https://doi.org/10.3389/fimmu.2020.570993. PMID: 33329533; PMCID: PMC7734084

25. RECOVERY Collaborative Group. Tocilizumab in patients admitted to hospital with COVID-19 (RECOVERY): a randomised, controlled, open-label, platform trial. Lancet. 2021;397(10285):1637–45. https://doi.org/10.1016/S0140-6736(21)00676-0. PMID: 33933206; PMCID: PMC8084355

26. Gordon AC, Mouncey PR, Al-Beidh F, Rowan KM, Nichol AD, Arabi YM, et al. Interleukin-6 receptor antagonists in critically ill patients with Covid-19. N Engl J Med. 2021;384(16):1491–502. https://doi.org/10.1056/NEJMoa2100433. Epub 2021 Feb 25. PMID: 33631065; PMCID: PMC7953461

27. Del Valle DM, Kim-Schulze S, Huang HH, Beckmann ND, Nirenberg S, Wang B, et al. An inflammatory cytokine signature predicts COVID-19 severity and survival. Nat Med. 2020;26(10):1636–43. https://doi.org/10.1038/s41591-020-1051-9. Epub 2020 Aug 24. PMID: 32839624; PMCID: PMC7869028

28. Ruan H, Lodish HF. Insulin resistance in adipose tissue: direct and indirect effects of tumor necrosis factor-alpha. Cytokine Growth Factor Rev. 2003;14(5):447–55. https://doi.org/10.1016/s1359-6101(03)00052-2.

29. Virdis A, Colucci R, Bernardini N, Blandizzi C, Taddei S, Masi S. Microvascular endothelial dysfunction in human obesity: role of TNF-α. J Clin Endocrinol Metab. 2019;104(2):341–8. https://doi.org/10.1210/jc.2018-00512.

30. Sperber K, Quraishi H, Kalb TH, Panja A, Stecher V, Mayer L. Selective regulation of cytokine secretion by hydroxychloroquine: inhibition of interleukin 1 alpha (IL-1-alpha) and IL-6 in human monocytes and T cells. J Rheumatol. 1993;20(5):803–8.

31. Gautret P, Lagier JC, Parola P, Hoang VT, Meddeb L, Mailhe M, et al. Hydroxychloroquine and azithromycin as a treatment of COVID-19: results of an open-label non-randomized clinical trial. Int J Antimicrob Agents. 2020;56(1):105949. https://doi.org/10.1016/j.ijantimicag.2020.105949. Epub 2020 Mar 20. PMID: 32205204; PMCID: PMC7102549

32. Mercuro NJ, Yen CF, Shim DJ, Maher TR, McCoy CM, Zimetbaum PJ, et al. Risk of QT interval prolongation associated with use of hydroxychloroquine with or without concomitant azithromycin among hospitalized patients testing positive for coronavirus disease 2019 (COVID-19). JAMA Cardiol. 2020;5(9):1036–41. https://doi.org/10.1001/jamacardio.2020.1834. Erratum in: JAMA Cardiol. 2020;5(9):1071. PMID: 32936252; PMCID: PMC7195692

33. Cook JR, Ausiello J. Functional ACE2 deficiency leading to angiotensin imbalance in the pathophysiology of COVID-19 [published online ahead of print, 2021 Jul 1]. Rev Endocr Metab Disord. 2021:1–20. https://doi.org/10.1007/s11154-021-09663-z.
34. de Kloet AD, Krause EG, Woods SC. The renin angiotensin system and the metabolic syndrome. Physiol Behav. 2010;100(5):525–34. https://doi.org/10.1016/j.physbeh.2010.03.018. Epub 2010 Apr 8. PMID: 20381510; PMCID: PMC2886177
35. Müller JA, Groß R, Conzelmann C, Krüger J, Merle U, Steinhart J, et al. SARS-CoV-2 infects and replicates in cells of the human endocrine and exocrine pancreas. Nat Metab. 2021;3(2):149–65. https://doi.org/10.1038/s42255-021-00347-1. Epub 2021 Feb 3
36. de Frel DL, Atsma DE, Pijl H, Seidell JC, Leenen PJM, Dik WA, et al. The impact of obesity and lifestyle on the immune system and susceptibility to infections such as COVID-19. Front Nutr. 2020;7:597600. https://doi.org/10.3389/fnut.2020.597600. PMID: 33330597; PMCID: PMC7711810
37. de Heredia FP, Gómez-Martínez S, Marcos A. Obesity, inflammation and the immune system. Proc Nutr Soc. 2012;71(2):332–8. https://doi.org/10.1017/S0029665112000092. Epub 2012 Mar 20
38. Huizinga GP, Singer BH, Singer K. The collision of meta-inflammation and SARS-CoV-2 pandemic infection. Endocrinology. 2020; https://doi.org/10.1210/endocr/bqaa154.
39. Feng M, Li J, Wang J, Ma C, Jiao Y, Wang Y, et al. High glucose increases LPS-induced DC apoptosis through modulation of ERK1/2, AKT and Bax/Bcl-2. BMC Gastroenterol. 2014;14:98. https://doi.org/10.1186/1471-230X-14-98. PMID: 24885625; PMCID: PMC4081508
40. Shaath H, Vishnubalaji R, Elkord E, Alajez NM. Single-cell transcriptome analysis highlights a role for neutrophils and inflammatory macrophages in the pathogenesis of severe COVID-19. Cell. 2020;9(11):2374. https://doi.org/10.3390/cells9112374. PMID: 33138195; PMCID: PMC7693119
41. Wong SL, Demers M, Martinod K, Gallant M, Wang Y, Goldfine AB, et al. Diabetes primes neutrophils to undergo NETosis, which impairs wound healing. Nat Med. 2015;21(7):815–9. https://doi.org/10.1038/nm.3887. Epub 2015 Jun 15. PMID: 26076037; PMCID: PMC4631120
42. Yu KK, Fischinger S, Smith MT, Atyeo C, Cizmeci D, Wolf CR, et al. Comorbid illnesses are associated with altered adaptive immune responses to SARS-CoV-2. JCI Insight. 2021;6(6):e146242. https://doi.org/10.1172/jci.insight.146242. PMID: 33621211; PMCID: PMC8026190
43. Šestan M, Marinović S, Kavazović I, Cekinović Đ, Wueest S, Turk Wensveen T, et al. Virus-induced interferon-γ causes insulin resistance in skeletal muscle and derails Glycemic control in obesity. Immunity. 2018;49(1):164–177.e6. https://doi.org/10.1016/j.immuni.2018.05.005. Epub 2018 Jun 26
44. Frauwirth KA, Riley JL, Harris MH, Parry RV, Rathmell JC, Plas DR, et al. The CD28 signaling pathway regulates glucose metabolism. Immunity. 2002;16(6):769–77. https://doi.org/10.1016/s1074-7613(02)00323-0.
45. Karki R, Sharma BR, Tuladhar S, Williams EP, Zalduondo L, Samir P, et al. Synergism of TNF-α and IFN-γ triggers inflammatory cell death, tissue damage, and mortality in SARS-CoV-2 infection and cytokine shock syndromes. Cell. 2021;184(1):149–168.e17. https://doi.org/10.1016/j.cell.2020.11.025. Epub 2020 Nov 19. PMID: 33278357; PMCID: PMC7674074
46. Xu G, Qi F, Wang H, Liu Y, Wang X, Zou R, et al. The transient IFN response and the delay of adaptive immunity feature the severity of COVID-19. Front Immunol. 2022;12:816745. https://doi.org/10.3389/fimmu.2021.816745. PMID: 35095917; PMCID: PMC8795972
47. Wu H, Ballantyne CM. Metabolic inflammation and insulin resistance in obesity. Circ Res. 2020;126(11):1549–64. https://doi.org/10.1161/CIRCRESAHA.119.315896. Epub 2020 May 21. PMID: 32437299; PMCID: PMC7250139
48. Grant RW, Dixit VD. Adipose tissue as an immunological organ. Obesity (Silver Spring). 2015;23(3):512–8. https://doi.org/10.1002/oby.21003. Epub 2015 Jan 22. PMID: 25612251; PMCID: PMC4340740

49. Kiernan K, MacIver NJ. The role of the adipokine leptin in immune cell function in health and disease. Front Immunol. 2021;11:622468. https://doi.org/10.3389/fimmu.2020.622468. PMID: 33584724; PMCID: PMC7878386

50. Radigan KA, Morales-Nebreda L, Soberanes S, Nicholson T, Nigdelioglu R, Cho T, et al. Impaired clearance of influenza a virus in obese, leptin receptor deficient mice is independent of leptin signaling in the lung epithelium and macrophages. PLoS One. 2014;9(9):e108138. https://doi.org/10.1371/journal.pone.0108138. PMID: 25232724; PMCID: PMC4169489

51. Neidich SD, Green WD, Rebeles J, Karlsson EA, Schultz-Cherry S, Noah TL, et al. Increased risk of influenza among vaccinated adults who are obese. Int J Obes. 2017;41(9):1324–30. https://doi.org/10.1038/ijo.2017.131.

52. Stefan N. Metabolic disorders, COVID-19 and vaccine-breakthrough infections. Nat Rev Endocrinol. 2022;18(2):75–6. https://doi.org/10.1038/s41574-021-00608-9. PMID: 34873287; PMCID: PMC8647056

53. Wang SY, Singh A, Eder MD, Vadlamani L, Lee AI, Chun HJ, Desai NR. Association of obesity with venous thromboembolism and myocardial injury in COVID-19. Obes Res Clin Pract. 2021;15(5):512–4. https://doi.org/10.1016/j.orcp.2021.07.003. Epub 2021 Jul 16. PMID: 34281793; PMCID: PMC8283573

54. Pasquarelli-do-Nascimento G, Braz-de-Melo HA, Faria SS, Santos IO, Kobinger GP, Magalhães KG. Hypercoagulopathy and adipose tissue exacerbated inflammation may explain higher mortality in COVID-19 patients with obesity. Front Endocrinol (Lausanne). 2020;11:530. Published 2020 Jul 28. https://doi.org/10.3389/fendo.2020.00530.

55. Zhang H, Park Y, Wu J, Xp C, Lee S, Yang J, et al. Role of TNF-alpha in vascular dysfunction. Clin Sci (Lond). 2009;116(3):219–30. https://doi.org/10.1042/CS20080196. PMID: 19118493; PMCID: PMC2620341

56. Wassmann S, Stumpf M, Strehlow K, Schmid A, Schieffer B, Böhm M, et al. Interleukin-6 induces oxidative stress and endothelial dysfunction by overexpression of the angiotensin II type 1 receptor. Circ Res. 2004;94(4):534–41. https://doi.org/10.1161/01.RES.0000115557.25127.8D.

57. De Jong A, Wrigge H, Hedenstierna G, Gattinoni L, Chiumello D, Frat JP, et al. How to ventilate obese patients in the ICU. Intensive Care Med. 2020;46(12):2423–35. https://doi.org/10.1007/s00134-020-06286-x. Epub 2020 Oct 23. PMID: 33095284; PMCID: PMC7582031

58. Paul V, Patel S, Royse M, Odish M, Malhotra A, Koenig S. Proning in non-intubated (PINI) in times of COVID-19: case series and a review. J Intensive Care Med. 2020;35(8):818–24. https://doi.org/10.1177/0885066620934801. PMID: 32633215; PMCID: PMC7394050

59. Aminian A, Bena J, Pantalone KM, Burguera B. Association of obesity with postacute sequelae of COVID-19. Diabetes Obes Metab. 2021;23(9):2183–8. https://doi.org/10.1111/dom.14454. Epub 2021 Jun 15. PMID: 34060194; PMCID: PMC8239834

Part III
Clinical Management

Chapter 8
Overview of Inpatient Management of Diabetes and COVID-19

Fuad Benyaminov, Patricia Garnica, and Alyson K. Myers

Introduction

Diabetes is one of the leading causes of inpatient hospitalization in the United States. It is also one of the diseases associated with an increased risk of hospitalization in persons with novel coronavirus 2019 (COVID-19). During the first surge in 2020, persons with diabetes (PWD) and COVID-19 also had increased mortality when hospitalized. Inpatient management of diabetes was further complicated by the ten-day use of steroids for persons with hypoxia. For inpatients with diabetes and COVID-19, insulin is the treatment of choice as it is effective for both hyperglycemia and inflammation.

F. Benyaminov
Department of Medicine, North Shore University Hospital, Northwell Health, Manhasset, NY, USA
e-mail: fbenyaminov@northwell.edu

P. Garnica
Department of Medicine, Division of Endocrinology, North Shore University Hospital, Northwell Health, Manhasset, NY, USA
e-mail: Pgarnica@northwell.edu

A. K. Myers (✉)
Donald and Barbara Zucker School of Medicine at Hofstra/Northwell, Hempstead, NY, USA

Division of Endocrinology, Department of Medicine, North Shore University Hospital, Northwell Health, Manhasset, NY, USA

Department of Medicine, Division of Endocrinology, Montefiore Medical Center/Einstein Albert Einstein College of Medicine, Bronx, NY, USA
e-mail: alymyers@montefiore.org

A. K. Myers (ed.), *Diabetes and COVID-19*, Contemporary Endocrinology,
https://doi.org/10.1007/978-3-031-28536-3_8

An Overview of Inpatient Admissions for Diabetes

Several studies have demonstrated that people with diabetes have hospital admission rates that are 2–6 times higher than people without diabetes, as well as an increased length of stay when compared to people without diabetes [1, 2]. According to the National Hospital Ambulatory Medical Care Survey in 2018, 8.25 million hospital discharges, diabetes was a diagnosis among US adults aged 18 years or older. These admissions were mostly for cardiovascular diseases such as ischemic heart disease, stroke, or lower-extremity amputation followed by hyperglycemic crisis and hypoglycemia [3]. Lower socioeconomic status, older age, obesity, tobacco smoking, physical inactivity, poor glycemic control plus clinical indicators including elevated Hemoglobin A1c (HbA1c), insulin use, longer duration of diabetes, and presence of complications have also been associated with increased rates of hospitalization and longer length of stay [4–6].

The Sax Institute's 45 and Up Study in Australia is one of the largest cohort studies regarding the rates of hospital admission and length of stay among a general population aged 45 years or older. The study showed that participants with diabetes were more likely (32% vs. 24%) to have a hospital admission for any reason within the year following their recruitment to the study than participants without diabetes [7].

Hyperglycemia has also been associated with adverse outcomes in several different hospital populations. An observational study by Martin et al. showed that admission glucose levels were independently associated with increased mortality in patients without a diagnosis of diabetes and that glycemic variability was associated with increased length of hospital stay in patients with type 2 diabetes (T2D) [8]. In a retrospective review of persons admitted to the hospital for a variety of diagnoses, those with lactate greater than 4 and glucose greater than 173 mg/dL had the greatest risk of mortality [9]. In both studies, those with hyperglycemia did not have a previous diagnosis of diabetes.

Diabetes and COVID-19 Requiring Inpatient Admission

Hyperglycemia was also seen as a risk factor for inpatient admission and worse health outcomes in those with COVID-19. Most people infected with the virus will experience mild to moderate respiratory illness and recover. However, older people and those with underlying medical conditions like cardiovascular disease, diabetes, chronic respiratory disease, or cancer are more likely to develop a serious illness with complications [10]. The relationship between COVID-19 and diabetes mellitus is complicated by an underlying compromised immune system.

COVID-19 infection directly affects glucose homeostasis by the increased release of cytokines and inflammatory mediators, which leads to increased insulin resistance and the associated hyperglycemia. Hyperglycemia in turn induces inflammation, endothelial dysfunction, and thrombosis via the generation of oxidative stress driving the dysregulation of glucose metabolism [11]. This dysregulation induces platelets to release prothrombotic factors such as thromboxane A2, increasing the risk for cardiovascular complications, multi-organ failure, and increased mortality rates [12]. When comparing COVID-19 patients with and without T2D, those with diabetes tend to develop more severe forms of the disease and have a significant increase in inflammatory markers (i.e., C-reactive protein, pro-calcitonin, ferritin, lactate dehydrogenase, and d-dimer) compared to patients without diabetes [13]. Another identified reason that diabetes worsens COVID-19 outcomes is that in human monocytes, elevated glucose levels directly increase SARS-CoV-2 replication by targeting the angiotensin-converting enzyme 2 (ACE2) receptors located in pancreatic islets (see Chap. 2 for more detail).

Diabetes and Increased Mortality in the Setting of COVID-19

Poorly controlled diabetes is known to increase the risk for severity of viral infections and mortality as seen with previous outbreaks of other viral illnesses including Severe Acute Respiratory Syndrome (SARS) [14], Middle East respiratory syndrome [15], and H1N1 influenza virus [16]. This has also been seen with COVID-19, as higher blood glucose levels at the time of COVID-19 illness have been associated with worse outcomes. Vargas-Vázquez et al. identified both prediabetes and undiagnosed T2D as risk factors for more severe illness [17]. In several studies, plasma glucose was the better predictor for severe COVID-19 compared to HbA1c [17–20] and intra-hospital hyperglycemia predicted severe COVID-19 independent of diabetes status [17]. In a meta-analysis of studies from around the world, diabetes with comorbid hypertension or chronic kidney disease increased the risk of death even further [21].

Initial studies examining health outcomes in patients with COVID-19 were limited to data from China, where the rates of persons with diabetes and COVID-19 have been lower than when examined in non-Asian populations in other parts of the world [22]. The other downside of this data is that it was homogenous, as it only captured outcomes in mainly Chinese patients. In both Asian and non-Asian patients with COVID-19, hyperglycemia at admission has been identified as a risk factor for increased mortality for patients with and without diabetes. In a retrospective chart review from China, PWD who presented with an admission serum glucose of 7 mmol/L (126 mg/dL) or higher were 2.3 times more likely to have mortality at 28 days when compared to those with an admission serum glucose of 6.1 mmol/L (110 mg/dL) [23]. This study was limited by the fact that HbA1c was not measured, so it is unclear if some of the patients with hyperglycemia may have had undiagnosed diabetes [23].

Large cohorts from Europe and the United States have provided more racial and ethnic diversity for patients, thus allowing for a better chance of generalizability. In an Italian cohort, those with hyperglycemia had a two-fold increased risk of mortality than those with normoglycemia and 30% greater mortality when compared to those with a history of diabetes [24]. Interestingly enough, those with diabetes had a higher mean average glucose on admission: 165 mg/dL vs. 154 mg/dL [24]. A Spanish cohort found no difference in mortality between those with or without diabetes if the admission serum glucose was greater than 180 mg/dL.

Mortality in Type 1 Versus Type 2 Diabetes

The difference in mortality among those with type 1 (T1D) versus type 2 diabetes is not clear as few studies have explored this. The findings of an English population study showed that those with T1D had a greater risk of in-hospital mortality when compared to those with T2D or those without diabetes [25]. A multicenter study from the United Kingdom compared those with T1D with a confirmed diagnosis of COVID-19 to those with suspected COVID-19. In both groups, the rates of hyperglycemia were high, with diabetic ketoacidosis rates higher in those with confirmed COVID-19—45.5% vs. 13.3% [26]. Diabetic keto-acidosis (DKA) rates varied from 13% to 45% in a systematic review of COVID-19 and T1DM, but it should be noted that the sample size of these studies was 58 persons or less [27]. In the national data set from the Cerner Electronic Health Record, variables such as the use of a continuous glucose monitor or insulin pump decreased the risk of DKA [28]. Those with a previous diagnosis of T1D had a 126% increased risk of having DKA [28]. Large clinical studies are required to identify the differences in outcomes for patients with T1D and those with T2D.

Emerging data showed the rates of mortality of persons with diabetes and COVID-19 can vary depending on variables such as age and comorbid conditions. The Coronavirus SARS-CoV-2 and Diabetes Outcomes (CORONADO) study found that older age, micro and macrovascular complications, and treated sleep apnea were all associated with increased mortality during the first surge in the Spring of 2020. With the administration of vaccines and the now endemic nature of the disease, mortality has declined in subsequent surges (see Chapters 12 and 13).

New-Onset Diabetes in Persons with COVID-19

Some cases of hyperglycemia were due to newly diagnosed diabetes associated with COVID-19. It has been noted that COVID-19 enters cells via the ACE2 receptors, which are expressed on the pancreatic beta cells [29]. Autopsy studies of persons who have died from Severe Acute Respiratory Syndrome (SARS) due to Coronavirus have shown "hydropic degeneration, fatty degeneration, and interstitial cell proliferation involving the liver, heart, kidney, and pancreas" [30]. These patients with new-onset diabetes can have higher levels of inflammatory marker expression (i.e.,

C-Reactive Protein, Erythrocyte Sedimentation Rate) when compared to those with pre-existing diabetes, thus leading to higher rates of mortality as compared to those with diabetes [31, 32].

Glycemic Control During Admission

Hyperglycemia during admission is also associated with worsening outcomes. In a retrospective review of 1129 patients at 88 hospitals, those with hyperglycemia with or without diabetes were nearly five times (28.8% versus 6.2%) as likely to die from COVID-19 as compared to those without hyperglycemia or diabetes [33]. In addition, those with hyperglycemia without a diagnosis of diabetes had a higher rate of mortality than those with diabetes (41.7% vs. 14.8%, $P < 0.001$), suggesting that hyperglycemia itself increases mortality regardless of diabetes diagnosis [8]. Hyperglycemia was defined as two blood glucose values greater than 180 mg/dL within a 24-h period during inpatient admission; persistence of hyperglycemia to days 2 and 3 of the admission was also associated with increased mortality [34].

Hypoglycemia has been relatively understudied as a risk factor for poor health outcomes in persons with COVID-19 and diabetes. In a multicenter, retrospective analysis, hypoglycemia was associated with a two-fold increased risk of mortality in those who were non-ICU, but not in those who went to the ICU.

Management of Diabetes and COVID-19

Steroids have been used as adjunctive therapy for patients with hypoxia. Various steroids have been tried in patients with COVID-19 including hydrocortisone, prednisone, methylprednisolone, and dexamethasone. Methylprednisolone and dexamethasone were initially favored due to better lung bioavailability compared to other steroids such as prednisone or hydrocortisone [35]. The RECOVERY trial assessed whether adjunctive steroid use with 6 mg of oral or IV dexamethasone would improve the 28-day survival of inpatients when compared to care as usual [36]; 24% of those enrolled in the study had diabetes. They found that only patients who required supplemental oxygen by invasive or non-invasive means benefit from dexamethasone therapy [36].

The downside of steroid use is the precipitation of hyperglycemia. Risk factors for the development of steroid-induced hyperglycemia in those without diabetes include high dosage, long-term use, older age, history of gestational diabetes or impaired fasting glucose, family history of diabetes, abdominal obesity, and belonging to a high-risk ethnic group for diabetes [37]. For persons with pre-existing diabetes, their glycemic control can be exacerbated by the initiation of steroid therapy. Steroids cause direct β-cell destruction, increased hepatic release of glucose, decreased glycogenesis, and increased insulin resistance [35]. In addition, hyperglycemia is further precipitated by decreased physical activity, β-cell dysfunction, and an influx of inflammatory markers, which are further magnified by COVID-19 illness. For inpatients, hyperglycemia is best managed with insulin as opposed to oral antidiabetic agents (OAD) [38]. The advantage of using insulin is that its dosing can be adjusted for changes in nutritional status or renal function. Insulin also decreases inflammation and platelet aggregation, which balances the increased inflammation and prothrombotic nature of COVID-19 [39].

There have been few studies examining the inpatient management of steroid-induced hyperglycemia in patients with COVID-19. One study in London found that men with pre-existing diabetes were 2.55 times more likely to have hyperglycemia than women with diabetes; however, there was no sex difference in patients without pre-existing diabetes [40]. Another study done in Saudi Arabia randomized patients to control versus an insulin algorithm with correctional scale insulin with or without basal insulin [41]. Those in the algorithm group had a greater proportion of target blood sugars (70–180 mg/dL), lower inpatient mortality, and were more likely to survive [41]. It was noted that those in the algorithm group took 2 days to achieve euglycemia, which was likely due to the use of basal insulin at a rate of 0.1 units/kg or the patient's home dose of basal insulin [41]. This is to be expected as past studies have shown that insulin requirements are often higher with steroid-induced hyperglycemia, with basal rates needing to be increased by 20–40% [42]. Basal insulin options include long-acting insulin analogs or intermediate insulin. The National Diabetes Inpatient COVID-19 Response Group suggests that Neutral Protamine Hagedorn (NPH) is the better option as its shorter length of action allows for more flexibility in dosing as compared to a 24-h analog [42]. For those who are insulin naïve, the insulin should be dosed at a total daily dose (TDD) of 0.3 units/kg; whereas those over the age of 70 or who have a creatinine clearance of 30 or less, the TDD should be 0.15 units/kg [42]. This dose needs to be titrated by increases or decreases of 10–20% if the glucose is outside of the range 6.1 mmol/L–12 mmol/L (110 mg/dL–216 mg/dL).

COVID-19 and Oral Agents for Inpatient Diabetes Management

Non-insulin therapies have been under investigation as a possible treatment option for patients hospitalized with COVID-19. Sodium-glucose cotransporter-2 inhibitors (SGLT2i) have been shown to have a protective effect on the heart and the kidneys in patients with T2D, as well as cardiovascular disease and kidney disease [43–49]. Patients hospitalized with COVID-19 can develop multi-organ failure, thus it was surmised that SGLT2i may prevent multi-organ damage and improve recovery in patients with COVID-19. A randomized control trial titled "Dapagliflozin in

Respiratory Failure in Patients with COVID-19" (DARE-19) tested this hypothesis. The DARE-19 trial was a randomized, double-blind, placebo-controlled trial of non-hypoxic patients hospitalized with COVID-19 and with at least one cardio-metabolic risk factor (hypertension, T2D, chronic kidney disease, heart failure, or cardiovascular disease). The patients were randomly assigned 1:1 to dapagliflozin (10 mg daily orally) or matched placebo for 30 days. This study had two primary outcomes: time until new or worsened organ (renal, cardiac, or pulmonary) dysfunction or death. The study found that patients with cardiometabolic risk factors who were hospitalized with COVID-19 and treated with dapagliflozin did not result in a statistically significant risk reduction in organ dysfunction, death, or improvement in clinical recovery, that is, hospital days [50]. There was also no statistically significant risk reduction in any of the secondary outcomes, including composite kidney outcome; death from any cause through day 30; the total number of days alive and free from mechanical ventilation through day 30; the total number of days alive, not in an intensive care unit and free from mechanical ventilation through day 30; and time to hospital discharge. Only two patients, both of whom had pre-existing diabetes, developed DKA in the treatment arm; whereas none had DKA in the placebo arm [50].

CORONADO, an observational study of inpatients with diabetes and COVID-19, found that outpatient metformin use was associated with decreased mortality at 7 days. In contrast, insulin therapy was found to be associated with death on day 7 [20]. This is likely due to the fact that insulin use is required in the more severe cases of diabetes. Metformin has shown anti-inflammatory properties as well as reduced the circulating levels of inflammatory biomarkers in people with type 2 diabetes [51]. In a retrospective study that compared the outcomes in hospitalized Chinese patients with COVID-19 and diabetes mellitus (mean age 64 years, 53% men), in-hospital mortality was significantly lower in those receiving metformin (2.9% versus 12.3%; $P = 0.01$) [52]. It has been suggested that the anti-inflammatory properties of metformin may help in treating COVID-19. Further prospective trials need to be done to study this further. Despite this, guidelines suggest discontinuing metformin on admission because of the risk of lactic acidosis in the event of renal or hepatic failure [53].

Other agents for diabetes have been studied for their use in COVID-19 and diabetes. CORONADO found that dipeptidyl peptidase 4 inhibitor (DPP4i), sulfonylurea, and glucagon-like peptide 1 receptor agonist (GLP1RA) use before admission was not associated with improvement in clinical outcomes such as the need for tracheal intubation and/or death within 7 days of admission [20]. This was surprising as GLP1RA-based treatments have been shown to reduce the production of various inflammatory cytokines and infiltration of immune cells in the liver, kidney, lung, brain, and cardiovascular system [54–56].

There had been some potential buzz about the use of DPP4i, which functions by preventing the DPP4-mediated enzymatic degradation of incretins such as glucagon-like protein (GLP-1), which leads to inhibition of glucagon release, the stimulation of insulin secretion, and the decrease of blood glucose. DPP4 is a transmembrane glycoprotein that was coincidentally identified as a functional receptor for the spike protein of the SARS-CoV-2 [57]. It is suspected that DPP4i may play a role in treating patients hospitalized for COVID-19 by possibly reducing SARS-CoV-2 entry into cells. A meta-analysis was conducted to assess if DPP4i was associated with decreased mortality in patients with COVID-19. The types of studies included in this meta-analysis were prospective or retrospective observational studies, case series, and randomized controlled trials. The intervention group was patients receiving DPP4i, while the control group was patients that did not receive DPP4i. There were 11 studies consisting of 5950 patients in this meta-analysis. DPP4i use was associated with reduced mortality [OR 0.75 (0.56, 0.99), $p = 0.043$] compared to those that did not receive DPP4i [58]. Interestingly enough, this effect was lost in patients who were also taking metformin, angiotensin receptor blockers, or angiotensin-converting enzyme inhibitors [58].

Since this initial meta-analysis was published, two other studies have been completed examining the impact of linagliptin on the need for mechanical ventilation and improving clinical outcomes. One parallel double-blind randomized clinical study was done to evaluate the effect of the combination of linagliptin and insulin on the need for mechanical ventilation in hospitalized patients with severe SARS-CoV-2 infection and hyperglycemia [59]. A total of 73 patients were randomized to the linagliptin and insulin (LI) group or the insulin-only (I) group. The study found that patients in the insulin-only group had a statistically significant higher incidence and risk of needing assisted mechanical ventilation than those in the LI group (HR 4.09; 95% CI 1.13–14.7; $p = 0.030$). Mortality was 5.9% ($n = 2$) in the LI group and 17.1% ($n = 6$) in the I group (RR 0.34; 95% CI 0.07–1.58; $p = 0.196$). Although the mortality reduction was not statistically significant, assisted mechanical ventilation was significantly associated with mortality since 53% ($n = 8$) of the patients requiring mechanical ventilation died, while patients not requiring a mechanical ventilator all survived ($p < 0.001$) [59]. The secondary outcomes of the study were glucose levels and insulin requirements, which were both decreased in the LI group versus the I group. This study was limited by the small sample size and the inadequate study power, which was not enough to identify differences in mortality.

Another randomized clinical trial with a similar sample size was designed to assess the effect of linagliptin compared to standard therapy in improving clinical outcomes in patients hospitalized with diabetes and COVID-19 [60]. Clinical outcome was defined as a reduction of 2 points or more on the 9 point WHO scale (see Fig. 8.1) after 28 days. A total of 64 patients were divided into two groups (32 in each group) and were randomized to receive 5 mg of linagliptin per os daily and basal/bolus insulin or just basal/bolus insulin. The study found that patients who were hospitalized with COVID-19 and treated with linagliptin did not result in a statistically significant time to clinical improvement compared with standard of care (7 days versus 8 days, hazard ratio, 1.22; 95% CI, 0.70–2.15; $p = 0.49$) [60].

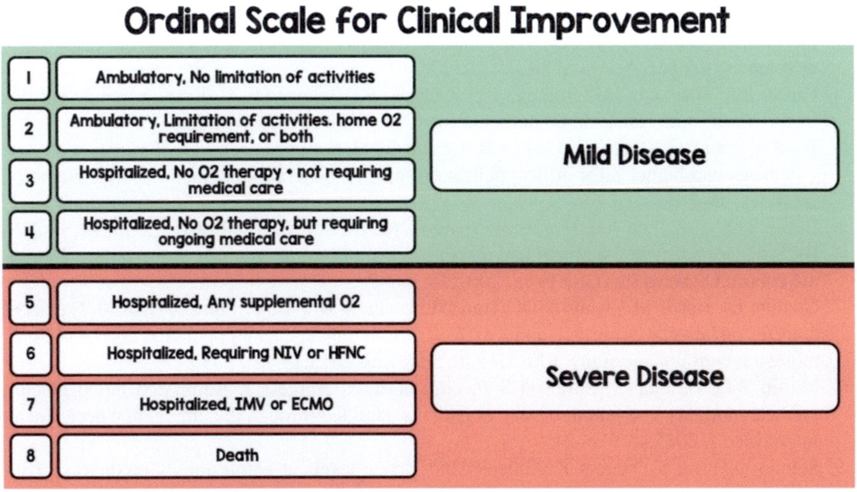

Fig. 8.1 Clinical Spectrum of SARS-CoV-2 Infection. Source: https://rebelem.com/wp-content/uploads/2020/05/COVID-19-Ordinal-Scale-of-Clinical-Improvement.png

Conclusions

Diabetes is one of the leading causes of inpatient admission and is a risk factor for hospitalization for those with COVID-19. Poor glycemic control increases mortality in this population, so achieving euglycemia is imperative. There have been some benefits noted with some of the oral agents – metformin and DPP4i – as they too have anti-inflammatory properties. The risk of lactic acidosis from both COVID-19 and metformin makes its use cautionary. Studies with DPP4i have not shown any benefit in outcomes. SGLT2i also seemed promising in having benefit as adjunctive therapy but that was not proven by the DARE trial, and their use in patients with COVID-19 can potentially lead to diabetic ketoacidosis. More randomized controlled trials are needed in determining the best therapies for glycemic control in persons with COVID-19 and diabetes. For now, insulin is the best option due to its anti-inflammatory properties as well as its ease of dose adjustment in the setting of profound hyperglycemia.

References

1. Carral F, Olveira G, Salas J, Garcia L, Sillero A, Aguilar M. Care resource utilization and direct costs incurred by people with diabetes in a Spanish hospital. Diabetes Res Clin Pract. 2002;56:27–34.
2. Aro S, Kangas T, Reunanen A, Salinto M, Koivisto V. Hospital use among diabetic patients and the general population. Diabetes Care. 1994;17:1320–9.

3. cdc.gov (2018) National Hospital Ambulatory Medical Care Survey: 2018 Emergency Department Summary Tables. https://www.cdc.gov/nchs/data/nhamcs/web_tables/2018-ed-web-tables-508.pdf. Accessed 20 Jul. 2022.

4. Panser LA, Naessens JM, Nobrega FT, Palumbo PJ, Ballard DJ. Utilization trends and risk factors for hospitalization in diabetes mellitus. Mayo Clin Proc. 1990;65:1171–84.

5. Bo S, Ciccone G, Grassi G, Gancia R, Rosato R, Merletti F, Pagano GF. Patients with type 2 diabetes had higher rates of hospitalization than the general population. J Clin Epidemiol. 2004;5:1196–201.

6. Burke V, Zhao Y, Lee AH, Hunter E, Spargo RM, Gracey M, Smith RM, Beilin LJ, Puddey IB. Predictors of type 2 diabetes and diabetes-related hospitalisation in an Australian aboriginal cohort. Diabetes Res Clin Pract. 2007;78:360–8.

7. Comino EJ, Harris MF, Islam MDF, Tran DT, Jalaludin B, Jorm L, Flack J, Haas M. Impact of diabetes on hospital admission and length of stay among a general population aged 45 year or more: a record linkage study. BMC Health Serv Res. 2015;15:12.

8. Martin WG, Galligan J, Simpson S Jr, Greenaway T, Burgess J. Admission blood glucose predicts mortality and length of stay in patients admitted through the emergency department. Intern Med J. 2015;45:916–24.

9. Sotello D, Yang S, Nugent K. Glucose and lactate levels at admission as predictors of in-hospital mortality. Cureus. 2019;11:e6027.

10. Coronavirus. In: World Health Organization. https://www.who.int/health-topics/coronavirus#tab=tab_1. Accessed 19 Jul 2022.

11. Ceriello A. Hyperglycemia and COVID-19: what was known and what is really new? Diabetes Res Clin Pract. 2020;167:108383.

12. Ulutas KT, Dokuyucu R, Sefil F, et al. Evaluation of mean platelet volume in patients with type 2 diabetes mellitus and blood glucose regulation: a marker for atherosclerosis? Int J Clin Exp Med. 2014;7:955–61.

13. Wang X, et al. Impacts of type 2 diabetes on disease severity, therapeutic effect, and mortality of patients with COVID-19. J Clin Endocrinol Metab. 2020;105:dgaa535.

14. Booth CM. Clinical features and short-term outcomes of 144 patients with SARS in the greater Toronto area. JAMA. 2003;289:2801–9.

15. Garbati MA, Fagbo SF, Fang VJ, Skakni L, Joseph M, Wani TA, Cowling BJ, Peiris M, Hakawi A. A comparative study of clinical presentation and risk factors for adverse outcome in patients hospitalised with acute respiratory disease due to MERS coronavirus or other causes. PLoS One. 2016;11:e0165978.

16. Schoen K, Horvat N, Guerreiro NFC, de Castro I, de Giassi KS. Spectrum of clinical and radiographic findings in patients with diagnosis of H1N1 and correlation with clinical severity. BMC Infect Dis. 2019;19:964.

17. Vargas-Vázquez A, Bello-Chavolla OY, Ortiz-Brizuela E, et al. Impact of undiagnosed type 2 diabetes and pre-diabetes on severity and mortality for SARS-CoV-2 infection. BMJ Open Diabetes Res Care. 2021;9:e002026.

18. Myers AK, Kim TS, Zhu X, Liu Y, Qiu M, Pekmezaris R. Predictors of mortality in a multiracial urban cohort of persons with type 2 diabetes and novel coronavirus 19. J Diabetes. 2021;13:430–8.

19. Agarwal S, Schechter C, Southern W, Crandall JP, Tomer Y. Preadmission diabetes-specific risk factors for mortality in hospitalized patients with diabetes and coronavirus disease 2019. Diabetes Care. 2020;43:2339–44.

20. Cariou B, Hadjadj S, Wargny M, Pichelin M, Al-Salameh A, Allix I, Amadou C, Arnault G, Baudoux F, Bauduceau B, Borot S. Phenotypic characteristics and prognosis of inpatients with COVID-19 and diabetes: the CORONADO study. Diabetologia. 2020;63:1500–15.

21. Corona G, Pizzocaro A, Vena W, Rastrelli G, Semeraro F, Isidori AM, Pivonello R, Salonia A, Sforza A, Maggi M. Diabetes is the most important cause for mortality in COVID-19 hospitalized patients: systematic review and meta-analysis. Rev Endocr Metabol Disord. 2021;22:275–96.

22. Mantovani A, Byrne CD, Zheng M-H, Targher G. Diabetes as a risk factor for greater COVID-19 severity and in-hospital death: a meta-analysis of observational studies. Nutr Metab Cardiovasc Dis. 2020;30:1236–48.
23. Wang S, Ma P, Zhang S, Song S, Wang Z, Ma Y, et al. Fasting blood glucose at admission is an independent predictor for 28-day mortality in patients with COVID-19 without previous diagnosis of diabetes: a multi-Centre retrospective study. Diabetologia. 2020;63:2102–11.
24. Coppelli A, Giannarelli R, Aragona M, Penno G, Falcone M, Tiseo G, et al. Hyperglycemia at hospital admission is associated with severity of the prognosis in patients hospitalized for COVID-19: the Pisa COVID-19 study. Diabetes Care. 2020;43:2345–8.
25. Barron E, Bakhai C, Kar P, Weaver A, Bradley D, Ismail H, Knighton P, Holman N, Khunti K, Sattar N, Wareham NJ, Young B, Valabhji J. Associations of type 1 and type 2 diabetes with COVID-19-related mortality in England: a whole-population study. Lancet Diabetes Endocrinol. 2020;8:813–22.
26. Ebekozien OA, Noor N, Gallagher MP, Alonso GT. Type 1 diabetes and COVID-19: preliminary findings from a Multicenter surveillance study in the U.S. Diabetes Care. 2020;43:e83–5.
27. Nassar M, et al. The association between COVID-19 and type 1 diabetes mellitus: a systematic review. Diabetes Metab Syndr. 2021;15:447–54.
28. Qeadan F, Tingey B, Egbert J, Pezzolesi MG, Burge MR, Peterson KA, Honda T. The associations between COVID-19 diagnosis, type 1 diabetes, and the risk of diabetic ketoacidosis: a nationwide cohort from the US using the Cerner real-world data. PLoS One. 2022;17:e0266809.
29. Rubino F, Amiel SA, Zimmet P, Alberti G, Bornstein S, Eckel RH, et al. New-onset diabetes in Covid-19. N Engl J Med. 2020;383:789–90.
30. Yang JK, Lin SS, Ji XJ, Guo LM. Binding of SARS coronavirus to its receptor damages islets and causes acute diabetes. Acta Diabetol. 2010;47:193–9.
31. Li H, Tian S, Chen T, Cui Z, Shi N, Zhong X, et al. Newly diagnosed diabetes is associated with a higher risk of mortality than known diabetes in hospitalized patients with COVID-19. Diabetes Obes Metab. 2020;22:1897–906.
32. Carrasco-Sánchez FJ, López-Carmona MD, Martínez-Marcos FJ, Pérez-Belmonte LM, Hidalgo-Jiménez A, Buonaiuto V, et al. Admission hyperglycaemia as a predictor of mortality in patients hospitalized with COVID-19 regardless of diabetes status: data from the Spanish SEMI-COVID-19 registry. Ann Med. 2021;53:103–16.
33. Bode B, Garrett V, Messler J, McFarland R, Crowe J, Booth R, et al. Glycemic characteristics and clinical outcomes of COVID-19 patients hospitalized in the United States. J Diabetes Sci Technol. 2020;14:813–21.
34. Klonoff DC, Messler JC, Umpierrez GE, Peng L, Booth R, Crowe J, Garrett V, McFarland R, Pasquel FJ. Association between achieving inpatient glycemic control and clinical outcomes in hospitalized patients with COVID-19: a multicenter, retrospective hospital-based analysis. Diabetes care. 2021;44(2):578–85.
35. Czock D, Keller F, Rasche FM, Häussler U. Pharmacokinetics and pharmacodynamics of systemically administered glucocorticoids. Clin Pharmacokinet. 2005;44:61–98.
36. Horby P, Lim WS, Emberson J, et al. Dexamethasone in hospitalized patients with Covid-19 — preliminary report. N Engl J Med. 2020;384:693–704.
37. Das S, Rastogi A, Harikumar KVS, Dutta D, Sahay R, Kalra S, et al. Diagnosis and management considerations in steroid-related Hyperglycemia in COVID-19: a position statement from the Endocrine Society of India. Indian J Endocrinol Metab. 2021;25:4–11.
38. American Diabetes Association Professional Practice Committee. 16. Diabetes Care in the Hospital: standards of medical Care in Diabetes—2022. Diabetes Care. 2020;45:S244–53.
39. Dandona P, Chaudhuri A, Mohanty P, Ghanim H. Anti-inflammatory effects of insulin. Curr Opin Clin Nutr Metabol Care. 2007;10:511–7.
40. Younes YR, Stockley S, Keegan L, O'Donoghue L, Yohannan E, Read L, et al. COVID-19 and dexamethasone-induced hyperglycaemia: workload implications for diabetes inpatient teams. Diabet Med. 2022;39:e14716.

41. Asiri AA, Alguwaihes AM, Jammah AA, Alfadda AA, Al-Sofiani ME. Assessment of the effectiveness of a protocol to manage dexamethasone-induced Hyperglycemia among hospitalized patients with COVID-19. Endocr Pract. 2021;27:1232–41.
42. Rayman G, Lumb A, Kennon B, Cottrell C, Nagi D, Page E, et al. New guidance on managing inpatient hyperglycaemia during the COVID-19 pandemic. Diabet Med. 2020;37:1210–3.
43. Packer M, Anker SD, Butler J, et al. Cardiovascular and renal outcomes with empagliflozin in heart failure. N Engl J Med. 2020;383:1413–24.
44. Heerspink HJL, Stefánsson BV, Correa-Rotter R, et al. Dapagliflozin in patients with chronic kidney disease. N Engl J Med. 2020;383:1436–46.
45. Perkovic V, Jardine MJ, Neal B, et al. Canagliflozin and renal outcomes in type 2 diabetes and nephropathy. N Engl J Med. 2019;380:2295–306.
46. McMurray JJV, Solomon SD, Inzucchi SE, et al. Dapagliflozin in patients with heart failure and reduced ejection fraction. N Engl J Med. 2019;381:1995–2008.
47. Zinman B, Wanner C, Lachin JM, et al. Empagliflozin, cardiovascular outcomes, and mortality in type 2 diabetes. N Engl J Med. 2015;373:2117–28.
48. Neal B, Perkovic V, Mahaffey KW, et al. Canagliflozin and cardiovascular and renal events in type 2 diabetes. N Engl J Med. 2017;377:644–57.
49. Wiviott SD, Raz I, Bonaca MP, et al. Dapagliflozin and cardiovascular outcomes in type 2 diabetes. N Engl J Med. 2019;380:347–57.
50. Kosiborod MN, Esterline R, Furtado RHM, et al. Dapagliflozin in patients with cardiometabolic risk factors hospitalised with COVID-19 (DARE-19): a randomised, double-blind, placebo-controlled, phase 3 trial. Lancet Diabet Endocrinol. 2021;9:586–94.
51. Cameron AR, et al. Anti-inflammatory effects of metformin irrespective of diabetes status. Circ Res. 2016;119:652–65.
52. Luo P, et al. Metformin treatment was associated with decreased mortality in COVID-19 patients with diabetes in a retrospective analysis. Am J Trop Med Hygiene. 2020;103:69–72.
53. Bornstein SR, Rubino F, Khunti K, et al. Practical recommendations for the management of diabetes in patients with COVID-19. Lancet Diabet Endocrinol. 2020;8:546–50.
54. Drucker DJ. The biology of incretin hormones. Cell Metab. 2006;3:153–65.
55. Lim S, Kim KM, Nauck MA. Glucagon-like peptide-1 receptor agonists and cardiovascular events: class effects versus individual patterns. Trends Endocrinol Metab. 2018;29:238–48.
56. Liu H, Dear AE, Knudsen LB, Simpson RW. A long-acting glucagon-like peptide-1 analogue attenuates induction of plasminogen activator inhibitor type-1 and vascular adhesion molecules. J Endocrinol. 2009;201:59–66.
57. Raj VS, Mou H, Smits SL, Dekkers DH, Muller MA, Dijkman R, et al. Dipeptidyl peptidase 4 is a functional receptor for the emerging human coronavirus-EMC. Nature. 2013;495:251–4.
58. Zein AFMZ, Raffaello WM. Dipeptidyl peptidase-4 (DPP-IV) inhibitor was associated with mortality reduction in COVID-19 - a systematic review and meta-analysis. Prim Care Diabetes. 2022;16:162–7.
59. Guardado-Mendoza R, Garcia-Magaña MA, Martínez-Navarro LJ, et al. Effect of linagliptin plus insulin in comparison to insulin alone on metabolic control and prognosis in hospitalized patients with SARS-CoV-2 infection. Sci Rep. 2022;12:536.
60. Abuhasira R, Ayalon-Dangur I, Zaslavsky N, et al. A randomized clinical trial of linagliptin vs. standard of care in patients hospitalized with diabetes and COVID-19. Front Endocrinol. 2021;12:794382.

Chapter 9
Management of Critically Ill Persons with COVID-19 and Diabetes

Justin Mathew and Hanna J. Lee

Introduction

Diabetic ketoacidosis (DKA) and hyperosmolar hyperglycemic state (HHS) are life-threatening hyperglycemic emergencies of diabetes mellitus (DM) that often necessitate intensive care unit (ICU) admissions. With the spread of the 2019 novel coronavirus (COVID-19), early case series soon revealed the increased risk for critical illness among individuals with diabetes who contracted the virus. Important questions promptly followed: How does COVID-19 trigger and impact the development of hyperglycemia and hyperglycemic emergencies? How can these complications be effectively managed while securing the safety of both the patients and the healthcare providers? This chapter will review the unique challenges and the novel initiatives implemented in the treatment of DKA and HHS during the COVID-19 pandemic.

Hyperglycemia and Diabetes Mellitus in the ICU

Hyperglycemia is a well-known common complication among hospitalized patients. Individuals with a history of DM are more prone to be hospitalized for acute illnesses, often requiring longer courses of hospital stay, and are at increased risk for infection-related mortality [1]. It has also been shown that hyperglycemia at admission, regardless of prior diagnosis of DM, is an independent predictor of mortality [2, 3].

J. Mathew · H. J. Lee (✉)
Division of Endocrinology, Department of Medicine, The Fleischer Institute for Diabetes and Metabolism, Albert Einstein College of Medicine and Montefiore Medical Center, Bronx, NY, USA
e-mail: jusmathew@montefiore.org; hlee8@montefiore.org

A. K. Myers (ed.), *Diabetes and COVID-19*, Contemporary Endocrinology,
https://doi.org/10.1007/978-3-031-28536-3_9

These tendencies have been especially amplified among COVID-19 patients; hyperglycemia itself and pre-existing diabetes are predictors of more severe COVID-19 disease [4]. Elevations in inflammatory markers such as interleukin-6 (IL6) and D-dimer were detected to be more persistent among COVID-19 patients with hyperglycemia [5]. In DM patients with COVID-19 disease, significantly higher incidences of in-hospital death and the need for renal replacement therapy as well as mechanical ventilation were noted [5, 6]. An early observational study among COVID-19 patients estimated that, compared to matched controls without DM, a fasting plasma glucose of ≥ 7 mmol/L (approximately equivalent to 126 mg/dL) translated into an odds ratio of 14.6 ($p < 0.01$) for an ICU admission [7]. A meta-analysis estimated that pre-existing DM increased the risk for severe COVID-19 disease by approximately two-fold and the mortality risk by three-fold [8].

Potential Mechanisms of Hyperglycemia by SARS-CoV-2

Severe acute respiratory syndrome coronavirus 2 (SARS-CoV-2) may uniquely trigger severe hyperglycemia, hyperglycemic emergencies, and possibly DM through various pathological mechanisms; these are discussed in greater detail in Chap. 2. In brief, these have been categorized into factors that cause direct pancreatic damage and those that cause peripheral insulin resistance. A number of these elements are likely at play simultaneously.

A link between the SARS-CoV-2 virus and the angiotensin-converting enzyme 2 (ACE2) receptor, present in pancreatic islet cells, has been established [9–11]. In vitro studies have shown that SARS-CoV-2 can directly infect cultured human islet cells [12, 13]. One group demonstrated increased endoplasmic reticulum stress, Golgi body swelling, and a trend toward reduced glucose-stimulated insulin secretion by the infected pancreatic cells, suggestive of a virus-driven functional impairment of pancreatic cells [13]. Other groups describe ACE2 expression in the microvasculature and ductal epithelium of the pancreas; histological analysis of tissue from SARS-CoV-2-infected patients demonstrated pancreatic fibrosis and microthrombi, suggesting potential pancreatic ischemic damage [10, 11]. Other indirect pancreatic impairment may result from the local intense inflammatory response and aberrant regulation of the renin-angiotensin-aldosterone and angiotensin (1–7) pathways leading to a decrease in glucose uptake [14, 15].

The generalized hyperinflammatory state of COVID-19 disease can mechanistically also potentiate systemic insulin resistance, as can some COVID-19 therapies. In fact, anti-inflammatory treatments including glucocorticoids and monoclonal antibodies targeting specific cytokines, such as the anti-IL6 therapies tocilizumab and sarilumab, have been incorporated into the treatment algorithms of COVID-19 infections [16]. The high-dose dexamethasone [6 mg oral or intravenous (IV)] therapy administered to quell the hyperinflammatory response can unfortunately further exacerbate the metabolic derangements of hyperglycemia, lipolysis, and peripheral insulin resistance [17].

Stress Hyperglycemia in Critically Ill Patients

In addition to the pathological mechanisms of hyperglycemia that are specific to the SARS-CoV-2 infection, multiple factors lead to stress hyperglycemia in critical illness. These include a complex web of increased counter-regulatory hormones such as glucagon, catecholamines, and cortisol that enhance hepatic gluconeogenesis and drive peripheral insulin resistance, perpetuating the intense pro-inflammatory state [18]. Furthermore, hyperglycemia weakens immune function and wound healing and amplifies oxidative stress and a prothrombotic state, all of which exacerbate the acute illness [19]. Therapeutic interventions frequently administered in critically ill patients, including glucocorticoids, vasopressors, enteral feeds, and parenteral feeds, further complicate the dysglycemia. Although there is a lack of studies specifically addressing how to uniquely manage DM and hyperglycemic emergencies in critically ill patients with COVID-19 disease, evidence-based consensus guidelines for the ICU and critically ill patients have been extended to the COVID-19 patient population.

Glycemic Targets in the ICU

Earlier landmark studies investigating the relationship between inpatient dysglycemia and clinical outcomes highlight the benefits of glycemic control among the ICU population. The consensus guidelines generally recommend a glucose target of 140–180 mg/dL in the ICU setting [20, 21]. One randomized control trial (RCT) demonstrated an astounding 32% risk reduction in mortality in critically ill surgical ICU patients with and without diabetes when glucoses were targeted to 80–110 mg/dL with intensive insulin therapy, compared to conventional targets of less than 215 mg/dL [22]. This benefit was primarily driven by reductions in septicemia and sepsis-related multi-organ failure.

Not all studies have shown clear-cut benefits to intensive glycemic control in the ICU in those with and without diabetes. When the same group applied the interventions to medical ICU patients, morbidity was likewise significantly reduced with earlier discharge from the ICU and hospital, less acute kidney injury, and accelerated weaning from mechanical ventilation. In-hospital mortality, however, was not decreased for all patients [23]. In fact, intensive insulin therapy and stricter glycemic targets were associated with significantly more hypoglycemia, an independent risk factor for mortality. In a subsequent large RCT, the Normoglycemia in Intensive

Care Evaluation and Survival Using Glucose Algorithm Regulation (NICE-SUGAR) trial, both surgical and medical ICU patients were either targeted for an intensive glucose goal of 81–108 mg/dL or a conventional glucose goal of less than 180 mg/dL [24]. Mortality was significantly increased in the intensive-treatment group with an adjusted odds ratio of 1.14 ($p = 0.04$); median survival time was also lower in the intensive group (HR, 1.11; 95% CI, 1.01 to 1.23; $P = 0.03$). The intensive therapy group did not show additional benefits in the length of stay in the ICU or other complications. Other meta-analyses have corroborated the mortality risks with tighter glycemic goals [25, 26]. Therefore, the general recommendation for most critically ill patients is a glucose target of ~140–180 mg/dL [20, 21].

Hyperglycemia Management in the Critically Ill

Continuous insulin infusions that follow a validated infusion algorithm are the standard of therapy in the ICU setting for management of hyperglycemia. This standard was derived from prior studies, particularly in the cardiac ICU, in which insulin infusion therapy, compared to subcutaneous insulin injections alone, reached glycemic targets more effectively and safely in patients with hyperglycemia with or without diabetes [20, 21]. This is likely due to the ideal pharmacokinetics of IV insulin, which both acts and is cleared rapidly to allow for immediate dose adjustments while avoiding extremes in hyperglycemia or hypoglycemia. These patients who were predominantly post-coronary artery bypass grafting or post-myocardial infarction also demonstrated significantly lower mortality rates. One observational study estimated that the odds of mortality were reduced by 57% with insulin infusion when compared to using subcutaneous insulin [27]. Another RCT of persons with diabetes showed long-term benefits in patients who were treated with insulin drips, with a 28% relative reduction in mortality observed over a follow-up period of up to 3.4 years [28]. Those who were insulin-naïve and had low cardiac risk were most likely to demonstrate a benefit.

Hyperglycemic Emergencies in COVID-19 Disease

DKA and HHS are life-threatening medical emergencies that carry considerable morbidity and mortality. In the past decade, an overall uptrend has been observed in the event rates for DKA and HHS; for instance, the annual percentage increase in non-admitted emergency department visits in the United States was 13.5% for DKA and 16.5% for HHS from 2009 to 2015 [29]. Mortality can be as high as 15–20% in patients with HHS [30] and ten-fold higher than those with DKA alone [31]. The in-hospital mortality rate has been noted to be significantly higher in combined DKA-HHS with an odds ratio of 2.7 versus isolated DKA or HHS [32]. Frequently and especially with HHS, the patients are acutely and critically ill with symptoms ranging from severe dehydration to altered mental status, requiring ICU admissions.

While it was promptly established that patients with diabetes were at increased risk for mortality from COVID-19 disease, a clear causal relationship between COVID-19 infection and DKA is less well established. Several case reports have described DKA and HHS as a presenting complication of COVID-19 disease [33, 34]. Although earlier reports hinted toward increased rates of DKA due to SARS-CoV-2, most studies have been limited by small numbers of patients, lack of pre-COVID-19 comparator groups, or variable diagnostic definitions of DKA [35, 36]. A larger American database review of COVID-19 admissions from March to November 2020 found that 37.3% of 1849 patients with type 1 diabetes (T1D) presented in DKA, as did 3.2% of 110,843 patients with type 2 diabetes (T2D) [37]. Another study from the United Kingdom of more than 8500 hospitalized patients with COVID-19 disease demonstrated a 6–7% increase in DKA admissions during the first and second pandemic surges, compared to the same months during pre-pandemic years between 2017 and 2020. Furthermore, DKA admissions during the early pandemic, among patients with a documented diagnosis of T2D, increased by 30–50% from pre-pandemic years. Likewise, DKA admissions increased up to 61% in those labeled as newly diagnosed DM compared to the preceding 3 years before the pandemic [38].

Data on mortality rates in COVID-19-related DKA is likewise limited. In-hospital DKA mortality rates in COVID-19 disease were reported to be as high as 40–50% in early case series [39, 40]. In a larger study based on a national database of 175 hospitals and 5029 inpatients diagnosed with DKA, of which 210 patients were confirmed positive for SARS-CoV-2, the mortality rate was significantly increased with COVID-19 disease [41]. Among patients younger than 45 years old with DKA, the mortality rate was up to 19% in COVID-19 disease versus 2% in patients without COVID-19 infections. Among patients older than 65 years old with DKA, the mortality rate was 45% in COVID-19 disease versus 13% without COVID-19 infections. In comparison, the Agency for Healthcare and Research Quality National Inpatient Sample report corresponding to more than 35 million annual hospitalizations from 2000 to 2014 reported an in-hospital DKA-fatality rate of 0.4% in 2014 [42].

The mortality risk specifically attributable to DKA rather than the COVID-19 disease itself and its systemic complications remains unclear. There are a number of other potential limitations of these retrospective studies investigating DKA mortality and COVID-19 disease. Many of these studies rely heavily on database documentation and clinical coding for case inclusion and outcomes data. The diagnosis of DKA itself may be challenging due to the many biochemical aberrations induced by severe systemic COVID-19 disease. Significant dehydration, hypotension, severe GI symptoms leading to poor oral intake, vomiting, and diarrhea, as well as renal dysfunction can result in mixed acid-base disorders and ketosis that can be difficult to differentiate from DKA. Moreover, it is unclear if and how hospital avoidance during the pandemic affected reported rates of DKA. Despite these limitations, the overall data indicates increased rates of DKA due to COVID-19 disease with higher mortality rates.

Data on HHS is even more limited, mostly consisting of case series [43, 44]. While there may be an increased incidence of HHS in patients with COVID-19 infection, it is difficult to draw any definitive conclusions from the current data.

Management of Hyperglycemic Emergencies in Critically Ill Patients

Standard treatment guidelines for DKA focus on the core principles of insulin infusion therapy: treatment of the absolute or relative insulin deficiency, fluid repletion, and electrolyte normalization. A typical water deficit of approximately 100 mL/kg body weight can be seen in DKA, and can be as high as 200 mL/kg in HHS. Classically, aggressive fluid hydration with initial 500–1000 mL hourly boluses followed by a continuous infusion at 250–500 mL/hr is recommended [30, 31, 45]. Isotonic fluids, including balanced crystalloids, are usually utilized [45, 46] unless otherwise dictated by electrolyte abnormalities. Hydration leads to intravascular volume repletion, adequate renal perfusion, and reduction in concentration of counter-regulatory hormones and hyperglycemia.

In critically ill patients, continuous insulin infusion therapy is the gold standard for DKA management and effectively suppresses hepatic gluconeogenesis, lipolysis, and ketogenesis. Frequent monitoring and normalization of electrolytes is another cornerstone in the management of DKA and HHS. In particular, potassium, phosphate, and potentially bicarbonate abnormalities need to be regularly monitored and adequately repleted in ICU patients who often have severe metabolic acidosis, acute renal failure, and respiratory or cardiac distress.

Management of Diabetic Ketoacidosis/Hyperosmolar Hyperglycemic State in the Setting of COVID-19 Disease

Unfortunately, the treatment of DKA and HHS in critically ill patients with COVID-19 has been a challenge, especially early in the pandemic when there was a national shortage of personal protective equipment (PPE), hospital (especially ICU) beds, and staffing. There was a profound need for standardized management protocols to adapt to the pandemic and a concern for staff exposure to the virus, insufficient clinical staffing relative to patient volume, and a limited capacity to accommodate all patients requiring ICU-level care for hourly glucose monitoring and insulin infusion adjustments. Furthermore, a prominent risk for acute respiratory distress syndrome (ARDS) and high-dose glucocorticoids [16] complicated optimal treatment. A more flexible approach with modifications to the standard treatment and monitoring protocols for DKA and HHS was required.

In response to these challenges, multiple institutions developed subcutaneous (SQ) insulin protocols for the management of mild to moderate DKA (defined as acidemia with a pH $\geq$ 7 and a serum bicarbonate $\geq$10 mEq/L in the setting of a glucose $\geq$250 mg/dL, positive urine and/or serum ketones, and a high anion gap metabolic acidosis) [47]. The goal of these protocols was to safely minimize the frequency of insulin dosing and point of care (POC) glucose checks to every 2–4 h, thereby limiting healthcare workers' exposure to SARS-CoV-2 and allowing for patient care in non-ICU settings. Additional advantages of using SQ insulin were the ability to provide an effect of continuous insulin in those patients with tenuous and inconsistent intravenous access, as well as allowing for the treatment of critically ill patients in non-ICU beds during times when there was limited ICU capacity. During the first pandemic surge at institutions in which insulin infusions were continued or for those patients who did not meet specific criteria for SQ insulin, long intravenous tubing connecting the patient to IV poles, located outside of the patient room, were utilized. This strategy permitted healthcare workers to adjust intravenous medications and infusion rates without the need to frequently re-enter patient rooms, minimizing the risk for SARS-CoV-2 transmission. Fortunately, many hospitals have phased out this practice due to increased vaccination rates, increased PPE availability, and decreased inpatient volume of COVID-19 cases.

Subcutaneous Insulin Protocols

Subcutaneous insulin protocols for the management of mild to moderate DKA have existed since the 1970s, with studies supporting their safety and efficacy [48, 49]. With the advent of rapid-acting insulin analogs in the 1990s, small trials were conducted to determine the efficacy of these new insulins, administered subcutaneously, in the management of DKA [50, 51]. A 2016 Cochrane review of five randomized trials with a total of 201 patients found SQ insulin lispro/aspart to be comparable to intravenous regular insulin infusions in time to DKA resolution and in the number of hypoglycemic events, although the evidence was determined to be suboptimal due to the limited number and heterogeneity of the studies and participants included [52]. One healthcare system retrospectively evaluated mortality and readmission rates as well as the length of hospital stay and the need for ICU care before and after implementation of a SQ insulin DKA protocol from 2010 to 2019, pre-pandemic [53]. Post-implementation of the SQ DKA protocol, they noted a 57% decrease in ICU admissions and a 50% reduction in 30-day hospital readmissions. However, no significant differences in mortality or length of stay were observed. Based on the overall evidence, the American Diabetes Association's annual Standards of Medical Care in Diabetes guidelines propose that subcutaneous insulin may be used safely in mild to moderate, uncomplicated DKA [20].

Subcutaneous insulin protocols for the management of mild to moderate DKA were developed early in the SARS-CoV-2 pandemic at Montefiore Medical Center, Mount

Sinai Hospital in New York, and the organization Diabetes UK to uniquely address the need for safe and effective DKA management during the first pandemic surge [54–56]. The specific clinical patient scenario for whom the SQ insulin protocol is indicated slightly varies among the three protocols. For instance, the Montefiore and UK Diabetes protocols recommend against the treatment with SQ insulin in DKA patients who are pregnant or with acute mental status change, acute coronary syndrome, and/or advanced renal dysfunction, among other significant comorbidities. Mount Sinai's primary exclusion criteria is pregnant patients. Like the pre-pandemic SQ protocols, all protocols recommend rapid-acting insulin to be dosed frequently to achieve a sufficient "stacking" effect. However, instead of dosing the insulin every 1–2 hours, in the newer protocols the frequency is modified to every 3–4 hours. Also unique to the new protocols is the immediate initiation of basal insulin therapy. Consequently, once the DKA resolves, the timing and dosing of the SQ rapid-acting insulin are simply adjusted without the need for a "bridging" transition, as is usually the case for patients on IV insulin infusions, as patients are already on a basal-bolus insulin regimen.

Insulin Dosing

The details of insulin dosing for each of the protocols are shown in Table 9.1. The protocols differ slightly in their recommended insulin doses, but they do share commonalities [54–56]. Each protocol recommends starting a basal insulin dose

Table 9.1 Insulin dosing for subcutaneous insulin COVID-19 DKA protocols

	Basal insulin	Rapid-acting insulin	Rapid-acting insulin frequency	Special considerations
Montefiore Medical Center	0.15–0.2 U/kg	Mild DKA: • 0.2 U/kg if FSG ≥250 mg/dL • 0.1 U/kg if FSG <250 mg/dL Moderate DKA: • 0.25 U/kg if FSG ≥250 mg/dL • 0.15 U/kg if FSG <250 mg/dL	Every 4 h	Transition to IV insulin infusion if not resolved within 24 h
Mount Sinai Hospital	0.2 U/kg	Initial: 0.2 U/kg • 0.1 U/kg if glucose drops >75 mg/dL • 0.1 U/kg if glucose <250 mg/dL	Every 3 h	Increase SQ insulin doses by 50% if on glucocorticoids. Decrease SQ insulin doses by 50% if ESRD.
Diabetes UK	0.15 U/kg or home dose	Initial: 0.4 U/kg • 0.2 U/kg if glucose <14 mmol/L[a]	Every 4 h	Increase rapid-acting insulin to 0.5 U/kg if ketones are not downtrending.

[a]14 mmol/L is ~equivalent to 252 mg/dL

of 0.15–0.2 U/kg; the Diabetes UK algorithm also allows initiating the patient's home dose of the long-acting insulin, as an alternative [56]. Likewise, the strategies regarding the specific frequency of administration and dosing of the rapid-acting insulin vary among the three protocols but all agree on the reduction of the weight-based rapid-acting insulin dose once the glucose reaches ≤250 mg/dL. More specifically, the Montefiore protocol differentiates weight-based insulin doses between mild DKA (pH >7.15, bicarbonate >12 mEq/L) and moderate DKA (pH 7.0–7.14, bicarbonate >10 mEq/L) [54]. The rapid-acting insulin dose starts at 0.2 U/kg for mild DKA while the dose starts at 0.25 U/kg for moderate DKA, dosed at 4-hour intervals. The Mount Sinai protocol's rapid-acting insulin dose starts at 0.2 U/kg and is either maintained at the same rate if the change in POC glucose is <75 mg/dL or is reduced to 0.1 U/kg if the change is >75 mg/dL, dosed at 3-hour intervals [55]. The Diabetes UK algorithm recommends initiating the rapid-acting insulin at 0.4 U/kg and to decrease the dose to 0.2 U/kg once the POC glucose falls to <14 mmol/L (equivalent to ~252 mg/dL), dosed at 4-hour intervals [56].

Fluid and Electrolyte Management

Each of the COVID DKA protocols advises judicious IV fluid hydration due to the risk for respiratory decompensation and ARDS in COVID pneumonia. The Montefiore protocol advises 200–400 mL/hr of isotonic fluids if the corrected sodium is <135 mEq/L or hypotonic saline at 200–400 mL/hr if the corrected sodium is ≥135 mEq/L [54]. The Mount Sinai protocol recommends 500–1000 mL of Plasma-Lyte for the first hour, followed by a continuous infusion at 125 mL/hr [55]. The Diabetes UK team similarly advises an initial 1 L bolus of 0.9% sodium chloride followed by a stepwise reduction in the infusion rate. For more tenuous patients, a weight- and pH-dependent volume resuscitation algorithm is additionally provided [56]. Similar to standard DKA management, all protocols endorse frequent assessment of volume status as well as the addition of a dextrose-containing fluid once glucoses drop to <250 mg/dL until DKA resolution.

Close monitoring and repletion of electrolytes, especially potassium, remains a standard part of the subcutaneous insulin DKA protocols. However, electrolyte management may be more challenging in COVID-19 disease due to concomitant severe renal dysfunction. The protocols all endorse holding insulin until serum potassium ranges within 3.3–3.5 mEq/L or higher. Providers are also advised to check plasma electrolytes frequently to reassess the sodium, potassium, magnesium, and phosphorous levels [54–56].

Safety and efficacy of these subcutaneous protocols in COVID-19 disease have not yet been studied, although efforts remain underway. The protocols provide general guidelines and need to be tailored for individual patients and modified based on clinical judgment. For example, patients receiving high-dose glucocorticoids and enteral tube feeds will be expected to have greater insulin requirements. Subcutaneous insulin will likely be suboptimally absorbed and less effective in patients with significant edema or vasoconstriction, or in patients treated with vasopressors. For critically ill patients with complicated or severe DKA, continuous insulin infusions remain the standard of care.

Glucose Monitoring

Continuous glucose monitoring (CGM) in critically ill patients, including patients with DKA, has not been well studied. A clinical advantage to the CGM is the potential ability to remotely monitor glucoses, thereby reducing exposure and transmission risk of SARS-CoV-2 from bedside POC glucose checks. A number of pilot studies have been conducted investigating CGM utilization in critically ill COVID-19-positive patients, some of whom were on continuous insulin infusions. All have shown acceptable accuracy and feasibility [57–60]. The largest study included 19 patients, of whom nine were in the ICU, eight were on hemodialysis, and seven were on vasopressors. It reported an overall MARD (mean absolute relative difference) of 13.5% on days 2–7 of sensor wear [59]. A similar study of 11 critically ill patients, of whom eight were on vasopressors and six were on renal replacement therapy, reported a MARD of 12.58% [57]. While the MARD found in these studies is higher than the standard 8–10% reported in clinical trials for the latest CGMs, it is significantly lower than what was described in the earliest FDA-approved CGM devices [61]. Furthermore, two studies demonstrated, through Clarke Error Grid analysis, that approximately 98–100% of CGM-reported values would have resulted in appropriate medical treatment [59, 60]. While larger studies are needed, these data support the potential role of continuous glucose monitoring in DKA management of critically ill patients with COVID-19 disease (see Chap. 11 for more on diabetes technology).

Conclusion

Severe acute respiratory syndrome coronavirus 2 has proven to be an unprecedented challenge in the management of critically ill patients with diabetes, necessitating a rapidly adaptive response from healthcare providers. Subcutaneous insulin protocols and inpatient continuous glucose monitor usage represent some of the pivotal efforts undertaken to manage hyperglycemic emergencies in the unique setting of the COVID-19 pandemic. More robust data is still needed to confirm their efficacy and safety to support their ongoing use in the post-pandemic world.

References

1. Bertoni AG, Saydah S, Brancati FL. Diabetes and the risk of infection-related mortality in the U.S. Diabetes Care. 2001;24(6):1044–9. https://doi.org/10.2337/diacare.24.6.1044.
2. Umpierrez GE, Isaacs SD, Bazargan N, You X, Thaler LM, Kitabchi AE. Hyperglycemia: an independent marker of in-hospital mortality in patients with undiagnosed diabetes. J Clin Endocrinol Metab. 2002;87(3):978–82. https://doi.org/10.1210/jcem.87.3.8341.
3. Roberts GW, Quinn SJ, Valentine N, Alhawassi T, O'Dea H, Stranks SN, et al. Relative hyperglycemia, a marker of critical illness: introducing the stress hyperglycemia ratio. J Clin Endocrinol Metab. 2015;100(12):4490–7. https://doi.org/10.1210/jc.2015-2660.
4. Sathish T, Kapoor N, Cao Y, Tapp RJ, Zimmet P. Proportion of newly diagnosed diabetes in COVID-19 patients: a systematic review and meta-analysis. Diabetes Obes Metab. 2021;23(3):870–4. https://doi.org/10.1111/dom.14269.
5. Vasbinder A, Anderson E, Shadid H, Berlin H, Pan M, Azam TU, et al. Inflammation, hyperglycemia, and adverse outcomes in individuals with diabetes mellitus hospitalized for COVID-19. Diabetes Care. 2022;45(3):692–700. https://doi.org/10.2337/dc21-2102.
6. Pazoki M, Keykhaei M, Kafan S, Montazeri M, Mirabdolhagh Hazaveh M, Sotoodehnia M, et al. Risk indicators associated with in-hospital mortality and severity in patients with diabetes mellitus and confirmed or clinically suspected COVID-19. J Diabetes Metab Disord. 2021;20(1):59–69. https://doi.org/10.1007/s40200-020-00701-2.
7. Alahmad B, Al-Shammari AA, Bennakhi A, Al-Mulla F, Ali H. Fasting blood glucose and COVID-19 severity: nonlinearity matters. Diabetes Care. 2020;43(12):3113–6. https://doi.org/10.2337/dc20-1941.
8. Mantovani A, Byrne CD, Zheng MH, Targher G. Diabetes as a risk factor for greater COVID-19 severity and in-hospital death: a meta-analysis of observational studies. Nutr Metab Cardiovasc Dis. 2020;30(8):1236–48. https://doi.org/10.1016/j.numecd.2020.05.014.
9. Yang JK, Lin SS, Ji XJ, Guo LM. Binding of SARS coronavirus to its receptor damages islets and causes acute diabetes. Acta Diabetol. 2010;47(3):193–9. https://doi.org/10.1007/s00592-009-0109-4.
10. Coate KC, Cha J, Shrestha S, Wang W, Goncalves LM, Almaca J, et al. SARS-CoV-2 cell entry factors ACE2 and TMPRSS2 are expressed in the microvasculature and ducts of human pancreas but are not enriched in beta cells. Cell Metab. 2020;32(6):1028–40 e4. https://doi.org/10.1016/j.cmet.2020.11.006.
11. Kusmartseva I, Wu W, Syed F, Van Der Heide V, Jorgensen M, Joseph P, et al. Expression of SARS-CoV-2 entry factors in the pancreas of Normal organ donors and individuals with COVID-19. Cell Metab. 2020;32(6):1041–51 e6. https://doi.org/10.1016/j.cmet.2020.11.005.
12. Wu CT, Lidsky PV, Xiao Y, Lee IT, Cheng R, Nakayama T, et al. SARS-CoV-2 infects human pancreatic beta cells and elicits beta cell impairment. Cell Metab. 2021;33(8):1565–76 e5. https://doi.org/10.1016/j.cmet.2021.05.013.
13. Muller JA, Gross R, Conzelmann C, Kruger J, Merle U, Steinhart J, et al. SARS-CoV-2 infects and replicates in cells of the human endocrine and exocrine pancreas. Nat Metab. 2021;3(2):149–65. https://doi.org/10.1038/s42255-021-00347-1.
14. Eskandarani RM, Sawan S. Diabetic ketoacidosis on hospitalization with COVID-19 in a previously nondiabetic patient: a review of pathophysiology. Clin Med Insights Endocrinol Diabetes. 2020;13:1179551420984125. https://doi.org/10.1177/1179551420984125.
15. Boddu SK, Aurangabadkar G, Kuchay MS. New onset diabetes, type 1 diabetes and COVID-19. Diabetes Metab Syndr. 2020;14(6):2211–7. https://doi.org/10.1016/j.dsx.2020.11.012.
16. COVID-19 Treatment Guidelines Panel Coronavirus Disease 2019 (COVID-19) Treatment Guidelines. https://www.covid19treatmentguidelines.nih.gov/ (2022). Accessed April 15 2022.
17. Kahn CRFH, O'Neill BT. Williams textbook of endocrinology. In: Pathophysiology of type 2 diabetes mellitus. 14th ed. Elsevier; 2020.

18. Dungan KM, Braithwaite SS, Preiser JC. Stress hyperglycaemia. Lancet. 2009;373(9677):1798–807. https://doi.org/10.1016/S0140-6736(09)60553-5.
19. Inzucchi SE. Clinical practice. Management of hyperglycemia in the hospital setting. N Engl J Med. 2006;355(18):1903–11. https://doi.org/10.1056/NEJMcp060094.
20. American Diabetes Association Professional Practice C, American Diabetes Association Professional Practice C, Draznin B, Aroda VR, Bakris G, Benson G, et al. 16. Diabetes Care in the Hospital: standards of medical Care in Diabetes-2022. Diabetes Care. 2022;45(Suppl 1):S244–S53. https://doi.org/10.2337/dc22-S016.
21. Moghissi ES, Korytkowski MT, DiNardo M, Einhorn D, Hellman R, Hirsch IB, et al. American Association of Clinical Endocrinologists and American Diabetes Association consensus statement on inpatient glycemic control. Diabetes Care. 2009;32(6):1119–31. https://doi.org/10.2337/dc09-9029.
22. van den Berghe G, Wouters P, Weekers F, Verwaest C, Bruyninckx F, Schetz M, et al. Intensive insulin therapy in critically ill patients. N Engl J Med. 2001;345(19):1359–67. https://doi.org/10.1056/NEJMoa011300.
23. Van den Berghe G, Wilmer A, Hermans G, Meersseman W, Wouters PJ, Milants I, et al. Intensive insulin therapy in the medical ICU. N Engl J Med. 2006;354(5):449–61. https://doi.org/10.1056/NEJMoa052521.
24. Investigators N-SS, Finfer S, Chittock DR, Su SY, Blair D, Foster D, et al. Intensive versus conventional glucose control in critically ill patients. N Engl J Med. 2009;360(13):1283–97. https://doi.org/10.1056/NEJMoa0810625.
25. Kansagara D, Fu R, Freeman M, Wolf F, Helfand M. Intensive insulin therapy in hospitalized patients: a systematic review. Ann Intern Med. 2011;154(4):268–82. https://doi.org/10.7326/0003-4819-154-4-201102150-00008.
26. Sathya B, Davis R, Taveira T, Whitlatch H, Wu W-C. Intensity of peri-operative glycemic control and postoperative outcomes in patients with diabetes: a meta-analysis. Diabetes Res Clin Pract. 2013;102(1):8–15. https://doi.org/10.1016/j.diabres.2013.05.003.
27. Furnary AP, Gao G, Grunkemeier GL, Wu Y, Zerr KJ, Bookin SO, et al. Continuous insulin infusion reduces mortality in patients with diabetes undergoing coronary artery bypass grafting. J Thorac Cardiovasc Surg. 2003;125(5):1007–21. https://doi.org/10.1067/mtc.2003.181.
28. Malmberg K. Prospective randomised study of intensive insulin treatment on long term survival after acute myocardial infarction in patients with diabetes mellitus. DIGAMI (Diabetes Mellitus, Insulin Glucose Infusion in Acute Myocardial Infarction) Study Group. BMJ. 1997;314(7093):1512–5. https://doi.org/10.1136/bmj.314.7093.1512.
29. Benoit SR, Hora I, Pasquel FJ, Gregg EW, Albright AL, Imperatore G. Trends in emergency department visits and inpatient admissions for hyperglycemic crises in adults with diabetes in the U.S., 2006-2015. Diabetes Care. 2020;43(5):1057–64. https://doi.org/10.2337/dc19-2449.
30. Scott AR. Joint British diabetes societies for inpatient C, group Jhhg. Management of hyperosmolar hyperglycaemic state in adults with diabetes. Diabet Med. 2015;32(6):714–24. https://doi.org/10.1111/dme.12757.
31. Umpierrez G, Korytkowski M. Diabetic emergencies - ketoacidosis, hyperglycaemic hyperosmolar state and hypoglycaemia. Nat Rev Endocrinol. 2016;12(4):222–32. https://doi.org/10.1038/nrendo.2016.15.
32. Pasquel FJ, Tsegka K, Wang H, Cardona S, Galindo RJ, Fayfman M, et al. Clinical outcomes in patients with isolated or combined diabetic ketoacidosis and hyperosmolar hyperglycemic state: a retrospective, Hospital-Based Cohort Study. Diabetes Care. 2020;43(2):349–57. https://doi.org/10.2337/dc19-1168.
33. Palermo NE, Sadhu AR, McDonnell ME. Diabetic ketoacidosis in COVID-19: unique concerns and considerations. J Clin Endocrinol Metab. 2020;105(8):2819. https://doi.org/10.1210/clinem/dgaa360.
34. Reddy PK, Kuchay MS, Mehta Y, Mishra SK. Diabetic ketoacidosis precipitated by COVID-19: a report of two cases and review of literature. Diabetes Metab Syndr. 2020;14(5):1459–62. https://doi.org/10.1016/j.dsx.2020.07.050.

35. Li J, Wang X, Chen J, Zuo X, Zhang H, Deng A. COVID-19 infection may cause ketosis and ketoacidosis. Diabetes Obes Metab. 2020;22(10):1935–41. https://doi.org/10.1111/dom.14057.
36. Cariou B, Hadjadj S, Wargny M, Pichelin M, Al-Salameh A, Allix I, et al. Phenotypic characteristics and prognosis of inpatients with COVID-19 and diabetes: the CORONADO study. Diabetologia. 2020;63(8):1500–15. https://doi.org/10.1007/s00125-020-05180-x.
37. Barrett CE, Park J, Kompaniyets L, Baggs J, Cheng YJ, Zhang P, et al. Intensive care unit admission, mechanical ventilation, and mortality among patients with type 1 diabetes hospitalized for COVID-19 in the U.S. Diabetes Care. 2021;44(8):1788–96. https://doi.org/10.2337/dc21-0604.
38. Misra S, Barron E, Vamos E, Thomas S, Dhatariya K, Kar P, et al. Temporal trends in emergency admissions for diabetic ketoacidosis in people with diabetes in England before and during the COVID-19 pandemic: a population-based study. Lancet Diabetes Endocrinol. 2021;9(10):671–80. https://doi.org/10.1016/S2213-8587(21)00208-4.
39. Chamorro-Pareja N, Parthasarathy S, Annam J, Hoffman J, Coyle C, Kishore P. Letter to the editor: unexpected high mortality in COVID-19 and diabetic ketoacidosis. Metabolism. 2020;110:154301. https://doi.org/10.1016/j.metabol.2020.154301.
40. Stevens JS, Bogun MM, McMahon DJ, Zucker J, Kurlansky P, Mohan S, et al. Diabetic ketoacidosis and mortality in COVID-19 infection. Diabetes Metab. 2021;47(6):101267. https://doi.org/10.1016/j.diabet.2021.101267.
41. Pasquel FJ, Messler J, Booth R, Kubacka B, Mumpower A, Umpierrez G, et al. Characteristics of and mortality associated with diabetic ketoacidosis among US patients hospitalized with or without COVID-19. JAMA Netw Open. 2021;4(3):e211091-e. https://doi.org/10.1001/jamanetworkopen.2021.1091.
42. Benoit SRZY, Geiss LS, Gregg EW, Albright A. Trends in diabetic ketoacidosis hospitalizations and in-hospital mortality — United States, 2000–2014. MMWR Morb Mortal Wkly Rep. 2018;67(12):362–5. https://doi.org/10.15585/mmwr.mm6712a3.
43. Armeni E, Aziz U, Qamar S, Nasir S, Nethaji C, Negus R, et al. Protracted ketonaemia in hyperglycaemic emergencies in COVID-19: a retrospective case series. Lancet Diabetes Endocrinol. 2020;8(8):660–3. https://doi.org/10.1016/S2213-8587(20)30221-7.
44. Shah A, Deak A, Allen S, Silfani E, Koppin C, Zisman-Ilani Y, et al. Some characteristics of hyperglycaemic crisis differ between patients with and without COVID-19 at a safety-net hospital in a cross-sectional study. Ann Med. 2021;53(1):1642–5. https://doi.org/10.1080/07853890.2021.1975042.
45. Tran TTT, Pease A, Wood AJ, Zajac JD, Martensson J, Bellomo R, et al. Review of evidence for adult diabetic ketoacidosis management protocols. Front Endocrinol (Lausanne). 2017;8:106. https://doi.org/10.3389/fendo.2017.00106.
46. Self WH, Evans CS, Jenkins CA, Brown RM, Casey JD, Collins SP, et al. Clinical effects of balanced crystalloids vs saline in adults with diabetic ketoacidosis: a subgroup analysis of cluster randomized clinical trials. JAMA Netw Open. 2020;3(11):e2024596. https://doi.org/10.1001/jamanetworkopen.2020.24596.
47. Kitabchi AE, Umpierrez GE, Miles JM, Fisher JN. Hyperglycemic crises in adult patients with diabetes. Diabetes Care. 2009;32(7):1335–43. https://doi.org/10.2337/dc09-9032.
48. Heber D, Molitch ME, Sperling MA. Low-dose continuous insulin therapy for diabetic ketoacidosis. Prospective comparison with "conventional" insulin therapy. Arch Intern Med. 1977;137(10):1377–80.
49. Fisher JN, Shahshahani MN, Kitabchi AE. Diabetic ketoacidosis: low-dose insulin therapy by various routes. N Engl J Med. 1977;297(5):238–41. https://doi.org/10.1056/NEJM197708042970502.
50. Umpierrez GE, Cuervo R, Karabell A, Latif K, Freire AX, Kitabchi AE. Treatment of diabetic ketoacidosis with subcutaneous insulin aspart. Diabetes Care. 2004;27(8):1873–8. https://doi.org/10.2337/diacare.27.8.1873.

51. Umpierrez GE, Latif K, Stoever J, Cuervo R, Park L, Freire AX, et al. Efficacy of subcutaneous insulin lispro versus continuous intravenous regular insulin for the treatment of patients with diabetic ketoacidosis. Am J Med. 2004;117(5):291–6. https://doi.org/10.1016/j.amjmed.2004.05.010.

52. Andrade-Castellanos CA, Colunga-Lozano LE, Delgado-Figueroa N, Gonzalez-Padilla DA. Subcutaneous rapid-acting insulin analogues for diabetic ketoacidosis. Cochrane Database Syst Rev. 2016;1:CD011281. https://doi.org/10.1002/14651858.CD011281.pub2.

53. Rao P, Jiang SF, Kipnis P, Patel DM, Katsnelson S, Madani S, et al. Evaluation of outcomes following hospital-wide implementation of a subcutaneous insulin protocol for diabetic ketoacidosis. JAMA Netw Open. 2022;5(4):e226417. https://doi.org/10.1001/jamanetworkopen.2022.6417.

54. Agarwal SCJ, Tomer Y Montefiore Subcutaneous Insulin DKA Protocol. https://professional.diabetes.org/sites/professional.diabetes.org/files/media/ada-montefiore_dka_protcol_version_3.0_5_22_20.pdf. Accessed April 15 2022.

55. Lam DLE, Leter A, Levy C, O'Malley G, Radparvar S, Shah N: MSHS COVID-19 DKA Protocol. https://professional.diabetes.org/sites/professional.diabetes.org/files/media/mshs_covid_dka_protocol.pdf (2022). Accessed April 15 2022.

56. Group NIDC-R: Guideline for managing DKA using subcutaneous insulin. https://www.diabetes.org.uk/resources-s3/public/2020-04/COvID_DKA_SC_v3.2.pdf (2022). Accessed April 15 2022.

57. Agarwal S, Mathew J, Davis GM, Shephardson A, Levine A, Louard R, et al. Continuous glucose monitoring in the intensive care unit during the COVID-19 pandemic. Diabetes Care. 2021;44(3):847–9. https://doi.org/10.2337/dc20-2219.

58. Sadhu AR, Serrano IA, Xu J, Nisar T, Lucier J, Pandya AR, et al. Continuous glucose monitoring in critically ill patients with COVID-19: results of an emergent pilot study. J Diabetes Sci Technol. 2020;14(6):1065–73. https://doi.org/10.1177/1932296820964264.

59. Faulds ER, Boutsicaris A, Sumner L, Jones L, McNett M, Smetana KS, et al. Use of continuous glucose monitor in critically ill COVID-19 patients requiring insulin infusion: an observational study. J Clin Endocrinol Metab. 2021;106(10):e4007–e16. https://doi.org/10.1210/clinem/dgab409.

60. Davis GM, Faulds E, Walker T, Vigliotti D, Rabinovich M, Hester J, et al. Remote continuous glucose monitoring with a computerized insulin infusion protocol for critically ill patients in a COVID-19 medical ICU: proof of concept. Diabetes Care. 2021;44(4):1055–8. https://doi.org/10.2337/dc20-2085.

61. Bailey TS, Alva S. Landscape of continuous glucose monitoring (CGM) and integrated CGM: accuracy considerations. Diabetes Technol Ther. 2021;23(S3):S5–S11. https://doi.org/10.1089/dia.2021.0236.

Chapter 10
Managing Outpatient Diabetes in Persons with COVID-19 and Diabetes

Celia Lu and Lyndonna Marrast

Introduction

Severe acute respiratory syndrome coronavirus 2 (SARS-CoV-2), the novel coronavirus, was identified in late 2019 and noted to cause a new respiratory illness, coronavirus 2019 (COVID-19). This disease was declared a pandemic in March 2020 by the World Health Organization [1]. As of November 8, 2022, over 97 million people have been infected with COVID-19 in the United States (U.S.) and over 1,072,749 have died [2]. COVID-19 resulted in a shutdown of global economies and the closure or reduced capacity of many ambulatory health-care offices. Much of the focus of health-care delivery shifted to inpatient care as many affected persons required hospitalization and intensive care unit admission [3]. A profile of populations most at risk for COVID-19 disease was outlined: older age, male gender, comorbidities like coronary artery disease, obesity, as well as both type 1 diabetes (T1D) and type 2 diabetes (T2D) [4].

T2D may be considered its own pandemic as over 37.3 million people in the U.S. carry this diagnosis [5]. Patients with T2D are at increased risk of infection,

C. Lu
St. John's University College of Pharmacy and Health Sciences, Queens, NY, USA

Department of Medicine, Division of General Internal Medicine, Northwell Health, New Hyde Park, NY, USA

Donald and Barbara Zucker School of Medicine at Hofstra/Northwell, Hempstead, NY, USA
e-mail: CLu1@northwell.edu

L. Marrast (✉)
Department of Medicine, Division of General Internal Medicine, Northwell Health, New Hyde Park, NY, USA

Donald and Barbara Zucker School of Medicine at Hofstra/Northwell, Hempstead, NY, USA
e-mail: Lmarrast@northwell.edu

A. K. Myers (ed.), *Diabetes and COVID-19*, Contemporary Endocrinology, https://doi.org/10.1007/978-3-031-28536-3_10

generally, because of hyperglycemia-induced immune dysfunction. Persons living with T2D are at risk for severe illness from COVID-19 as well as hospitalization and death [6–8]. Diabetes care in the hospital has been well described previously (see Chaps. 8 and 9) [9].

Still, there is a need for guidance in ambulatory settings on the management of T2D for those who are not infected but remain at increased risk, who are ill at home, and who are newly diagnosed with T2D and return home after hospitalization for COVID-19 infection. Patients with T2D need continuation of care, given diabetes management can be complex with cross-disciplinary interactions with diabetes educators, endocrinologists, and pharmacists as well as medications with varying mechanisms of actions that can impact a patient who is ill with COVID-19. The social, economic, and geopolitical factors that influence health need to be considered as we look to the future management of persons living with T2D in the era of the COVID-19 pandemic.

Preventing COVID-19 Among Those Not Infected

Patients with diabetes must be encouraged to maintain precautions to prevent infection. Standard precautions such as social distancing, mask wearing, and hand washing are encouraged. In addition, providers can make recommendations to work from home, if possible and feasible, for the individual patient.

Vaccinations

Vaccines for COVID-19 represent a primary prevention strategy and became available late in 2020. Since then, multiple pharmaceutical companies have distributed vaccines worldwide. Evidence show that they reduce inpatient hospitalization and death [10]. Though neutralizing antibodies are present for only a few months, they are worthwhile as a prevention strategy. For patients with diabetes with an increased risk of contracting COVID-19, vaccination is encouraged. The primary care physician can approach these conversations with curiosity and invite a shared decision-making discussion about vaccination. Many patients have doubts about the need for vaccination because of the speed at which the vaccine was made as well as questions about unknown risks and side effects from taking the vaccine. Lastly, for immunocompromised patients who may not develop an adequate immune response from vaccines, or patients who are unable to get vaccinated as a result of allergies, tixagevimab and cilgavimab (Evusheld™) has been approved for emergency use authorization (EUA) in the U.S [11]. This medication is considered pre-exposure prophylaxis and is delivered intramuscularly (For more on vaccines, see Chaps. 12 and 13).

Ambulatory Management of Patients with COVID-19

After testing positive for COVID-19, an ambulatory provider has several factors to consider for a person with diabetes; this includes their medication regimen and illness severity (i.e., mild, moderate, severe). The most common symptoms are mild symptoms and can include fever, body aches, malaise, etc. [12]. Severe symptoms include dyspnea, in the setting of low oxygen saturation, and confusion. Hyperglycemia can contribute to illness severity and thus having an urgency to improve and maintain glucose control is an essential goal for primary care physicians.

Symptomatic Management

Patients can take antipyretics and/or antitussives to relieve fever and cough [13]. Patients' comorbidities should be taken into consideration when choosing therapies for symptom management. To avoid increasing blood glucose further, patients with diabetes should review the labels of over-the-counter (OTC) products and avoid cough and cold formulations that contain sugar. Those who use continuous glucose monitor (CGM) should be mindful that acetaminophen can falsely elevate glucose readings for older models [14]. Affected models include Dexcom G4 and G5 as well as Medtronic Guardian Connect and Medtronic iPro2 [15, 16]. Dexcom G6 is also affected by acetaminophen if the patient takes more than the maximum dose of 4 grams per day [15]. Vitamin C at doses exceeding 500 mg daily can also falsely elevate glucose readings for the Freestyle Libre CGM systems [17]. Nonsteroidal anti-inflammatory drugs (NSAIDs) were previously thought to worsen COVID-19 infection due to their potential suppression of the immune response, though studies have not shown this to be the case [18]. However, patients with diabetes and chronic kidney disease are at risk of acute kidney injury when taking NSAIDs, especially if the patient is dehydrated during acute illness [19]. Drinking 4–6 oz. of sugar-free liquids such as water or Gatorade Zero ™ every half hour can help prevent dehydration [20]. In addition to maintaining hydration, patients should monitor temperature and if possible, oxygen saturation. If oxygen saturation consistently falls below 95%, the patient should be evaluated in person [13].

Medical Treatment

By 2021, medications to treat COVID-19 were available in the form of monoclonal antibodies (mAb) and antiviral agents [21]. These therapeutics received EUA for non-hospitalized patients at elevated risk for progression to severe disease, which included patients with diabetes mellitus [22]. The National Institute of Health (NIH) developed guidelines that provided recommendations on selecting appropriate treatments for non-hospitalized patients with COVID-19 [13]. In addition to symptom management, the NIH Panel recommends ritonavir-boosted nirmatrelvir, or remdesivir if ritonavir-boosted nirmatrelvir is not available. If neither of the preferred options are available or appropriate for the patient, molnupiravir or bebtelovimab can be used as alternative options.

Steroids such as dexamethasone are not recommended for patients with mild to moderate COVID-19 unless they need to be hospitalized or need supplemental oxygen. In the unusual case where the lack of resources limits the hospital's ability to admit the patient, dexamethasone 6 mg daily can be prescribed for up to 10 days. Pulse oximetry and blood glucose should be monitored closely during this period. Steroids should be discontinued upon discharge unless the patient has a prior indication for steroids [13].

Ritonavir-Boosted Nirmatrelvir

A 5-day course of ritonavir-boosted nirmatrelvir (Paxlovid™) is recommended for high-risk non-hospitalized patients at least 12 years of age and over 40 kg, who have moderate-to-severe COVID-19 infection [13]. It has been found to be safe and effective in reducing the risk of hospitalization and death in this population [23]. The safety of using nirmatrelvir in pregnant patients has not been determined since data from human studies is not yet available. In some cases, the benefits of treating COVID-19 may outweigh the risks of the medication [24]. Ritonavir-boosted nirmatrelvir should be started immediately after diagnosis if symptoms have occurred within 5 days since onset [24]. It is contraindicated in patients with eGFR <30 mL/min/1.73 m^2 and those with severe liver disease. Dose adjustments are required for patients with eGFR ≥30 to 59 mL/min/1.73 m^2. Since ritonavir-boosted nirmatrelvir is a CYP3A4 inhibitor and substrate, providers should review the patient's medications and herbal supplements for drug interactions including statins, which are commonly used in patients with diabetes. Depending on the statin, the patient may need to temporarily hold the statin before, during, and after treatment. In addition to using the Food & Drug Administration (FDA) Fact Sheet for Health Care Providers: EUA for Paxlovid™, providers can also check for drug interactions using the Liverpool COVID-19 Drug Interaction Website [24, 25]. Some patients may experience Paxlovid rebound, which is the phenomenon of developing COVID-19 symptoms for a second time after treatment or having a positive test within two to 8 days of therapy [26]. Despite this possibility, the medication is still recommended, and retreatment is not recommended (at the time of this writing), though maintaining isolation is.

Remdesivir

If ritonavir-boosted nirmatrelvir is not available, remdesivir (Veklury™) is recommended as a second preferred option [13]. Remdesivir, an intravenous antiviral agent, has also been found to be safe and effective in reducing the risk of hospitalization or death in outpatients [27]. Remdesivir is noted to increase blood glucose in a small percentage of patients [28]. The three-day course should be administered within 7 days of symptom onset in a setting where the patient can be monitored for anaphylaxis after the infusion.

Alternative Options

If neither ritonavir-boosted nirmatrelvir nor remdesivir are available, bebtelovimab and molnupiravir (Lagevrio™) are recommended as alternative options [13]. Monoclonal antibodies (mAbs) such as bebtelovimab work by binding to the spike protein and preventing entry into the cells of the host. Over time as variants developed, some mAbs were found to be less effective and were removed from the market in the U.S. by the FDA [29]. Bebtelovimab may have activity against the Omicron variant and the BA.1, BA.1.1, and BA.2 subvariants based on in vitro studies [30]. However, more data is needed to determine its safety and efficacy in reducing the risk of hospitalizations or death. Molnupiravir is an oral antiviral medication that works by inhibiting the replication of the SARS-COV-2 virus [31]. Compared to ritonavir-boosted nirmatrelvir or remdesivir, molnupiravir has lower efficacy rates in lowering the risk of hospitalization and death [23, 27, 32]. Since molnupiravir was found to have teratogenic effects in animal studies, it should not be used in pregnant women and contraception should be advised [33].

Non-approved Therapies

During the pandemic, medications used to treat other health conditions were evaluated for potential repurposing as COVID-19 treatment. Hydroxychloroquine, indicated for autoimmune disorders such as systemic lupus erythematosus and rheumatoid arthritis, was initially thought to have potential benefits against COVID-19 based on preliminary but low-quality studies. As data from more robust clinical trials became available, the evidence did not show hydroxychloroquine to be effective for treating or preventing COVID-19 [34]. Furthermore, patients taking hydroxychloroquine were at higher risk for adverse cardiac events such QTc prolongation especially when taken with azithromycin [35]. For these reasons, the FDA revoked the EUA for using hydroxychloroquine in hospitalized patients outside of clinical trials in June 2020 [36]. Ivermectin, a medication used to treat parasitic infections, also sparked interest for its potential in treating COVID-19. Like hydroxychloroquine, ivermectin has not been shown to be safe and effective for preventing or treating COVID-19 [37–40]. High doses of ivermectin, which were indicated for veterinary use, were found to cause dangerous neurologic effects and death [41]. Due to the lack of efficacy and risk of harm, the NIH Panel recommends against the use of hydroxychloroquine or ivermectin for treating or preventing COVID-19 [13, 42].

Managing Diabetes During COVID-19 Infection

Adjustment of medications in the outpatient setting depends on the patient's symptoms, the severity of COVID-19 infection, and dietary changes [43]. Patients should be advised to follow sick-day management guidelines with the goal of preventing hypoglycemia, hyperglycemia, and diabetic ketoacidosis (DKA). Those on insulin, especially those with T1D, are at risk of developing severe hyperglycemia as either DKA or hyperosmolar hyperglycemic syndrome (HHS). Sick-day management strategies include continuing or temporarily stopping medications as clinically appropriate, glucose monitoring, maintaining hydration and nutrition, and checking one's temperature [20, 44].

Sick-day management begins when one is well; patients should keep at least a one-month supply of medications as well as glucose and ketone testing supplies [45]. During sick days, patients should monitor their glucose more frequently, every 2–4 h, as the insulin needs may change. If glucose values are above 250 mg/dL, the patient should check urine or blood ketones [45]. If the patient has moderate or large ketones, they may need to take additional doses of rapid-acting insulin and seek emergency medical care if ketone levels do not improve. Figure 10.1 illustrates the above sick-day management recommendations. Due to potential insulin resistance during COVID-19 infection (see Chap. 2), insulin requirements may increase [46].

For patients who take other anti-glycemic medications, they may continue their medications as usual if they have no or mild COVID-19 symptoms, which may include fever, body aches, and malaise [12, 44]. However, adjustments for certain medications may be needed if patients have more severe symptoms, which can include dyspnea and confusion [12, 43]. Table 10.1 summarizes recommendations for diabetes medications during COVID-19 infection. After the infection has been resolved, it is important for the patient to maintain glycemic control to prevent further complications. This includes keeping fasting blood glucose between 80 and 130 mg/dL and 2-h post-prandial blood glucose less than 180 mg/dL [47]. Patients using a CGM should aim for a time-in-range of more than 70% or more than 50% for older adults [48].

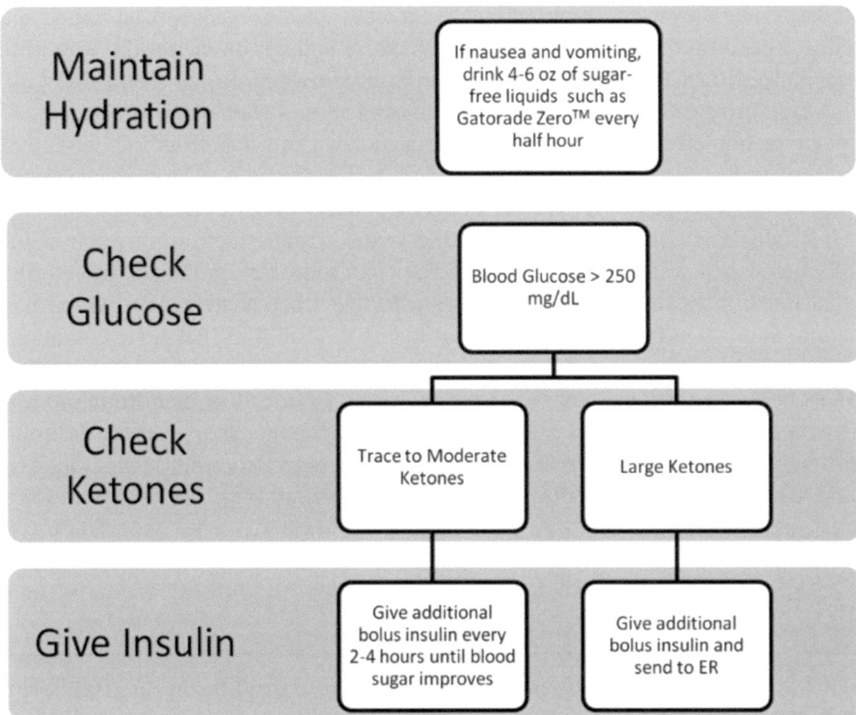

Fig. 10.1 Sick-day management recommendations [46]

Table 10.1 Anti-glycemic medication adjustments during COVID-19 infection

	Medication classes
Continue to take during COVID-19 infection	• DPP-4 inhibitors • Insulin
Monitor renal function and consider stopping if the patient has respiratory distress, dehydration, or acute kidney injury	• Metformin • SGLT-2 inhibitors • Sulfonylureas
Consider stopping in patients who have severe gastrointestinal symptoms	• Metformin • GLP-1 receptor agonists
Consider stopping if patient has poor oral intake	• Sulfonylureas (if hypoglycemic) • Metformin (need to be taken with food)

Metformin

Metformin is generally considered first-line therapy for patients with T2D due to its efficacy in HbA1c lowering, safety profile, affordability, and possible reduction in cardiovascular mortality [49]. In addition to lowering glucose by improving insulin sensitivity, metformin may also exert anti-inflammatory, antithrombotic, and antiviral effects that may help patients with COVID-19 infection [50]. Retrospective studies have shown favorable clinical outcomes such as reduced mortality and reduced need for intensive care unit admission for patients on metformin who were hospitalized for COVID-19 compared to those who were not on metformin [50]. However, prospective studies are needed to confirm these beneficial effects.

A rare side effect of metformin, lactic acidosis, can occur from the buildup of metformin during impaired renal elimination. In patients with existing renal impairment, it is usually advised to reduce metformin dose to 500 mg twice daily when the eGFR falls below 45 mL/min/1.73m^2 and to discontinue metformin when eGFR falls below 30 mL/min/1.73m^2 [51]. Expert consensus recommends monitoring renal function closely during COVID-19 infection since acute kidney injury may require the patient to temporarily discontinue metformin [43]. Hypoxic conditions such as acute respiratory failure can also predispose a patient to develop lactic acidosis. In hospitalized patients with severe COVID-19 infection, metformin use was associated with an increased risk of lactic acidosis [52]. In cases of severe gastrointestinal symptoms or severe COVID-19 infection especially with respiratory distress, discontinuation of metformin should be considered [43].

SGLT-2 Inhibitors

SGLT-2 inhibitors (SGLT2i) include canagliflozin, dapagliflozin, empagliflozin, and ertuglifozin. SGLT2i with proven cardioprotective benefits are generally recommended for patients with T2D who have comorbid atherosclerotic cardiovascular disease (ASCVD), heart failure (HF), and/or chronic kidney disease (CKD) [49]. These medications have also been shown to reduce HbA1c, weight, and blood pressure in patients when used in addition to insulin in patients with T1D. However, these are not FDA-approved for diabetes use in those with T1D [53, 54]. Cases of euglycemic diabetic ketoacidosis (euDKA) and DKA have been reported in patients with both T1D and T2D who are on SGLT2i. Since acute infection can predispose patients on SGLT2i to euDKA, SGLT2i may need to be stopped if the patient has severe COVID-19 infection [43]. These have not been found to improve outcomes in those who are hospitalized (see Chap. 8).

GLP-1 Receptor Agonists

GLP-1 receptor agonists (GLP-1 RAs) include liraglutide, exenatide, dulaglutide, semaglutide, and lixisenatide. Like SGT2i, GLP-1 RAs with proven cardiovascular benefits are generally recommended for patients with T2D who have comorbid obesity, ASCVD, and/or CKD [49]. These medications are also beneficial for weight loss [49]. They also have anti-inflammatory and insulin-sensitizing properties which may be beneficial during COVID-19 illness [46]. Since GLP-1 RAs work by slowing gastric emptying, adverse effects include nausea and vomiting. Discontinuation of GLP-1 RA may be considered in patients with severe COVID-19 infection and gastrointestinal symptoms to reduce the risk of further dehydration [46].

DPP-4 Inhibitors

DPP-4 inhibitors include sitagliptin, saxaglitpin, linagliptin, and alogliptin. They have not been shown to negatively or positively affect outcomes in patients with diabetes and COVID-19 infection [55]. Since these are well tolerated, DDP-4 inhibitors can be considered for continuation during COVID-19 infection [43, 46].

Sulfonylureas

Sulfonylureas, such as glipizide, glimepiride, and glyburide, work by stimulating insulin secretion from the pancreas, which can put the patient at risk of hypoglycemia if the patient is not eating [56]. Discontinuation of sulfonylureas may be considered if the patient is experiencing hypoglycemia from poor nutritional intake or if the patient has acute kidney injury [46].

Thiazolidinediones

As an agonist for peroxisome proliferator-activated receptor gamma, thiazolidinediones help improve insulin sensitivity in patients with diabetes. Based on animal studies, pioglitazone may reduce lung injury by attenuating inflammation [57, 58]. Therefore, it is theorized that pioglitazone may have a beneficial effect during COVID-19 infection and so it may be safe to continue the medication in patients who do not have contraindications such as HF [59, 60].

Angiotensin-Converting Enzyme Inhibitors

Angiotensin-converting enzyme inhibitors (ACEi) were previously thought to increase the risk of severe COVID-19 infection. In response to the medication, more angiotensin-converting enzyme 2 (ACE2) receptors are expressed in patients taking ACE inhibitors. These receptors can be found in the heart, kidney, gastrointestinal system, and the lungs. Since the SARS-COV-2 virus attaches to the ACE2 receptor for viral host entry, it was theorized that this could lead to enhanced viral activity in the lungs [61]. However, it was determined that this risk was unfounded. In March 2022, the American Heart Association, the Heart Failure Society of America, and the American College of Cardiology advised that patients infected with COVID-19 should continue their antihypertensive medications including ACEi and angiotensin receptor blockers (ARB) [62].

While we may emphasize medications in diabetes management, this is but one part of the comprehensive care of patients with this condition. Lifestyle factors such as physical activity and nutrition also play an important role. Lifestyles changed dramatically as some patients worked from home and others were no longer able to work i.e., job loss, and these factors contribute to well-being medically. Thinking holistically, health-care providers must also consider how patients are impacted socially by the events of the COVID-19 pandemic.

The Impact of Social Determinants of Health Among Persons with Type 2 Diabetes in the Era of COVID-19

The social determinants of health are the conditions in which people are born, live, work, and grow that play a larger role in contributing to health [63]. These factors can include education, employment, access to insurance, transportation, financial security, and food insecurity. Health-care providers need to recognize that health care represents only 20% of the factors that contribute to one's health. The COVID-19 pandemic has resulted in increased job loss, and financial and food insecurity that can affect patients with diabetes and their ability to optimally manage their disease.

Financial and Food Insecurity

Patients who are unemployed or underemployed must make decisions about purchasing food and necessities versus medications. This can result in hyperglycemia due to the high glycemic index of the foods they select. In addition, they are at risk of hypoglycemia, should they limit food intake while taking medications like sulfonylureas or insulin where hypoglycemia is a side effect.

Food insecurity is defined as having limited access to food because of high costs. Food insecurity is associated with higher HbA1c [64, 65]. Patients with food insecurity and T2D have a high risk of hypoglycemia and its complications [66]. Though not officially recommended for adults, screening for food insecurity has been recommended for children [67]. Still, outpatient providers can consider incorporating questions about food and financial security for patients with diabetes and consider food insecurity in their "differential" for patients with poor glucose control.

Medication and Glucose Testing Supply Access

Patients may also face challenges with affording their medications and glucose testing supplies due to loss of insurance from their employer or high deductibles. To save money for other necessary expenses, patients may be forced to forgo or ration their medications. Insulin rationing can lead to dangerous consequences such as DKA and death [68]. In the U.S., health-care providers can help connect patients to resources to lower the cost of their medications and glucose testing supplies. Table 10.2 provides additional information on these resources. In addition to costs, lack of transportation or mobility may pose another barrier for patients in obtaining their medications. To overcome this barrier, patients can request that the pharmacy deliver their medications if the service is available or switch to mail-order pharmacies.

Table 10.2 Cost-saving resources for medications and glucose testing supplies

	Resource	Additional information
	NeedyMeds	• Provides information on brand and generic medication cost-savings programs such as patient assistance programs and manufacturer coupons • Drug discount card
Brand medications	Patient assistance programs: • NovoCare® • Sanofi Patient Connection® • Lilly Cares Foundation	Eligibility: • No insurance • May be eligible for Medicare part D patients with out-of-pocket costs • Additional requirements vary by program
	Manufacturer savings card	Eligibility: • Commercial insurance
Generic medications	Discount cards • GoodRx • SingleCare • ScriptSave WellRx	• Eligible for all insurance types or no insurance • Can use in lieu of insurance, cannot use both at the same time
	Pharmacy savings programs • Walmart $4 Prescriptions • Walgreens Prescription Savings Club	• Eligible for all insurance types or no insurance • Can use in lieu of insurance, cannot use both at the same time • Additional membership fee for Walgreens prescription savings Club
	Online pharmacy programs • Mark Cuban Cost Plus Drug Company • Amazon Prime Rx Savings • Blink Health	• Eligible for all insurance types or no insurance • Can use in lieu of insurance, cannot use both at the same time • Additional membership fee for Amazon prime Rx savings

(continued)

Table 10.2 (continued)

	Resource	Additional information
Medications under Medicare part D	Patient assistance programs	• See above
	Extra Help with Medicare	• Eligibility based on income and resource limits • Helps pay costs associated with Medicare prescription drug plan: Premiums, deductibles, and copayments
Insulin pump	Omnipod Financial Assistance Program	Eligibility: • Omnipod system user • No insurance • Omnipod system not covered under insurance • Inability to afford out-of-pocket insurance expenses • Order directly from Insulet corporation
	Medtronic Assurance	• Receive up to three months of glucose sensors, infusion sets, and reservoirs for no cost if lost job and health insurance • Defer payments for up to 3 months if you or a family member is laid off or furloughed from their job • Additional financial assistance may be available
CGM	Eversense CGM Patient Assistance Program	Eligibility: • Insurance coverage for Eversense E3 Cost with assistance • $99 for initial sensor and transmitter • No more than $600 for each sensor/transmitter
	Dexcom Patient Assistance Program	Eligibility: • Current users who lost insurance during the pandemic Cost with assistance: • $45 for two 90-day supply shipments: Each contains one transmitter, nine sensors.
	Medtronic CGM Access Discount	Eligibility: • Not have insurance coverage for Medtronic CGM Cost with assistance: • Transmitter: $180 • Five-pack sensors: $60
	Medtronic Assurance	See above
Glucometers	Low-cost glucometer systems	• Examples: Walmart Relion confirm micro, CVS advanced • Accuracy may differ among systems based on the results from the Diabetes Technology Society Blood Glucose Monitor System Surveillance Program [69]

Access to Care

In addition to access to medications and testing supplies, patients' access to medical care was also at risk during the pandemic. Patients' concerns with exposure to COVID-19 at outpatient practices threatened to disrupt the continuity of care essential for chronic disease management. A solution to this is telehealth, defined by the Health Resources and Services Administration as "the use of electronic information and telecommunications technologies to support and promote long-distance clinical health care, patient, and professional health-related education, and public health and health administration" [70]. These technologies include audio and video platforms, mobile applications, and remote monitoring devices [71].

Although the technology has been available for some time prior to the pandemic, its use in health care was limited to rural areas under Medicare due to provider shortages. When legislative changes granted the expansion of telehealth services, the use of telehealth accelerated during the pandemic. Telehealth enables healthcare providers to conduct virtual visits as well as enable health information exchange between the providers and patients. This can help overcome health-care disparities, especially for patients living in rural areas or those with transportation-related barriers. However, disparities still exist for patients who do not have internet access or for patients who are not familiar with using the technology, such as older adults [72]. Overall, telehealth has become a tool that can help close some gaps in care not just during the pandemic but going forward.

Virtual visits via audio and video platforms allow health-care providers to perform services that usually take place during in-person visits. These services include medication reconciliation, assessing adherence to medications and lifestyle modifications, and interpreting glucose readings for medication adjustments. Providers can also provide device education for injectable medications, such as GLP-1 agonists or insulin, or glucose monitoring devices such as blood glucose monitors or CGM. Despite the advances in technology, there are still limitations in the type of care that can be provided via telehealth. For example, providers are not able to perform certain physical assessments that require palpation or in-person screenings such as foot exams (see Chap. 11 for further details on diabetes telehealth).

Unanswered Questions

Many questions remain unanswered regarding people with diabetes and COVID-19. For example: (1) Are anti-glycemic drugs able to reduce or exacerbate COVID-19 transmission? (2) How does treatment with a monoclonal antibody or anti-viral agents impact persons with T2D? (3) What are the outcomes for patients with Long COVID-19 illness who have diabetes? (4) Is the progression of diabetes different for patients who developed the disease in the context of a COVID-19 infection? (5) Will rates of diabetes increase given the increase in sedentary lifestyle/weight gain/ obesity that can result from lifestyle changes during the pandemic?

Conclusions

Ambulatory care providers are well versed in managing diabetes mellitus as guidelines have been in place for years. But, with the COVID-19 pandemic, additional guidelines are needed to manage patients with diabetes affected by COVID-19. As the virus becomes endemic in the population, we must keep abreast of the need for medication adjustments as new therapies are produced. Ambulatory providers must also adapt to the increased use of technologies such as CGM and telehealth platforms that can be used to manage patients while they are home. Inquiring on social factors that impact health will remain important. These strategies contribute to the new normal that has developed in health-care systems in response to the SARS-CoV-2 virus.

References

1. WHO Director-General's opening remarks at the media briefing on COVID-19 - 11 March 2020 [Internet]. [cited 2022 May 12]. Available from: https://www.who.int/director-general/speeches/detail/who-director-general-s-opening-remarks-at-the-media-briefing-on-covid-19. 11 Mar 2020
2. Johns Hopkins Coronavirus Resource Center [Internet]. [cited 2022 Nov 7]. Available from: https://coronavirus.jhu.edu/
3. Richardson S, Hirsch JS, Narasimhan M, Crawford JM, McGinn T, Davidson KW, et al. Presenting Characteristics, Comorbidities, and Outcomes Among 5700 Patients Hospitalized With COVID-19 in the New York City Area. JAMA [Internet]. 2020 May 26 [cited 2022 Apr 23];323(20):2052–9. Available from: https://pubmed.ncbi.nlm.nih.gov/32320003/
4. Huang C, Wang Y, Li X, Ren L, Zhao J, Hu Y, et al. Clinical features of patients infected with 2019 novel coronavirus in Wuhan, China. Lancet [Internet]. 2020 Feb 15 [cited 2022 May 10];395(10223):497–506. Available from: https://pubmed.ncbi.nlm.nih.gov/31986264/
5. National Diabetes Statistics Report | Diabetes | CDC [Internet]. [cited 2022 May 12]. Available from: https://www.cdc.gov/diabetes/data/statistics-report/index.html
6. Shabto JM, Loerinc L, O'Keefe GA, O'Keefe J. Characteristics and outcomes of COVID-19 positive patients with diabetes managed as outpatients. Diabetes Res Clin Pract [Internet]. 2020 Jun 1 [cited 2022 May 12];164:108229. Available from: https://www.ncbi.nlm.nih.gov/pmc/articles/PMC7242203/
7. Myers AK, Kim TS, Zhu X, Liu Y, Qiu M, Pekmezaris R. Predictors of mortality in a multiracial urban cohort of persons with type 2 diabetes and novel coronavirus 19. J Diabetes. 2021;13(5):430–8.
8. Scheen AJ, Marre M, Thivolet C. Prognostic factors in patients with diabetes hospitalized for COVID-19: findings from the CORONADO study and other recent reports. Diabetes Metab [Internet] 2020 Sep 1 [cited 2022 May 12];46(4):265. Available from: https://www.ncbi.nlm.nih.gov/pmc/articles/PMC7241378/

9. Korytkowski M, Antinori-Lent K, Drincic A, Hirsch IB, McDonnell ME, Rushakoff R, et al. A pragmatic approach to inpatient diabetes management during the COVID-19 pandemic. J Clin Endocrinol Metab [Internet] 2020 [cited 2022 May 12];105(9):3076–87. Available from: https://www.ncbi.nlm.nih.gov/pmc/articles/PMC7313952/

10. Lin DY, Gu Y, Wheeler B, Young H, Holloway S, Sunny SK, et al. Effectiveness of Covid-19 vaccines over a 9-month period in North Carolina. New England J Med [Internet] 2022 Mar 10 [cited 2022 May 12];386(10):933–41. Available from: https://www.nejm.org/doi/full/10.1056/NEJMoa2117128

11. Fact Sheet for Healthcare Providers: Emergency Use Authorization for Evulsheld™ (tixagevimab co-packaged with cilgavimab). [cited 2022 May 12]; Available from: https://www.cdc.gov/vaccines/covid-19/clinical-considerations/covid-19-vaccines-

12. Coronavirus [Internet]. [cited 2022 Sep 15]. Available from: https://www.who.int/health-topics/coronavirus#tab=tab_3

13. Nonhospitalized Adults: Therapeutic Management | COVID-19 Treatment Guidelines [Internet]. [cited 2022 Nov 7]. Available from: https://www.covid19treatmentguidelines.nih.gov/management/clinical-management/nonhospitalized-adults%2D%2Dtherapeutic-management/

14. Maahs DM, Desalvo D, Pyle L, Ly T, Messer L, Clinton P, et al. Effect of Acetaminophen on CGM Glucose in an Outpatient Setting. Diabetes Care [Internet]. 2015 Oct 1 [cited 2022 May 12];38(10):e158. Available from: https://www.ncbi.nlm.nih.gov/pmc/articles/PMC4876736/

15. Interfering Substances and Risks | Dexcom [Internet]. [cited 2022 Jun 28]. Available from: https://www.dexcom.com/interference

16. Diabetes - Indications, Safety, and Warnings | Medtronic [Internet]. [cited 2022 Jun 28]. Available from: https://www.medtronic.com/us-en/healthcare-professionals/products/diabetes/indications-safety-warnings.html

17. Safety Information | The FreeStyle Libre System [Internet]. [cited 2022 Jun 28]. Available from: https://www.freestyle.abbott/us-en/safety-information.html

18. Moore N, Bosco-Levy P, Thurin N, Blin P, Droz-Perroteau C. NSAIDs and COVID-19: A Systematic Review and Meta-analysis. Drug Saf [Internet]. 2021 Sep 1 [cited 2022 May 12];44(9):929. Available from: https://www.ncbi.nlm.nih.gov/pmc/articles/PMC8327046/

19. Lim CC, Kadir HBA, Tan NC, Ang ATW, Bee YM, Lee PH, et al. Non-steroidal anti-inflammatory drugs and risk of acute adverse renal outcomes in diabetes and diabetic kidney disease. Int J Risk Safety in Med. 2022;33(1):27–36.

20. Managing Sick Days | Diabetes | CDC [Internet]. [cited 2022 Sep 18]. Available from: https://www.cdc.gov/diabetes/managing/flu-sick-days.html

21. Coronavirus (COVID-19) Update: FDA Authorizes Monoclonal Antibodies for Treatment of COVID-19 | FDA [Internet]. [cited 2022 May 12]. Available from: https://www.fda.gov/news-events/press-announcements/coronavirus-covid-19-update-fda-authorizes-monoclonal-antibodies-treatment-covid-19-0

22. Underlying Medical Conditions Associated with Higher Risk for Severe COVID-19: Information for Healthcare Professionals | CDC [Internet]. [cited 2022 May 12]. Available from: https://www.cdc.gov/coronavirus/2019-ncov/hcp/clinical-care/underlyingconditions.html

23. Hammond J, Leister-Tebbe H, Gardner A, Abreu P, Bao W, Wisemandle W, et al. Oral nirmatrelvir for high-risk, nonhospitalized adults with covid-19. N Engl J Med [Internet]. 2022 Apr 14 [cited 2022 May 12];386(15):1397–408. Available from: https://www.ncbi.nlm.nih.gov/pmc/articles/PMC8908851/

24. Fact Sheet for Healthcare Providers: Emergency Use Authorization for Paxlovid Highlights of Emergency Use Authorization (EUA). 2022 [cited 2022 May 12]; Available from: https://www.cdc.gov/coronavirus/2019-ncov/need-

25. Liverpool COVID-19 Interactions [Internet]. [cited 2022 May 12]. Available from: https://www.covid19-druginteractions.org/

26. CDC Health Alert Network. COVID-19 Rebound After Paxlovid Treatment. [cited 2022 Sep 18d]; Available from: https://doi.org/10.21203/rs.3.rs-1588371/v1.

27. Gottlieb RL, Vaca CE, Paredes R, Mera J, Webb BJ, Perez G, et al. Early remdesivir to prevent progression to severe covid-19 in outpatients. N Engl J Med [Internet]. 2022 Jan 27 [cited 2022 May 12];386(4):305–15. Available from: https://www.ncbi.nlm.nih.gov/pmc/articles/PMC8757570/

28. Beigel JH, Tomashek KM, Dodd LE, Mehta AK, Zingman BS, Kalil AC, et al. Remdesivir for the treatment of Covid-19 — final report. New England JMed [Internet]. 2020 Nov 5 [cited 2022 Jun 28];383(19):1813–26. Available from: https://www.nejm.org/doi/full/10.1056/nejmoa2007764

29. Coronavirus (COVID-19) Update: FDA limits use of certain monoclonal antibodies to treat COVID-19 due to the omicron variant | FDA [Internet]. [cited 2022 May 12]. Available from: https://www.fda.gov/news-events/press-announcements/coronavirus-covid-19-update-fda-limits-use-certain-monoclonal-antibodies-treat-covid-19-due-omicron

30. Westendorf K, Wang L, Žentelis S, Foster D, Vaillancourt P, Wiggin M, et al. LY-CoV1404 (bebtelovimab) potently neutralizes SARS-CoV-2 variants. bioRxiv [Internet]. 2022 Jan 7 [cited 2022 May 12]; Available from: https://pubmed.ncbi.nlm.nih.gov/33972947/

31. Kabinger F, Stiller C, Schmitzová J, Dienemann C, Kokic G, Hillen HS, et al. Mechanism of molnupiravir-induced SARS-CoV-2 mutagenesis. Nat Struct Mol Biol [Internet]. 2021 Sep 1 [cited 2022 May 12];28(9):740. Available from: https://www.ncbi.nlm.nih.gov/pmc/articles/PMC8437801/

32. Bernal AJ, Silva MMG da, Musungaie DB, Kovalchuk E, Gonzalez A, Reyes VD, et al. Molnupiravir for oral treatment of Covid-19 in nonhospitalized patients. N Engl J Med [Internet]. 2022 Feb 10 [cited 2022 May 12];386(6):509–20. Available from: https://www.ncbi.nlm.nih.gov/pmc/articles/PMC8693688/

33. Fact Sheet for Healthcare Providers: Emergency Use Authorization for Lagevrio™ (molnupiravir) Capsules. 2022.

34. Singh B, Ryan H, Kredo T, Chaplin M, Fletcher T. Chloroquine or hydroxychloroquine for prevention and treatment of COVID-19. Cochrane Database of Systematic Reviews [Internet]. 2021 Feb 12 [cited 2022 Sep 15];2021(2). Available from: https://www.cochranelibrary.com/cdsr/doi/10.1002/14651858.CD013587.pub2/full

35. FDA cautions against use of hydroxychloroquine or chloroquine for COVID-19 outside of the hospital setting or a clinical trial due to risk of heart rhythm problems | FDA [Internet]. [cited 2022 Sep 15]. Available from: https://www.fda.gov/drugs/drug-safety-and-availability/fda-cautions-against-use-hydroxychloroquine-or-chloroquine-covid-19-outside-hospital-setting-or

36. Coronavirus (COVID-19) Update: FDA revokes emergency use authorization for chloroquine and hydroxychloroquine | FDA [Internet]. [cited 2022 Sep 15]. Available from: https://www.fda.gov/news-events/press-announcements/coronavirus-covid-19-update-fda-revokes-emergency-use-authorization-chloroquine-and

37. Reis G, Silva EASM, Silva DCM, Thabane L, Milagres AC, Ferreira TS, et al. Effect of early treatment with ivermectin among patients with Covid-19. N Engl J Med [Internet]. 2022 May 5 [cited 2022 Sep 15];386(18):1721–31. Available from: https://www.ncbi.nlm.nih.gov/pmc/articles/PMC9006771/

38. Lim SCL, Hor CP, Tay KH, Jelani AM, Tan WH, Ker HB, et al. Efficacy of ivermectin treatment on disease progression among adults with mild to moderate COVID-19 and comorbidities: The I-TECH Randomized Clinical Trial. JAMA Intern Med [Internet]. 2022 Apr 1 [cited 2022 Sep 15];182(4):426–35. Available from: https://jamanetwork.com/journals/jamainternal-medicine/fullarticle/2789362

39. López-Medina E, López P, Hurtado IC, Dávalos DM, Ramirez O, Martínez E, et al. Effect of ivermectin on time to resolution of symptoms among adults with mild COVID-19: a randomized clinical trial. JAMA [Internet]. 2021 Apr 4 [cited 2022 Sep 15];325(14):1426. Available from: https://www.ncbi.nlm.nih.gov/pmc/articles/PMC7934083/

40. Vallejos J, Zoni R, Bangher M, Villamandos S, Bobadilla A, Plano F, et al. Ivermectin to prevent hospitalizations in patients with COVID-19 (IVERCOR-COVID19) a randomized, double-blind, placebo-controlled trial. BMC Infect Dis [Internet] 2021 Dec 1 [cited 2022 Sep 15];21(1). Available from: https://pubmed.ncbi.nlm.nih.gov/34215210/
41. HAN Archive - 00449 | Health Alert Network (HAN) [Internet]. [cited 2022 Sep 15]. Available from: https://emergency.cdc.gov/han/2021/han00449.asp?ACSTrackingID=USCDC_1052-DM74752&ACSTrackingLabel=Ivermectin%20Products%20are%20Not%20Approved%20by%20FDA%20to%20Prevent%20or%20Treat%20COVID-19&deliveryName=USCDC_1052-DM74752
42. Ivermectin | COVID-19 Treatment Guidelines [Internet]. [cited 2022 Jun 28]. Available from: https://www.covid19treatmentguidelines.nih.gov/therapies/antiviral-therapy/ivermectin/
43. Bornstein SR, Rubino F, Khunti K, Mingrone G, Hopkins D, Birkenfeld AL, et al. Practical recommendations for the management of diabetes in patients with COVID-19. Lancet Diabetes Endocrinol [Internet]. 2020 Jun 1 [cited 2022 Apr 27];8(6):546–50. Available from: http://www.thelancet.com/article/S2213858720301522/fulltext
44. Pettus J, Skolnik N. Importance of diabetes management during the COVID-19 pandemic. Postgrad Med [Internet]. 2021 [cited 2022 Apr 28];133(8):912–9. Available from: https://pubmed.ncbi.nlm.nih.gov/34602003/
45. Diabetic Ketoacidosis | Diabetes | CDC [Internet]. [cited 2022 May 12]. Available from: https://www.cdc.gov/diabetes/basics/diabetic-ketoacidosis.html
46. Koliaki C, Tentolouris A, Eleftheriadou I, Melidonis A, Dimitriadis G, Tentolouris N. Clinical Management of Diabetes Mellitus in the Era of COVID-19: Practical Issues, Peculiarities and Concerns. J Clin Med [Internet]. 2020 Jul 1 [cited 2022 Apr 28];9(7):1–25. Available from: https://www.ncbi.nlm.nih.gov/pmc/articles/PMC7408673/
47. Committee ADAPP. 6. Glycemic Targets: Standards of Medical Care in Diabetes—2022. Diabetes Care [Internet]. 2022 Jan 1 [cited 2022 Jun 28];45(Supplement_1):S83–96. Available from: https://diabetesjournals.org/care/article/45/Supplement_1/S83/138927/6-Glycemic-Targets-Standards-of-Medical-Care-in
48. Battelino T, Danne T, Bergenstal RM, Amiel SA, Beck R, Biester T, et al. Clinical Targets for Continuous Glucose Monitoring Data Interpretation: Recommendations from the International Consensus on Time in Range. Diabetes Care [Internet]. 2019 Aug 1 [cited 2022 Nov 7];42(8):1593–603. Available from: https://diabetesjournals.org/care/article/42/8/1593/36184/Clinical-Targets-for-Continuous-Glucose-Monitoring
49. Committee ADAPP. 9. Pharmacologic Approaches to Glycemic Treatment: Standards of Medical Care in Diabetes—2022. Diabetes Care [Internet]. 2022 Jan 1 [cited 2022 Apr 27];45(Supplement_1):S125–43. Available from: https://diabetesjournals.org/care/article/45/Supplement_1/S125/138908/9-Pharmacologic-Approaches-to-Glycemic-Treatment
50. Bailey CJ, Gwilt M. Diabetes, Metformin and the Clinical Course of Covid-19: Outcomes, Mechanisms and Suggestions on the Therapeutic Use of Metformin. Front Pharmacol [Internet]. 2022 Mar 9 [cited 2022 Apr 26];13. Available from: https://www.ncbi.nlm.nih.gov/pmc/articles/PMC8964397/
51. Lipska KJ, Bailey CJ, Inzucchi SE. Use of Metformin in the Setting of Mild-to-Moderate Renal Insufficiency. Diabetes Care [Internet]. 2011 Jun [cited 2022 Apr 27];34(6):1431. Available from: https://www.ncbi.nlm.nih.gov/pmc/articles/PMC3114336/
52. Cheng X, Liu YM, Li H, Zhang X, Lei F, Qin JJ, et al. Metformin Is Associated with Higher Incidence of Acidosis, but Not Mortality, in Individuals with COVID-19 and Pre-existing Type 2 Diabetes. Cell Metab [Internet]. 2020 Oct 6 [cited 2022 Apr 27];32(4):537. Available from: https://www.ncbi.nlm.nih.gov/pmc/articles/PMC7439986/
53. Dandona P, Mathieu C, Phillip M, Hansen L, Griffen SC, Tschöpe D, et al. Efficacy and safety of dapagliflozin in patients with inadequately controlled type 1 diabetes (DEPICT-1): 24 week results from a multicentre, double-blind, phase 3, randomised controlled trial. Lancet Diabetes Endocrinol [Internet]. 2017 Nov 1 [cited 2022 Apr 27];5(11):864–76. Available from: http://www.thelancet.com/article/S221385871730308X/fulltext

54. Rosenstock J, Marquard J, Laffel LM, Neubacher D, Kaspers S, Cherney DZ, et al. Empagliflozin as Adjunctive to Insulin Therapy in Type 1 Diabetes: The EASE Trials. Diabetes Care [Internet]. 2018 Dec 1 [cited 2022 Apr 27];41(12):2560–9. Available from: https://diabetesjournals.org/care/article/41/12/2560/36495/Empagliflozin-as-Adjunctive-to-Insulin-Therapy-in

55. Hariyanto TI, Kurniawan A. Dipeptidyl peptidase 4 (DPP4) inhibitor and outcome from coronavirus disease 2019 (COVID-19) in diabetic patients: a systematic review, meta-analysis, and meta-regression. J Diabetes Metab Disord [Internet]. 2021 Jun 1 [cited 2022 May 12];20(1):543. Available from: https://www.ncbi.nlm.nih.gov/pmc/articles/PMC8003892/

56. Sola D, Rossi L, Schianca GPC, Maffioli P, Bigliocca M, Mella R, et al. Sulfonylureas and their use in clinical practice. Arch Med Sci [Internet]. 2015 Aug 1 [cited 2022 May 12];11(4):840. Available from: https://www.ncbi.nlm.nih.gov/pmc/articles/PMC4548036/

57. Aoki Y, Maeno T, Aoyagi K, Ueno M, Aoki F, Aoki N, et al. Pioglitazone, a Peroxisome Proliferator-Activated Receptor Gamma Ligand, Suppresses Bleomycin-Induced Acute Lung Injury and Fibrosis. Respiration [Internet]. 2009 Apr [cited 2022 Sep 18];77(3):311–9. Available from: https://www.karger.com/Article/FullText/168676

58. Kutsukake M, Matsutani T, Tamura K, Matsuda A, Kobayashi M, Tachikawa E, et al. Pioglitazone attenuates lung injury by modulating adipose inflammation. J Surg Res. 2014;189(2):295–303.

59. Carboni E, Carta AR, Carboni E. Can pioglitazone be potentially useful therapeutically in treating patients with COVID-19? Med Hypotheses [Internet]. 2020 Jul 1 [cited 2022 Sep 18];140:109776. Available from: https://www.ncbi.nlm.nih.gov/pmc/articles/PMC7175844/

60. Jagat J M, Kalyan K G, Subir R. Use of pioglitazone in people with type 2 diabetes mellitus with coronavirus disease 2019 (COVID-19): Boon or bane? Diabetes Metab Syndr [Internet]. 2020 Sep 1 [cited 2022 Sep 18];14(5):829. Available from: https://www.ncbi.nlm.nih.gov/pmc/articles/PMC7836749/

61. Patel AB, Verma A. COVID-19 and angiotensin-converting enzyme inhibitors and angiotensin receptor blockers: what is the evidence? JAMA [Internet]. 2020 May 12 [cited 2022 Jul 4];323(18):1769–70. Available from: https://jamanetwork.com/journals/jama/fullarticle/2763803

62. Position Statement of the ESC Council on Hypertension on ACE-Inhibitors and Angiotensin Receptor Blockers [Internet]. [cited 2022 May 12]. Available from: https://www.escardio.org/Councils/Council-on-Hypertension-(CHT)/News/position-statement-of-the-esc-council-on-hypertension-on-ace-inhibitors-and-ang

63. Social Determinants of Health | Healthy People 2020 [Internet]. [cited 2022 May 10]. Available from: https://www.healthypeople.gov/2020/topics-objectives/topic/social-determinants-health/interventions-resources

64. Wang EA, McGinnis KA, Goulet J, Bryant K, Gibert C, Leaf DA, et al. Food insecurity and health: data from the veterans aging cohort study. Public Health Reports [Internet]. 2015 Jun 27 [cited 2022 May 12];130(3):261. Available from: https://www.ncbi.nlm.nih.gov/pmc/articles/PMC4388224/

65. Berkowitz SA, Karter AJ, Corbie-Smith G, Seligman HK, Ackroyd SA, Barnard LS, et al. Food insecurity, food "deserts," and glycemic control in patients with diabetes: A longitudinal analysis. Diabetes Care [Internet]. 2018 Jun 1 [cited 2022 Apr 27];41(6):1188–95. Available from: https://www.ncbi.nlm.nih.gov/pmc/articles/PMC5961388/

66. Seligman HK, Jacobs EA, Lopez A, Sarkar U, Tschann J, Fernandez A. Food Insecurity and Hypoglycemia Among Safety Net Patients with Diabetes. Arch Intern Med [Internet]. 2011 Jul 7 [cited 2022 Sep 18];171(13):1204. Available from: https://www.ncbi.nlm.nih.gov/pmc/articles/PMC4230711/

67. Barnidge E, La Barge G, Krupsky K, Arthur J. Screening for Food Insecurity in Pediatric Clinical Settings: Opportunities and Barriers. Journal of Community Health 2016 42:1 [Internet]. 2016 Aug 4 [cited 2022 May 12];42(1):51–7. Available from: https://link.springer.com/article/10.1007/s10900-016-0229-z

68. Findings From The 2018 T1International Patient Survey. [cited 2022 May 12]; Available from: https://www.t1international.com/media/assets/file/T1International_Report_-_Costs_and_Rationing_of_Insulin__Diabetes_Supplies_2.pdf
69. Diabetes Technology Society [Internet]. [cited 2022 May 12]. Available from: https://www.diabetestechnology.org/surveillance.shtml
70. What is Telehealth? | Official web site of the U.S. Health Resources & Services Administration [Internet]. [cited 2022 May 10]. Available from: https://www.hrsa.gov/rural-health/telehealth/what-is-telehealth
71. Johnson EL, Miller E. Remote patient monitoring in diabetes: how to acquire, manage, and use all of the data. Diabetes Spectrum [Internet]. 2022 Feb 15 [cited 2022 May 9];35(1):43–56. Available from: https://diabetesjournals.org/spectrum/article/35/1/43/139218/Remote-Patient-Monitoring-in-Diabetes-How-to
72. Lam K, Lu AD, Shi Y, Covinsky KE. Assessing Telemedicine Unreadiness Among Older Adults in the United States During the COVID-19 Pandemic. JAMA Intern Med [Internet]. 2020 Oct 1 [cited 2022 May 10];180(10):1389–91. Available from: https://jamanetwork.com/journals/jamainternalmedicine/fullarticle/2768772

Chapter 11
The Use of Diabetes Technology in Persons with Diabetes and Coronavirus 2019

Emily D. Szmuilowicz and Grazia Aleppo

Introduction

Diabetes is a major risk factor in the morbidity and mortality of COVID-19 [1], and people with preexisting diabetes who develop COVID-19 infection have an increased risk of multiple diabetes-related complications [2], including diabetic ketoacidosis (DKA) and hyperosmolar hyperglycemic state (HHS) [3]. Therefore, novel modes for glucose monitoring and diabetes care delivery were needed when COVID-19-related lockdowns, social distancing, and reduced in-person interactions became necessary. The use of telehealth has increased access to care during lockdowns and during times when reduced in-person exposure to the community and/or public health-care spaces is warranted among a community already at higher risk of serious COVID-19 complications. Continuous glucose monitoring (CGM) use has expanded rapidly in the outpatient setting [4], with well-established benefits on glycemic control and well-being [5–9]. CGM use during the COVID-19 era has thus afforded unique opportunities for remote data-driven diabetes management.

E. D. Szmuilowicz
Department of Medicine, Division of Endocrinology, Metabolism and Molecular Medicine, Northwestern University Feinberg School of Medicine, Chicago, IL, USA
e-mail: edszmuilowicz@northwestern.edu

G. Aleppo (✉)
Division of Endocrinology, Metabolism and Molecular Medicine, Department of Medicine, Northwestern University Feinberg School of Medicine, Chicago, IL, USA
e-mail: aleppo@northwestern.edu

A. K. Myers (ed.), *Diabetes and COVID-19*, Contemporary Endocrinology,
https://doi.org/10.1007/978-3-031-28536-3_11

Diabetes Technology and COVID-19 in the Outpatient Setting

Telehealth/Virtual Clinics

Telehealth refers to the provision of health care using electronic telecommunication tools when the provider and patient are in different locations, in the absence of an in-person office visit, typically using a computer, tablet, or smartphone connected through the internet [10]. Synchronous telehealth refers to healthcare visits in which patients communicate directly about their health with a provider in real-time over phone or video [10]. In contrast, asynchronous telehealth can be utilized when a provider reviews information (such as forms, photos, or prerecorded information) submitted previously by the patient, and the provider then uses the stored information to provide medical advice at a separate time [10].

Diabetes technologies, including cloud-based glucose monitors and insulin delivery systems which digitally store information about insulin dosing and delivery, have opened the door to many unique opportunities for virtual remote diabetes care. Virtual care models have the potential to introduce unique advantages to the provision of diabetes care in general, including increased access for patients who live in remote areas or have difficulty traveling to in-person appointments, reduced costs for travel and space utilization, and improved quality of life for people living with diabetes [11]. While telemedicine clinics carry many potential advantages, significant potential obstacles to widespread adoption remain, including restricted reimbursement to health-care providers, limitations on providing care to patients living in different states, and lack of uniform compatibility between devices and upload software programs from different manufacturers.

A survey of healthcare providers caring for people with type 1 diabetes (T1D) during the COVID-19 pandemic reported that the most common barriers to effective telemedicine care related to logistical problems with accessing the patient's data, patient limitations in interacting with digital technologies, and problems with the teleconferencing technology itself [12]. These findings raise particular concern, as obstacles relating to decreased patient digital literacy introduce the potential to widen preexisting health inequities. Digital health literacy has been defined as "the ability to seek, find, understand, and appraise health information from electronic sources and apply the knowledge gained to addressing or solving a health problem." [13] In addition to requiring access to devices and internet with sufficient connectivity and speed, consumption of health information via digital sources also requires the critical appraisal of the validity of online medical advice amid an overwhelming amount of information available online. Thus, with the increasing reliance on online information derived at home during the lockdown and growing utilization of virtual modalities of care, those either without access to devices compatible with video teleconferencing programs or without the digital literacy to effectively utilize digitally derived information have the potential to become even more disproportionately isolated from access to high-quality medical care [14]. Telehealth has been suggested as one way to increase the availability of medical care in underserved areas [15]. Perceptions regarding telehealth were assessed among underserved African Americans and Latinos [15]. Multiple perceived benefits were noted including decreased wait time and increased access, but multiple concerns were also noted, including concerns about confidentiality, privacy, and being physically separated from the provider [15]. When the effectiveness of telehealth care (including telephone calls, text messages, web-based portals, and virtual visits) was evaluated specifically among Black and Hispanic patients with diabetes, it was associated with improvements in glycemia (decrease in HbA1c of −0.465 ([CI: −0.648 to −0.282], $p = 0.000$) [16]. However, while the risk of developing diabetes and hypertension is higher in Black and Hispanic patients, marked disparities in internet access were reported among Black and Hispanic patients with hypertension or diabetes, with a median difference in internet use prevalence of −16.54% (interquartile range [IQR] −10.16, −20.22) for Black patients and −15.58% (−3.67, −24.12) for Hispanics patients compared with those who identify as White [17]. Thus, while telehealth is a promising means of increasing access to care for underserved populations, a significant limitation remains the lack of access to the technology needed to successfully implement such measures.

While telehealth predated the COVID-19 era, in many ways the COVID-19 pandemic compelled health-care systems and providers to rapidly adopt virtual platforms for care delivery that were far from mainstream in even the recent past. With the onset of the pandemic and associated public health emergency, the Centers for Medicare & Medicaid Services (CMS) expanded coverage for a wide range of inpatient and outpatient telehealth encounters, including emergency department visits, group psychotherapy, psychological and neuropsychological testing, office/outpatient evaluation and management, and lower-level home visits, among others [10].

Patient perceptions of telemedicine care among people with T1D have been very positive overall [18]. When a multidisciplinary diabetes clinical care program in Mexico was converted to a virtual format due to the COVID-19 pandemic, implementation of the virtual multidisciplinary clinic was not only feasible but also effective. The comprehensive program consisted of four intensive monthly 6-hour visits, followed by annual evaluations. Each visit included multidisciplinary evaluations targeting medical care (endocrinologists, ophthalmologists/optometrists, nurses, and dentists); mental health (psychologists/psychiatrists); lifestyle (dietitians, physical activity instructors); and diabetes education, noting that in the United States this is not always reimbursable. After the onset of the COVID-19 pandemic, the comprehensive program was converted to a virtual format (telephone and video were utilized) in which links to questionnaire-derived information were provided to patients via email. After the implementation of the virtual format, there was no change in self-monitoring of blood glucose, foot care practices, or metabolic parameters including hemoglobin A1c (HbA1c) [19]. It was noted in this study that the amount of exercise performed each week during the virtual program adopted during the pandemic decreased, and there was an increase in the frequency of anxiety, depression, and diabetes distress compared to those who had received in-person care in 2019. However, the two comparator groups differed not only in the mode of care delivery but also in time (before vs. after June 2020), and pre- versus post-pandemic, it is difficult to attribute these changes solely to the mode of care delivery.

One research group assessed perceptions among 500 people with T1D regarding the use of telehealth by disseminating an anonymous survey via social media platforms in 2021 which ascertained information about opinions and experiences with telehealth and diabetes therapy during the COVID-19 pandemic across 40 countries in Europe, North America, South America, Africa, and Asia. Interestingly, the study found that the proportion of people wishing to continue telemedicine in the future decreased from 75% to 45% from 2020 to 2021 [18]. Exploration of the differences in patient factors that predict greater acceptance of remote virtual care should be explored in future studies.

Interestingly, a survey of more than 2500 people with type 2 diabetes (T2D) in India showed that only approximately 15% of patients contacted their provider during the lockdown, and of those only approximately one-third utilized the structured telemedicine program that was available to them [20]. Despite the low rates of adoption, approximately 80% of those who did take advantage of the telemedicine program reported satisfaction with the system and a desire to continue to utilize the virtual platform. One study in the United States showed that among participants in a telehealth program for the treatment of T2D prior to the COVID-19 pandemic, there was a significant improvement in diabetes distress over an average of 6 months among those reporting moderate or high diabetes distress at baseline [21]. Telehealth has not only been used during the pandemic in the care of people with preexisting diabetes but also in the care of people with newly diagnosed diabetes. The feasibility of using telemedicine in the education and treatment of people with newly diagnosed T1D has been reported, including patient and family education as well as training on the use of CGM and insulin delivery by either multiple daily injections or continuous subcutaneous insulin infusion (CSII) [22, 23].

Thus while telehealth is a welcomed addition to the care armamentarium for many people with diabetes, these findings are not universal and individualized care plans must be devised between patients and their providers. It will be imperative in the years to come to identify any patient-related and clinical characteristics that can help to identify those most likely to benefit from and react positively to virtual diabetes care. One must also note that telehealth cannot substitute for many components of standard medical care, such as physical exam components, which cannot always be reproduced in a virtual format.

Continuous Glucose Monitoring

Continuous glucose monitoring use among people with T1D and T2D has expanded greatly [4], and its use has in many ways revolutionized diabetes care and monitoring for those living with diabetes. Well-established benefits, spanning from glycemic benefits to improved well-being, have been demonstrated [5–9], and CGM use has rapidly become a well-accepted component of modern diabetes care [24]. While HbA1c, a measure of average glycemia over the preceding 2–3 months, provides important information about overall glycemic control, it does not characterize daily glycemic patterns, glycemic responses to different foods and activities, and importantly provides no information about the frequency or timing of hyperglycemia or hypoglycemia, which remains the most serious adverse effect of insulin therapy. In contrast, CGM provides information about daily glycemic patterns and glucose variability that may guide therapeutic adjustments, and real-time CGM devices additionally can alarm the user to the occurrence of hypoglycemia or its impending occurrence. An additional important advantage of CGM use in the COVID-19 era is the ability for patients to remotely upload CGM data to cloud-based software programs which can be remotely accessed by members of the health-care team, without the need for an in-person visit to the clinic. The recommended report for CGM review and interpretation is the Ambulatory Glucose Profile or AGP report (Fig. 11.1). The dashboard on the AGP includes data reporting the number of days CGM was used (recommendation is at least 14 days) and the percentage of CGM use or wear (recommended is at least 70%). The report also includes the average glucose levels and the Glucose Management Indicator (GMI), which is a CGM-derived estimation of HbA1c. Furthermore, all the core glucometrics recommended by the International Consensus on Time in Range [25] are depicted in the AGP. These represent the various time in ranges and the percentage of time spent in each glucose range. The recommended targets have been outlined in Table 11.1. Finally, the AGP includes the actual profile which combines inputs from multiple days and displays CGM data over a single 24-hour period. Usually a 14-day composite glucose profile is shown, providing fundamental information to the provider and patient alike [26–28] to allow not only interpretation but also personalized therapy changes.

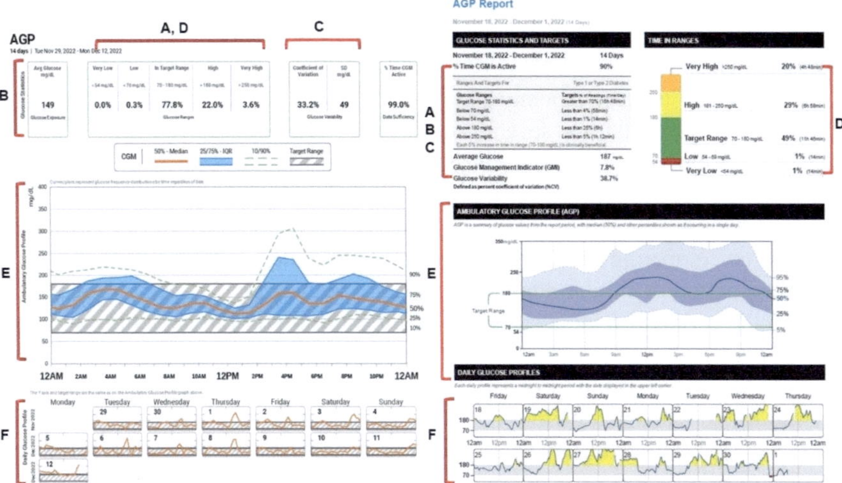

Fig. 11.1 CGM-based report – Ambulatory Glucose Profile. Legend. (**a**) glucose ranges; (**b**) average glucose; (**c**) glucose variability indexes; (**d**) time in ranges; (**e**) AGP (ambulatory glucose profile); (**f**) daily glucose trends

Table 11.1 CGM-based time in ranges for adults with diabetes [25]

Glucometrics for TIR with CGM		Recommended % of time (hours/day)
Time Above Range (TAR) >250 mg/dL	Hyperglycemia Level 2	<5% (1 h, 12 min)
Time above range (TAR) 181–250 mg/dL	Hyperglycemia level 1	<25% (<6 h, including % of values >250 mg/dL)
Time in range (TIR) 70–180 mg/dL	**In target range**	**>70% (>16 h, 48 m)**
Time below range (TBR) 54–69 mg/dL	Hypoglycemia level 1	<4% (<1 h, including % of values <54 mg/dL)
Time below range (TBR) <54 mg/dL	Hypoglycemia level 2	<1% (<15 min)

Many benefits of CGM use have become evident in the COVID-19 era. An analysis of the T1D Exchange COVID-19 Surveillance Registry, a multicenter observational study of people with T1D, reported that DKA and hospitalization rates were lower among users compared to non-users of any diabetes device, including those who used CGM only or insulin pump only, compared with those who used no devices [29]. In a report describing people with T1D and COVID-19 infection in Italy who used CGM, a deterioration in glycemic control during COVID-19 infection was manifested by increased glucose management index, glycemic variability, and time spent above 250 mg/dL [30]. As hyperglycemia is a known consequence of COVID-19 infection, this COVID-19-induced glycemic deterioration is not surprising. However, personal use of CGM uniquely bestows upon people with diabetes the ability to easily share their glycemic patterns with the health-care team, even during quarantine, so that effective treatment strategies can be implemented [23], alarming glycemic patterns requiring urgent care can be easily identified by a remote caregiver, and adverse glycemic outcomes can be more readily averted.

CGM use during the pandemic has also provided information about population-wide trends in glycemia, and several studies have reported improved Time in Range (TIR) among those using CGM during the pandemic [31, 32]. One analysis of CGM data from more than 60,000 CGM users interestingly showed improved TIR from 59% to 61% across three major counties in the Chicago, Los Angeles, and New York areas, when comparing an eight-week period before the pandemic predating lockdown to a period of similar duration in the early pandemic [32]. An observational study in the United Kingdom showed that a higher proportion of people with T1D achieved targets for TIR, Time Above Range (TAR), Time Below Range (TBR), as well as glycemic variability, comparing the pre-pandemic period to two time periods within the lockdown period [33]. While it is unclear if the reported improvements were causally related to CGM use, it is notable that glycemic control did not worsen amid the decreased health-care access and stressors which abounded during the early pandemic months among these real-time CGM users.

Table 11.1 describes optimal targets for adults with diabetes.

Continuous Subcutaneous Insulin Infusion

Continuous subcutaneous insulin infusion (CSII) therapy via an insulin pump is a cornerstone of therapy for people with T1D and also an important therapeutic modality for a substantial number of people with T2D [24]. Shortly after the onset of lockdown restrictions, many diabetes clinics rapidly converted from in-person to virtual formats for insulin pump training programs, to allow patients uninterrupted access to CSII during the lockdown measures.

Reassuringly, several studies are now available which have demonstrated comparable outcomes utilizing a virtual training platform [34–37]. Patient satisfaction and glycemic outcomes assessed shortly after CSII initiation were comparable among those who underwent virtual pump training during the COVID-19 era compared to in-person pump training in the pre-COVID-19 era for a commonly used hybrid-closed loop CSII system [35]. Interestingly, in this study, calls to the technical support team for pump education were lower after virtual training, though calls related to software support were higher. Another observational study of more than 20,000 trainings for another commonly used hybrid-closed loop pump system found that virtual trainings were associated with greater TIR, in addition to improved patient satisfaction and confidence, in comparison to in-person trainings [36]. While it is unclear if a causal relationship exists between virtual training and improved outcomes, the authors hypothesize that the requirements to complete software setup and required simulator tasks that were required for virtual training may have engendered more active participation and resultant better outcomes than the standard in-person training sessions. In an observational study of people with T1D in Spain using a sensor-augmented insulin pump, TIR and TAR both improved during the lockdown compared to the pre-COVID-19 era, without an increased time spent in the hypoglycemia range, consistent with overall improved glycemic control [38]. Again, these observational findings could be explained by other factors, such as a consistent daily routine while on lockdown at home, without the more typical variability in food intake, activity level, and other unpredictable stressors which occur outside of home quarantine. Notably, however, no apparent glycemic deterioration occurred in this population despite the decreased access to routine health-care facilities during the lockdown.

Overall, these studies provide reassurance that virtual training modalities for CSII were feasible and effective, and most likely can be relied upon when in-person training is not feasible or desired, whether due to COVID-19 risks or other physical or geographic barriers which impede in-person training. However, multiple barriers to technology adoption have been identified, particularly for individuals with T2D, Medicare beneficiaries, and those covered by Medicaid insurance. Minority racial or ethnic status as well as government insurance have been correlated to lower rates of CSII use. In particular, Medicare and Medicaid beneficiaries have limited access to CSII which further contributes to these disparities [28, 39]. While these observational findings do not prove a causal relationship between virtual training and improved outcomes, the findings provide reassuring evidence that the virtual training sessions necessitated by COVID-19 lockdown measures were both efficacious and feasible, and in the populations studied there was no apparent deterioration in clinical outcomes or patient acceptance during this unprecedented time.

Diabetes Technology and COVID-19 in the Inpatient Setting

Inpatient hyperglycemia, with or without a history of diabetes, is a major contributing factor to the increase in morbidity and mortality [40]. Furthermore, hyperglycemia increases the length of stay and health-care costs [40]. During the COVID-19 pandemic, hyperglycemia or exacerbation of hyperglycemia in the inpatient setting has been correlated with worse outcomes and increased risk for DKA, and as a result, the inpatient management of hyperglycemia has become much more complex and challenging overall. Hyperglycemia with COVID-19 infection may be due to high levels of stress inflammation, cytokine-mediated insulin resistance, or direct beta cell damage leading to insulin deficiency [41].

Insulin therapy has been the treatment of choice for critically ill patients with COVID-19 (see Chap. 9 for more information); similarly, non-critically ill patients with COVID-19 have responded better to insulin protocols to overcome the insulin resistance caused by the SARS-CoV-2 infection and other factors, such as continuous tube feeding and administration of systemic glucocorticoids. Intensive insulin therapy, whether via intravenous continuous infusion or via basal/bolus subcutaneous therapy, requires frequent glucose measurements, as often as once per hour to at least four times per day, respectively. This in turn caused further challenges to the healthcare workers caring for these patients in strict isolation, because of the frequent need to interact and measure glucose levels while at the same time facing the shortage of personal protective equipment (PPE) and trying to minimize exposure. These challenges offered a unique opportunity to use diabetes technology in the inpatient setting during COVID-19 hospitalizations. On April 1, 2020, the U.S. Food and Drug Administration announced it would not object to the use of CGM systems to assist with COVID-19 patient monitoring [42, 43], and several protocols were implemented both in the intensive care units (ICU) and in the non-critically ill patients admitted with COVID-19 infection who required insulin therapy.

Accuracy of Continuous Glucose Monitoring in the Hospital Setting

CGM systems have become increasingly accurate with lower mean absolute relative difference (MARD) levels. MARD is a measure that defines the accuracy of CGM. The smaller the MARD value, expressed as a percentage, the more accurate the device is when compared to the reference glucose value. Most currently available CGM in the world have a MARD value less than 10%, and today most do not need fingerstick confirmation for insulin dosing decisions; however, these systems have been tested mostly in the outpatient setting. When CGM use was being considered during the COVID-19 pandemic, data regarding their accuracy was still scarce [44], and it became necessary to better understand how these systems would perform in the inpatient setting. While many institutions across the country started using CGM in the inpatient setting to limit the shortage of PPE and to limit healthcare workers' exposure in early 2020, this unprecedented situation also generated a need for data regarding inpatient CGM accuracy. In early 2020, a prospective study from Galindo et al. compared the performance of the masked (i.e., where the values were not visible to the user) FreeStyle Libre Pro CGM to point-of-care capillary glucose testing (POC) in hospitalized patients with T2DM [45]. Data from 97 participants were analyzed and showed that the mean daily glucose was significantly higher by POC glucose measurements (188.9 ± 37.3 vs. 176.1 ± 46.9 mg/dL) with an estimated mean difference of 12.8 mg/dL (95% CI 8.3–17.2 mg/dL); the proportion of patients with glucose readings <70 mg/dL (14% vs. 56%) and < 54 mg/dL (4.1% vs. 36%) detected by POC blood glucose was lower than those detected by the blinded CGM (all $P < 0.001$). The overall MARD was 14.8%, ranging between 11.4% and 16.7% for glucose values between 70 and 250 mg/dL and higher for 51–69 mg/dL (MARD 28.0%). The percentages of glucose readings within ±15%/15 mg/dL, ±20%/20 mg/dL, and ± 30%/30 mg/dL were 62%, 76%, and 91%, respectively. The Clarke Error Grid (CEG) quantifies clinical accuracy of a glucose measuring system (either glucose meter or CGM); it considers the absolute and relative differences between the device reading and a reference value and addresses the clinical significance of this difference. There are five zones, A to E. For greater accuracy, CGM values should fall within zones A and/or B [46]. In this study [45], the CEG analysis showed 98.8% of glucose pairs within zones A and B. The authors concluded that this blinded CGM system showed lower than ideal accuracy in the inpatient setting.

The accuracy in the perioperative setting was evaluated in a prospective study that enrolled ten adults with diabetes undergoing surgery using blinded CGM Dexcom G6 Pro (Dexcom, San Diego, CA). Patients were treated with insulin both in the intraoperative and postoperative periods. In this small study the MARD was 9.4%, very close to the information in the package insert, and 89% of paired glucose values were within the no-risk surveillance error grid zone. The authors concluded that Dexcom G6 CGM could be used safely in the hospital for COVID-19-infected patients [47].

In a subsequent retrospective matched-pair CGM and capillary POC glucose data from three inpatient CGM studies with non-critically ill patients with diabetes treated with insulin, the accuracy of the real-time Dexcom G6 CGM system was evaluated. The authors investigated several accuracy metrics such as the MARD, median absolute relative difference (ARD), and proportion of CGM values within 15%, 20%, and 30% or 15, 20, and 30 mg/dL of POC reference values for blood glucose >100 mg/dL or <100 mg/dL, respectively. Clinical reliability was assessed with CEG. The analysis included 218 patients and the overall MARD was 12.8%

with a median ARD of 10.1%, both very close to the MARD levels reported by the device manufacturers (9%). In addition, the proportions of readings meeting FDA accuracy criteria for glucose levels compared to reference values (YSI, Yellow Spring Instrument) were reported. These are called % 15/15 (readings within 15 mg/dL or 15%), % 20/20 (readings within 20 mg/dL or 20%), and % 30/30 (readings within 30 mg/dL or 30%). In this study, the %15/15, %20/20, and %30/30 criteria were 68.7%, 81.7%, and 93.8%, respectively. Finally, the CEG analysis showed that 98.7% of all values were in zones A and B. These findings indicated that CGM technology could be a reliable tool for hospital use [48].

Continuous glucose monitoring accuracy may be a complex challenge when patients are acutely ill in the ICU, due to hemodynamic changes, possible reduction in peripheral perfusion due to hypoxemia, pressor use, and potential interfering medications that may affect the performance of CGM systems in this setting. Imaging studies and the need to remove the sensors for MRI, CT scans, or X-rays also contribute to the many challenges these acutely ill patients present. Nevertheless, interesting findings were reported in a study that investigated the accuracy of CGM in hospitalized patients on general floors and in ICU with COVID-19. The study aimed to decrease health-care professional exposure to COVID-19 and to improve glycemic management in hospitalized COVID-19 patients. POC and laboratory glucose values were matched with simultaneous CGM glucose values and measures of accuracy were performed to evaluate the safety and usability of CGM in this population. In 808 paired samples obtained from 28 patients (10 ICU, 18 general floor), overall MARD for all patients using either POC or the laboratory as reference was 13.2%. When using POC as the reference glucose, MARD was 13.9% and using the laboratory glucose as the reference 10.9%, respectively. Using both POC and laboratory reference glucose pairs, the overall MARD for critical care patients was 12.1% and for general floor patients 14%. The authors concluded that with proper protocols and safeguards in place, the use of CGM in the hospitalized patient would be a reasonable alternative to standard of care glucose measurement to achieve the goal of reducing health-care professional exposure [49].

Despite the initial limited knowledge of CGM accuracy in the hospital, many institutions started implementing its use in the hospital in the early pandemic months in 2020, when the U.S. Food and Drug Administration announced it would not object to the use of CGM systems to assist with COVID-19 patient monitoring [50, 51]. These institutions used the CGM systems in the hospital mostly under research protocols, and these efforts are now providing crucial information regarding the benefits and challenges of implementing this technology in the inpatient setting.

Use of CGM in the Inpatient Setting During COVID-19

One of the earliest published studies on the use of CGM in the hospital on COVID-19 patients was a pilot study ($n = 9$) conducted in non-ICU adults receiving subcutaneous insulin administration as well as POC glucose measurement; this study evaluated the feasibility of using CGM in non-critically ill patients. A Dexcom G6 sensor was placed on the abdomen and an iPhone 5S was used as a receiver and placed at the patient's door. The data were transmitted through the Dexcom Follow App on another smartphone at the nurses' station as well as the investigator smart devices. The frequency of glucose measurements by fingerstick was decreased from 4 to 2 times per day after 24 hours if the sensor and glucose correlated unless clinically indicated. The correlation coefficient between POC and sensor glucose values was 0.927, MARD was 9.77%, 84.8% of the sensor glucose values were in CEG zone A, 100% were in zone A or B, and CGM readings prompted five clinical interventions due to high or low glucose values (by alarm and trend glucose). This pilot study emphasized the importance of communication between the multidisciplinary team members, the education of the nursing staff in a short time, and their engagement in this new "method" of monitoring glucose levels [52].

A subsequent randomized controlled trial of real-time CGM compared with POC in a non-ICU hospital setting enrolled 110 adults with T2DM on a non-ICU floor who received Dexcom G6 CGM versus usual care of POC capillary glucose monitoring by fingerstick. CGM data were wirelessly transmitted from the bedside; in addition, hospital telemetry monitored CGM data and notified bedside nursing of glucose alerts and trends. Interventions for glucose management were made according to standardized protocols. The CGM group demonstrated significantly lower mean glucose (-18.5 mg/dL), percentage of time in hyperglycemia >250 mg/dL (-11.41%), and higher TIR 70–250 mg/dL ($+11.26\%$) compared to usual care ($P < 0.05$). This clinical trial demonstrated that CGM and standardized protocols for the management of acute hyper–/hypoglycemia improved mean glucose and TIR without increasing the percentage of time in hypoglycemia in patients with T2D. Of note, the number of hypoglycemic events were few, and the duration of hypoglycemic episodes was shorter in the CGM group [53].

Although multiple factors can affect the reliability and accuracy of CGM use in the ICU, a single-center study evaluated 11 patients with COVID-19 infection in the ICU and used Dexcom G6 with POC glucose-CGM matched pairs. In this study, considerable accuracy was reported, with a MARD of 12.58% and median ARD of 6.3%, respectively, and 98% of all sensor readings were in the CED zone A + B. In addition, CGM use reduced POC testing by ~60% for patients on intravenous continuous insulin infusion [54].

The results of another randomized controlled trial from Demark were recently published and included 64 participants with COVID-19 infection, randomized to either non-blinded telemetric CGM as the only method for glucose monitoring or traditional POC fingerstick with blinded CGM. The primary endpoint was TIR based on CGM in both groups and a questionnaire was provided to the health-care providers taking care of these patients. Even though in this cohort there was no improvement in glycemic outcomes in the CGM group, CGM use was associated with fewer POC measurements (P<0.001) and fewer patient-personnel contacts. In addition, health-care providers preferred CGM over POC measurements [55].

Finally, the use of CGM was employed to investigate the role of various glucose metrics and their relationship with the risk of acute complications in hospitalized patients with COVID-19 infection. In this prospective, single-center cohort study, 60 adults with T2DM or hyperglycemia admitted with COVID-19 infection and treated with basal/bolus insulin regimen were enrolled and Flash Libre CGM (Abbott, Diabetes Care, Alameda, CA) was used to monitor glucose levels during their hospital stay. The primary outcome was to determine the relationship between time in ranges (TIR, TAR, TBR) and glycemic variability and a composite of complications including ICU admission, acute respiratory distress syndrome (ARDS), and acute kidney injury. In this study, a total of 190,080 data points of CGM were available, with the majority of values (72.5%) within the target range of 70–180 mg/dL; in addition, coefficient of variation and TBR (<70 mg/L) were low at 30% and 3%, respectively. However, 22% of the values were above 180 mg/dL and were correlated with a higher rate of composite complications (22.5% vs. 16%, $P < 0.04$) emphasizing that time spent in hyperglycemia increases the risks of acute complications in hospitalized patients with COVID-19 [56].

Data regarding the benefits of CGM in the hospital for COVID-19-infected patients are growing, each substantiating the previous with reduction of hypoglycemia, improvement in TIR, and reduction of hyperglycemia. However, the implementation of CGM use in the hospital during the pandemic was mainly based on research protocols. Evaluation of benefits and barriers will need to occur for this technology to become standard of care in the future for COVID-19 or any patient admitted with hyperglycemia [57].

Telemedicine and Remote Patient Monitoring

Implementation of diabetes co-management service via telehealth was in its infancy prior to the COVID-19 pandemic. One academic institution, however, had already begun to implement a telehealth inpatient diabetes service in July 2019. With the advent of the COVID-19 pandemic, most of the diabetes service at the University of North Carolina was transitioned to a virtual care model as early as March 2020, with the institution of automatic consults for COVID-19 patients. Their evaluation of glycemic outcomes from before and after transition over a 15-week period showed that every hospital unit where the diabetes virtual service was utilized had more blood glucose readings within TIR goals with unchanged rates of hypoglycemia. This study showed that a virtual care model for inpatient diabetes/hyperglycemia management was not only feasible but also provided similar outcomes compared to face-to-face patient care [58].

Multiple additional institutions across the country (personal communications) implemented virtual consultation services for inpatient diabetes care in view of the immediate need for patient care in a time when PPE was limited, and efforts were made to reduce as much as possible the exposure of healthcare workers. Future data will show whether long-term inpatient virtual care can be successfully implemented or continued, especially in those healthcare facilities where endocrinologists' presence is limited and expert diabetes management may not be immediately available. Additional issues will need to be addressed in the future to determine how long-term virtual inpatient care can be provided. Among these, a crucial issue will be to define and structure reimbursement for this model of care by healthcare facilities as well as commercial and government insurers.

Health Disparities and Access to Diabetes Technology During the COVID-19 Pandemic

While providers and patients alike have derived multiple unique benefits from virtual interactions, and telehealth in the outpatient and inpatient setting has expanded access to health care in many vital ways, the increasing use of telehealth has at the same time amplified many preexisting health disparities [59]. COVID-19 has disproportionately impacted underserved communities, and it therefore becomes all the more crucial to ensure that inequitable access to the many diabetes technologies which have expanded care options amid the pandemic does not widen these preexisting health inequities [60].

During the lockdown imposed in the early months of the pandemic, internet usage increased coincident with increased needs for implementation of work and medical, shopping, and essential needs from home. However, many underserved communities in both rural and urban areas suffered from decreased internet connectivity, further decreasing access to these essential amenities and opportunities [61]. In addition, the increasing use of virtual health-care modalities has further amplified preexisting inequalities in health-care access. While telehealth utilization has increased significantly since the onset of the COVID-19 pandemic, the proportion of vulnerable populations utilizing telehealth decreased, including patients with public insurance and patients who do not speak English [62]. Furthermore, patients who were Black, Native American, men, older, or whose preferred language was not English were more likely to utilize telephone instead of video for virtual care, which could disproportionately lead to a more limited medical evaluation and potentially resultant less comprehensive care among some vulnerable populations [62]. During the pandemic, those who did not have consistent access to internet service, private space at home or work, and/or smartphones or laptops, as well as those who lacked the literacy or numeracy necessary to manage device uploads to cloud-based software programs may have been disproportionately isolated from the benefits afforded by these expanding technologies. One survey of more than 1200 people who had received subspecialty diabetes care between March and June 2020 found that a major impediment to participation in telehealth was a lack of familiarity with or access to a smartphone [63]. This study also found that older people, people reliant on public insurance, and people who required language interpretation utilized virtual care options less. As interpretation support may be less readily available during a virtual care encounter than through in-person clinics, those who do not speak English as a first language have the potential to be systematically excluded from virtual and remote care options. These findings are notable, as those with limited resources and/or lack of access/familiarity with these technologies may be disproportionately excluded from telemedicine services, which has the potential to further deepen preexisting societal health-care disparities.

Thus, historically vulnerable and underserved populations are more at risk for continued and magnified exclusion from virtual and digital care and their potential clinical benefits.

Racial disparities in the use of diabetes technology were strikingly evident in the T1D Exchange COVID-19 Surveillance Registry [29]. Non-Hispanic White persons used CGM devices significantly more than those who identify as non-Hispanic Black (67% vs. 10%; $P < 0.01$) or Hispanic (67% vs. 16%; $P < 0.01$). Furthermore, racial and ethnic minoritized groups are underrepresented in research studies evaluating diabetes technologies in the general diabetes population [64]. It is currently unknown to what extent implicit bias and biases in prescribing diabetes technologies contribute to these inequities [60], and these inequities only serve to further amplify preexisting health-care disparities. The clinical benefit derived from the use of diabetes technologies coupled with the racial disparities in access to and utilization of these beneficial technologies must serve as a call to action to ensure not only increasing access to diabetes technologies for people with diabetes but also equitable access to and utilization of these beneficial technologies [60]. As diabetes technologies have the capacity to expand healthcare access through cloud-based data-sharing for connected glucose monitoring devices, smart insulin pens, and insulin pumps, and telehealth-based care has the potential to widen the reach of clinical care providers and comprehensive diabetes programs, equitable access to these virtual care options and digital technologies must be ensured, particularly among underserved populations that are already disproportionately impacted by diabetes and decreased access to care.

Age has emerged as another factor which may impact access to and participation in telehealth. Interestingly, in one large survey of adults with diabetes, the youngest age group (age 18–29 years) most commonly reported delay in receiving medical care, which was strikingly reported in nearly 90% of survey respondents in this age group [65]. Alarmingly, most of this age group (96%) did not perceive themselves to be at high risk for severe COVID-19, a lower proportion of younger adults reported that they intended to be vaccinated, and fewer younger adults with DM reported health insurance coverage compared with older adults. In the large survey of people who had obtained subspecialty diabetes care referenced above, many responded that in-person care was preferred due to a belief that in-person care provides better care than virtual care, a belief that is thought to be more common among older adults [63]. It is important to note that physical impairments such as impaired vision, hearing, or dexterity, which may impede the use of computers and smartphones, may represent another barrier to the provision of virtual care to an older population.

Conclusion

In the face of access limitations imposed by the COVID-19 pandemic, the adoption of virtual care models has increased access to care for people with an increased risk of health complications from COVID-19 infection. Similarly, diabetes technologies, which allow remote assessment of glucose trends and therapeutic effects, have expanded the ability to provide virtual and remote care for people with diabetes. While these revolutionary diabetes technologies and virtual care models carry many potential advantages, significant potential obstacles remain, including inequitable access to these revolutionary technologies and a growing body of evidence regarding the potential benefits of inpatient CGM use among people hospitalized with COVID-19 infection. However, a larger and more systematic evaluation of the benefits and barriers of CGM use in the inpatient setting is needed before this becomes standard of care in caring for people with diabetes and COVID-19 in the hospital.

References

1. Fadini GP, Morieri ML, Longato E, Avogaro A. Prevalence and impact of diabetes among people infected with SARS-CoV-2. J Endocrinol Invest. 2020; https://doi.org/10.1007/s40618-020-01236-2.
2. Zhu L, She ZG, Cheng X, et al. Association of blood glucose control and outcomes in patients with COVID-19 and pre-existing type 2 diabetes. Cell Metab. 2020;31(6):1068–1077 e3. https://doi.org/10.1016/j.cmet.2020.04.021.
3. Kim NY, Ha E, Moon JS, Lee YH, Choi EY. Acute Hyperglycemic crises with coronavirus disease-19: case reports. Diabetes Metab J. 2020;44(2):349–53. https://doi.org/10.4093/dmj.2020.0091.
4. Hood KK, DiMeglio LA, Riddle MC. Putting continuous glucose monitoring to work for people with type 1 diabetes. Diabetes Care. 2020;43(1):19–21. https://doi.org/10.2337/dci19-0054.
5. Beck RW, Riddlesworth T, Ruedy K, et al. Effect of continuous glucose monitoring on glycemic control in adults with type 1 diabetes using insulin injections: the DIAMOND randomized clinical trial. JAMA. 2017;317(4):371–8. https://doi.org/10.1001/jama.2016.19975.
6. Lind M, Polonsky W, Hirsch IB, et al. Continuous glucose monitoring vs conventional therapy for glycemic control in adults with type 1 diabetes treated with multiple daily insulin injections: the GOLD randomized clinical trial. JAMA. 2017;317(4):379–87. https://doi.org/10.1001/jama.2016.19976.
7. Heinemann L, Freckmann G, Ehrmann D, et al. Real-time continuous glucose monitoring in adults with type 1 diabetes and impaired hypoglycaemia awareness or severe hypoglycaemia treated with multiple daily insulin injections (HypoDE): a multicentre, randomised controlled trial. Lancet. 2018;391(10128):1367–77. https://doi.org/10.1016/S0140-6736(18)30297-6.
8. Oliver N, Gimenez M, Calhoun P, et al. Continuous glucose monitoring in people with type 1 diabetes on multiple-dose injection therapy: the relationship between glycemic control and hypoglycemia. Diabetes Care. 2020;43(1):53–8. https://doi.org/10.2337/dc19-0977.
9. Polonsky WH, Hessler D, Ruedy KJ, Beck RW, Group DS. The impact of continuous glucose monitoring on markers of quality of life in adults with type 1 diabetes: further findings from the DIAMOND randomized clinical trial. Diabetes Care. 2017;40(6):736–41. https://doi.org/10.2337/dc17-0133.

10. Telehealth: health care from the safety of our homes. Updated June 29, 2022. https://telehealth. hhs.gov/. Accessed 16 Aug 2022.
11. Phillip M, Bergenstal RM, Close KL, et al. The digital/virtual diabetes clinic: the future is now-recommendations from an international panel on diabetes digital technologies introduction. Diabetes Technol Ther. 2021;23(2):146–54. https://doi.org/10.1089/dia.2020.0375.
12. Forde H, Choudhary P, Lumb A, Wilmot E, Hussain S. Current provision and HCP experiences of remote care delivery and diabetes technology training for people with type 1 diabetes in the UK during the COVID-19 pandemic. Diabet Med. 2022;39(4):e14755. https://doi.org/10.1111/dme.14755.
13. Digital Health Literacy. https://allofus.nnlm.gov/digital-health-literacy. Accessed 24 May 2022.
14. Anderson A, O'Connell SS, Thomas C, Chimmanamada R. Telehealth interventions to improve diabetes management among Black and Hispanic patients: a systematic review and meta-analysis. J Racial Ethn Health Disparities. 2022;9:1–2.
15. George S, Hamilton A, Baker RS. How do low-income urban African Americans and Latinos feel about telemedicine? A diffusion of innovation analysis. Int J Telemed Appl. 2012;2012:715194. https://doi.org/10.1155/2012/715194.
16. Anderson A, O'Connell SS, Thomas C, Chimmanamada R. Telehealth interventions to improve diabetes management among Black and Hispanic patients: a systematic review and meta-analysis. J Racial Ethn Health Disparities. 2022; https://doi.org/10.1007/s40615-021-01174-6.
17. Jain V, Al Rifai M, Lee MT, et al. Racial and geographic disparities in internet use in the U.S. among patients with hypertension or diabetes: implications for telehealth in the era of COVID-19. Diabetes Care. 2021;44(1):e15–7. https://doi.org/10.2337/dc20-2016.
18. Scott SN, Fontana FY, Helleputte S, et al. Use and perception of telemedicine in people with type 1 diabetes during the COVID-19 pandemic: a 1-year follow-up. Diabetes Technol Ther. 2022;24(4):276–80. https://doi.org/10.1089/dia.2021.0426.
19. Hernandez-Jimenez S, Garcia-Ulloa AC, Alcantara-Garces MT, et al. Feasibility and acceptance of a virtual multidisciplinary care programme for patients with type 2 diabetes during the COVID-19 pandemic. Ther Adv Endocrinol Metab. 2021;12:20420188211059882. https://doi.org/10.1177/20420188211059882.
20. Anjana RM, Pradeepa R, Deepa M, et al. Acceptability and utilization of newer technologies and effects on glycemic control in type 2 diabetes: lessons learned from lockdown. Diabetes Technol Ther. 2020;22(7):527–34. https://doi.org/10.1089/dia.2020.0240.
21. Polonsky WH, Layne JE, Parkin CG, et al. Impact of participation in a virtual diabetes clinic on diabetes-related distress in individuals with type 2 diabetes. Clin Diabetes. 2020;38(4):357–62. https://doi.org/10.2337/cd19-0105.
22. Garg SK, Rodbard D, Hirsch IB, Forlenza GP. Managing new-onset type 1 diabetes during the COVID-19 pandemic: challenges and opportunities. Diabetes Technol Ther. 2020;22(6):431–9. https://doi.org/10.1089/dia.2020.0161.
23. Carlson AL, Martens TW, Johnson L, Criego AB. Continuous glucose monitoring integration for remote diabetes management: virtual diabetes care with case studies. Diabetes Technol Ther. 2021;23(S3):S56–65. https://doi.org/10.1089/dia.2021.0241.
24. American Diabetes Association Professional Practice Committee, Draznin B, Aroda VR, et al. 7. Diabetes technology: standards of medical care in diabetes-2022. Diabetes Care. 2022;45(Suppl 1):S97–S112. https://doi.org/10.2337/dc22-S007.
25. Battelino T, Danne T, Bergenstal RM, et al. Clinical targets for continuous glucose monitoring data interpretation: recommendations from the international consensus on time in range. Diabetes Care. 2019;42(8):1593–603. https://doi.org/10.2337/dci19-0028.
26. Szmuilowicz ED, Aleppo G. Stepwise approach to continuous glucose monitoring interpretation for internists and family physicians. Postgrad Med. 2022; https://doi.org/10.1080/0032548 1.2022.2110507.
27. Aleppo G. Clinical application of time in range and other metrics. Diabetes Spectr. 2021;34(2):109–18. https://doi.org/10.2337/ds20-0093.

28. Forlenza GP, Carlson AL, Galindo RJ, Kruger DF, Levy CJ, McGill JB, Umpierrez G, Aleppo G. Real-world evidence supporting tandem control-IQ hybrid closed-loop success in the Medicare and Medicaid type 1 and type 2 diabetes populations. Diabetes Technol Ther. 2022; https://doi.org/10.1089/dia.2022.0206.
29. Noor N, Ebekozien O, Levin L, et al. Diabetes technology use for management of type 1 diabetes is associated with fewer adverse COVID-19 outcomes: findings from the T1D exchange COVID-19 surveillance registry. Diabetes Care. 2021;44(8):E160–2. https://doi.org/10.2337/dc21-0074.
30. Longo M, Scappaticcio L, Petrizzo M, et al. Glucose control in home-isolated adults with type 1 diabetes affected by COVID-19 using continuous glucose monitoring. J Endocrinol Investig. 2022;45(2):445–52. https://doi.org/10.1007/s40618-021-01669-3.
31. Garg S, Norman GJ. Impact of COVID-19 on health economics and technology of diabetes care: use cases of real-time continuous glucose monitoring to transform health care during a global pandemic. Diabetes Technol Ther. 2021;23(S1):S15–20. https://doi.org/10.1089/dia.2020.0656.
32. van der Linden J, Welsh JB, Hirsch IB, Garg SK. Real-time continuous glucose monitoring during the coronavirus disease 2019 pandemic and its impact on time in range. Diabetes Technol Ther. 2021;23(S1):S1–7. https://doi.org/10.1089/dia.2020.0649.
33. Prabhu Navis J, Leelarathna L, Mubita W, et al. Impact of COVID-19 lockdown on flash and real-time glucose sensor users with type 1 diabetes in England. Acta Diabetol. 2021;58(2):231–7. https://doi.org/10.1007/s00592-020-01614-5.
34. Bozzetto L, De Angelis R, Calabrese I, Giglio C, Annuzzi G. Clinical outcomes of remote training for advanced diabetes technologies during the COVID-19 pandemic. J Diabetes Sci Technol. 2022;16(1):264–5. https://doi.org/10.1177/19322968211050653.
35. Vigersky RA, Velado K, Zhong A, Agrawal P, Cordero TL. The effectiveness of virtual training on the MiniMed 670G system in people with type 1 diabetes during the COVID-19 pandemic. Diabetes Technol Ther. 2021;23(2):104–9. https://doi.org/10.1089/dia.2020.0234.
36. Pinsker JE, Singh H, McElwee Malloy M, et al. A virtual training program for the tandem t:slim X2 insulin pump: implementation and outcomes. Diabetes Technol Ther. 2021;23(6):467–70. https://doi.org/10.1089/dia.2020.0602.
37. Gomez AM, Henao D, Parra D, et al. Virtual training on the hybrid close loop system in people with type 1 diabetes (T1D) during the COVID-19 pandemic. Diabetes Metab Syndr. 2021;15(1):243–7. https://doi.org/10.1016/j.dsx.2020.12.041.
38. Vinals C, Mesa A, Roca D, et al. Management of glucose profile throughout strict COVID-19 lockdown by patients with type 1 diabetes prone to hypoglycaemia using sensor-augmented pump. Acta Diabetol. 2021;58(3):383–8. https://doi.org/10.1007/s00592-020-01625-2.
39. Forlenza GP, Carlson AL, Galindo RJ, et al. Real-world evidence supporting tandem control-IQ hybrid closed-loop success in the Medicare and Medicaid type 1 and type 2 diabetes populations. Diabetes Technol Ther. 2022; https://doi.org/10.1089/dia.2022.0206.
40. Umpierrez GE, Isaacs SD, Bazargan N, You X, Thaler LM, Kitabchi AE. Hyperglycemia: an independent marker of in-hospital mortality in patients with undiagnosed diabetes. J Clin Endocrinol Metab. 2002;87(3):978–82. https://doi.org/10.1210/jcem.87.3.8341.
41. Pasquel FJ, Umpierrez GE. Individualizing inpatient diabetes management during the coronavirus disease 2019 pandemic. J Diabetes Sci Technol. 2020;14(4):705–7. https://doi.org/10.1177/1932296820923045.
42. Abbott's Freestyle® Libre 14 day system now available in U.S. for hospitalized patients with diabetes during COVID-19 pandemic. https://abbott.mediaroom.com/2020-04-08-Abbotts-FreeStyle-R-Libre-14-Day-System-Now-Available-in-U-S-for-Hospitalized-Patients-with-Diabetes-During-COVID-19-Pandemic. Accessed 30 June 2022.
43. Fact sheet for healthcare providers: use of dexcom continuous glucose monitoring systems during the COVID-19 pandemic. https://www.dexcom.com/hospitalfacts. Accessed 30 June 2022.

44. Schierenbeck F, Franco-Cereceda A, Liska J. Accuracy of 2 different continuous glucose monitoring systems in patients undergoing cardiac surgery. J Diabetes Sci Technol. 2017;11(1):108–16. https://doi.org/10.1177/1932296816651632.
45. Galindo RJ, Migdal AL, Davis GM, et al. Comparison of the FreeStyle libre pro flash continuous glucose monitoring (CGM) system and point-of-care capillary glucose testing in hospitalized patients with type 2 diabetes treated with basal-bolus insulin regimen. Diabetes Care. 2020;43:2730–5. https://doi.org/10.2337/dc19-2073.
46. Clarke WL, Anderson S, Farhy L, et al. Evaluating the clinical accuracy of two continuous glucose sensors using continuous glucose-error grid analysis. Diabetes Care. 2005;28:2412–7. https://doi.org/10.2337/diacare.28.10.2412.
47. Nair BG, Dellinger EP, Flum DR, Rooke GA, Hirsch IB. A pilot study of the feasibility and accuracy of inpatient continuous glucose monitoring. Diabetes Care. 2020;43:e168–9. https://doi.org/10.2337/dc20-0670.
48. Davis GM, Spanakis EK, Migdal AL, et al. Accuracy of Dexcom G6 continuous glucose monitoring in non-critically ill hospitalized patients with diabetes. Diabetes Care. 2021;44(7):1641–6. https://doi.org/10.2337/dc20-2856.
49. Longo RR, Elias H, Khan M, Seley JJ. Use and accuracy of inpatient CGM during the COVID-19 pandemic: an observational study of general medicine and ICU patients. J Diabetes Sci Technol. 2021:19322968211008446. https://doi.org/10.1177/19322968211008446.
50. U.S. Food and Drug Administration. Coronavirus (COVID-19) Update: FDA allows expanded use of devices to monitor patients' vital signs remotely. https://www.fda.gov/news-events/press-announcements/coronavirus-covid-19-update-fda-allows-expanded-use-devices-monitor-patients-vital-signs-remotely. Accessed 12 June 2020.
51. U.S. Food and Drug Administration. Coronavirus (COVID-19) Update: FDA allows expanded use of devices to monitor patients' vital signs remotely, 2020. https://www.fda.gov/news-events/press-announcements/coronavirus-covid-19-update-fda-allows-expanded-use-devicesmonitor-patients-vital-signs-remotely. Accessed 12 June 2020.
52. Reutrakul S, Genco M, Salinas H, et al. Feasibility of inpatient continuous glucose monitoring during the COVID-19 pandemic: early experience. Diabetes Care. 2020;43:e137–8. https://doi.org/10.2337/dc20-1503.
53. Fortmann AL, Spierling Bagsic SR, Talavera L, et al. Glucose as the fifth vital sign: a randomized controlled trial of continuous glucose monitoring in a non-ICU hospital setting. Diabetes Care. 2020;43:2873–7. https://doi.org/10.2337/dc20-1016.
54. Agarwal S, Mathew J, Davis GM, et al. Continuous glucose monitoring in the intensive care unit during the COVID-19 pandemic. Diabetes Care. 2021;44(3):847–9. https://doi.org/10.2337/dc20-2219.
55. Klarskov CK, Windum NA, Olsen MT, et al. Telemetric continuous glucose monitoring during the COVID-19 pandemic in isolated hospitalized patients in Denmark: a randomized controlled exploratory trial. Diabetes Technol Ther. 2022;24(2):102–12. https://doi.org/10.1089/dia.2021.0291.
56. Gomez AM, Henao DC, Munoz OM, et al. Glycemic control metrics using flash glucose monitoring and hospital complications in patients with COVID-19. Diabetes Metab Syndr. 2021;15(2):499–503. https://doi.org/10.1016/j.dsx.2021.02.008.
57. Galindo RJ, Aleppo G, Klonoff DC, et al. Implementation of continuous glucose monitoring in the hospital: emergent considerations for remote glucose monitoring during the COVID-19 pandemic. J Diabetes Sci Technol. 2020;14(4):822–32. https://doi.org/10.1177/1932296820932903.
58. Jones MS, Goley AL, Alexander BE, Keller SB, Caldwell MM, Buse JB. Inpatient transition to virtual care during COVID-19 pandemic. Diabetes Technol Ther. 2020;22(6):444–8. https://doi.org/10.1089/dia.2020.0206.
59. Monaghan M, Marks B. Personal experiences with COVID-19 and diabetes technology: all for technology yet not technology for all. J Diabetes Sci Technol. 2020;14(4):762–3. https://doi.org/10.1177/1932296820930005.

60. Kerr D, Warshaw H. Clouds and silver linings: COVID-19 pandemic is an opportune moment to democratize diabetes care through telehealth. J Diabetes Sci Technol. 2020;14(6):1107–10. https://doi.org/10.1177/1932296820963630.
61. Holpuch A. US's digital divide 'is going to kill people' as Covid-19 exposes inequalities. https://www.theguardian.com/world/2020/apr/13/coronavirus-covid-19-exposes-cracks-us-digital-divide. Accessed 24 May 2022.
62. Sachs JW, Graven P, Gold JA, Kassakian SZ. Disparities in telephone and video telehealth engagement during the COVID-19 pandemic. JAMIA Open. 2021;4(3):ooab056. https://doi.org/10.1093/jamiaopen/ooab056.
63. Haynes SC, Kompala T, Neinstein A, Rosenthal J, Crossen S. Disparities in telemedicine use for subspecialty diabetes care during COVID-19 shelter-in-place orders. J Diabetes Sci Technol. 2021;15(5):986–92. https://doi.org/10.1177/1932296821997851.
64. Jang M, Johnson CM, D'Eramo-Melkus G, Vorderstrasse AA. Participation of racial and ethnic minorities in technology-based interventions to self-manage type 2 diabetes: a scoping review. J Transcult Nurs. 2018;29(3):292–307. https://doi.org/10.1177/1043659617723074.
65. Czeisler ME, Barrett CE, Siegel KR, et al. Health care access and use among adults with diabetes during the COVID-19 pandemic - United States, February-March 2021. MMWR Morb Mortal Wkly Rep. 2021;70(46):1597–602. https://doi.org/10.15585/mmwr.mm7046a2.

Part IV
Health Outcomes

Chapter 12
COVID-19 Vaccination in Persons with Diabetes: How to Approach Patients

Matthew T. Crow and Erica N. Johnson

Introduction

The syndrome caused by SARS-CoV-2 was designated by the World Health Organization (WHO) in February 2020 as novel coronavirus 2019 (COVID-19). Since that time there has been a global effort to better understand the virus and how to combat it. The symptoms of COVID-19 range from asymptomatic to multi-organ manifestations. Many cases are mild and can be characterized by cough, fever, headache, myalgia, vomiting, diarrhea, and loss of taste and smell. Early in the pandemic, mild cases could transition rapidly to severe illness with respiratory failure requiring ICU care and in the absence of effective therapeutics, could end in death [1, 2]. A more severe disease course can be characterized by organ damage, hypercoagulability, and inflammatory factors [3]. However, vaccination has dramatically altered the trajectory of the disease course. This chapter will discuss further the approach to vaccination among people living with diabetes—a population known to be at increased risk for severe disease courses in the absence of prior immunity to SARS-CoV-2.

M. T. Crow
Department of Medicine, Johns Hopkins Bayview Medical Center, Johns Hopkins University School of Medicine, Baltimore, MD, USA

E. N. Johnson (✉)
Department of Medicine, Division of Infectious Diseases, Johns Hopkins University School of Medicine, Baltimore, MD, USA
e-mail: ejohn144@jhmi.edu

A. K. Myers (ed.), *Diabetes and COVID-19*, Contemporary Endocrinology,
https://doi.org/10.1007/978-3-031-28536-3_12

General Approach to Vaccination

Theoretically, there is an increased risk of acquiring COVID-19 infection in individuals with diabetes as it is well established that in general, patients with diabetes are more at risk for many types of infections [4]. However, it is unclear if diabetes increases the risk of acquiring COVID-19 (see Chap. 3). An early meta-analysis of six studies summarizing the prevalence of cardiovascular diseases and diabetes in 1527 patients with COVID-19 that included 129 patients with diabetes did not find that disease prevalence in patients with diabetes was significantly different from the general population, and although the likelihood of severe disease or disease requiring ICU care was higher, it was not statistically significant [5]. A retrospective chart review in Italy also showed that individuals with diabetes may not be at increased risk of SARS-CoV-2, despite having worsened outcomes [6]. Despite whether there are differences in the risk of developing COVID-19 infection among patients with diabetes, worse prognosis with COVID-19, including higher mortality, has been well established in observational studies in those with diabetes [7]. Thus, people with diabetes have been a priority population for vaccination.

Most of the available COVID-19 vaccines and vaccines still under development target the spike protein expressed on the surface of the virus (Fig. 12.1) [8]. The SARS-CoV-2 virus uses this protein to bind to the angiotensin-converting enzyme 2 (ACE2) receptor on host cells and induces membrane fusion, allowing it to access the host cell [9]. Antibodies can neutralize the virus by binding to the receptor-binding domain of the SARS-CoV-2 spike protein, preventing attachment and entry to the host cell [10]. The available vaccines use a variety of different platforms, both traditional and novel, including inactivated vaccines, vector virus vaccines, recombinant protein vaccines, and mRNA vaccines. Some of the currently available vaccines are addressed in the previous chapter.

Most SARS-CoV-2 vaccines use the spike protein as an antibody target as the immune response to this target is the most protective against the disease [11]. The COVID-19 vaccine induces both innate and adaptive immunity. Adaptive immunity induction results in immunological memory. The process of producing memory involves antibody production by B cells that lead to the production of specific antibodies able to bind to the virus and inhibit viral entry into cells. The degree of immunological memory resulting from vaccination indicates the effectiveness of the vaccine.

At this time, there is limited clinical evidence elucidating the immune response specifically in people with diabetes after COVID-19 vaccination. However, vaccines such as hepatitis B and influenza are recommended for persons with diabetes as they have been shown to be efficacious. A study by Lampasona et al. demonstrated that the antibody response against several SARS-CoV-2 antigens in patients with diabetes showed only marginal differences in timing and titers when compared to individuals without diabetes [12]. The surprising results of this study may have been due to the fact that roughly half of those with diabetes were newly diagnosed at the time of COVID illness. This differed from a study by Karamese et al. which did demonstrate lower antibody levels in participants aged 65 and over with

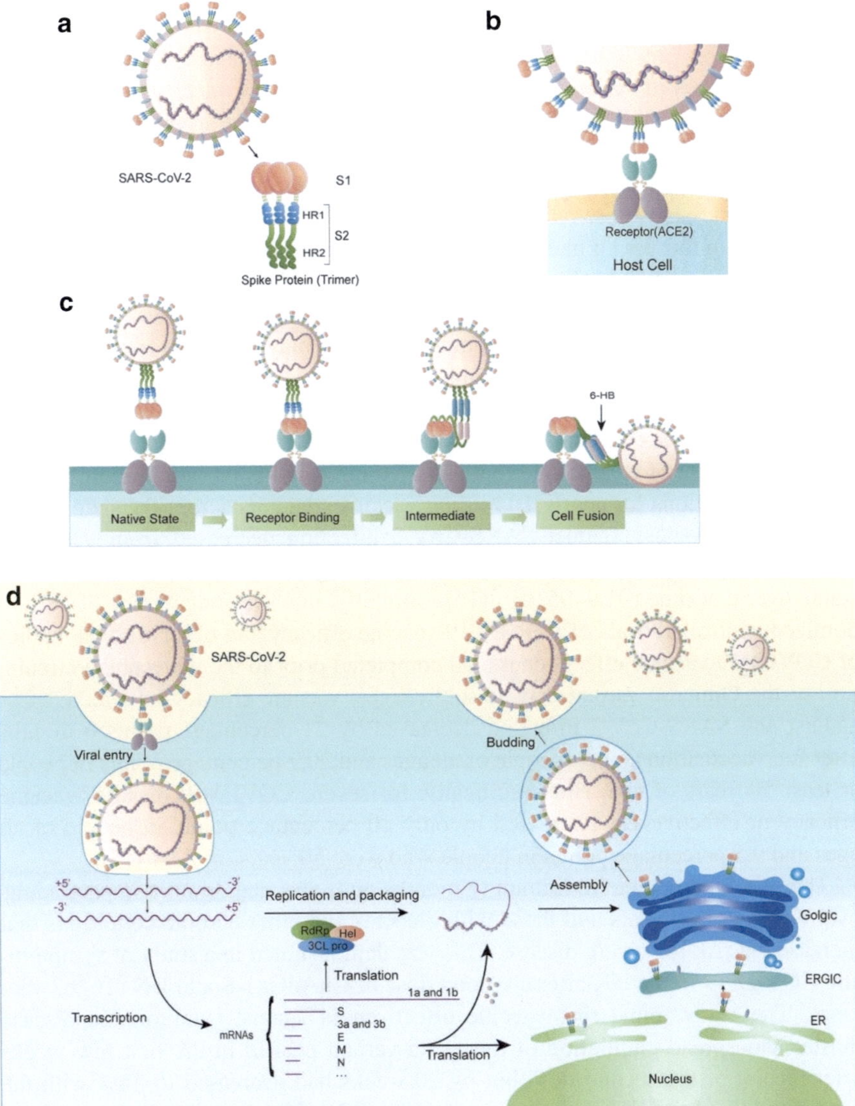

Fig. 12.1 Structure and function of SARS-CoV-2 spike protein [8]. (**a**) The schematic structure of the S protein. (**b**) The S protein binds to the receptor ACE2. (**c**) The binding and virus–cell fusion process mediated by the S protein. (**d**) The life cycle of SARS-CoV-2 in host cells. https://www.nature.com/articles/s41401-020-0485-4

diabetes compared with similarly aged participants without diabetes [13]. Another study showed that while a similar increase in anti-SARS-CoV-2 titers after vaccination was observed in both participants with and without type 1 diabetes (T1D), three-fourths of patients with T1D did not show any increase in the cytotoxic response to SARS-CoV-2 compared to the increase observed in patients without diabetes [14].

Duration of Vaccine Response

Published studies to date suggest that available COVID-19 vaccines remain effective against severe disease, hospitalization, and death but that protection against infection with SARS-CoV-2 wanes in the months following vaccination. This waning immunity was demonstrated in a study in Israel during circulation of the Delta (B.1.617.2) variant, where rates of infection in adults in all age groups in July 2021 were higher in those who had received a second dose of the BNT162b2 vaccine in the month they were first eligible compared with those who had received their second dose two months later, suggesting that immunity had waned after receipt of the second dose of vaccine [15]. The waning immunity may have also been due to the change in the dominant COVID strain from Alpha to Delta.

Despite waning immunity to infection, protection against severe disease and hospitalization after vaccination remains high, as shown in a study utilizing New York State Department of Health data that included information on vaccination, testing, and hospitalizations for nearly 10 million vaccinated adults across the state. While vaccine effectiveness against SARS-CoV-2 infection decreased from 91.7% to 79.8% during May–July 2021, the effectiveness against hospitalization remained stable over that time (91.9–95.3%) [16]. Similarly, in a systemic review of 18 randomized controlled trials of COVID-19 vaccine efficacy and observational studies of COVID-19 vaccine effectiveness, all completed prior to the widespread circulation of the Omicron variant and its sublineages, vaccine efficacy or effectiveness against any SARS-CoV-2 infection decreased by 21 percentage points 6 months after full vaccination among people of all ages and 20.7 percentage points in people at least 50 years of age. But specifically, for severe COVID-19 disease, vaccine efficacy or effectiveness decreased by only 10 percentage points in people of all ages and 9.5 percentage points in people who were 50 years or older [17].

The observed decline in immunity months after vaccination may impact adults over the age of 60 years and those with diabetes and other chronic conditions that increase the risk for severe disease. This was demonstrated in a study of symptomatic COVID-19 in the UK after a second dose of ChAdOx1-S and BNT162b2 vaccines. The study found that vaccine effectiveness against symptomatic disease during widespread circulation of the Delta variant peaked in the first few weeks after receipt of the second dose but by 20 weeks had decreased to 44% with the ChAdOx1-S (Astra-Zeneca) vaccine and 66% with the BNT162b2 (Pfizer, BioNTech) vaccine. Less protection against hospitalization was observed in persons over the age of 65 and those with underlying medical conditions such as diabetes [18].

Nonetheless, infection after vaccination remains less likely to cause severe disease in vaccinated adults than in unvaccinated adults. A study of over 1.2 million vaccinated adults from 465 facilities in the United States showed that rates of severe COVID-19 (0.00015%) or death (0.000033%) were extremely rare. Risk factors for severe outcomes included age $\geq$ 65 years, immunosuppressed status, or one of six other chronic conditions (chronic kidney, cardiac, pulmonary, neurologic, and liver disease) including diabetes mellitus. All cases of severe COVID-19 and all deaths occurred in participants who had at least one of these risk factors [19].

Additional attenuation in the effectiveness of COVID-19 vaccines against symptomatic infection while remaining highly effective against severe disease and hospitalization has been observed since the widespread circulation of the Omicron variant and its sublineages, including BA.1, BA.2, BA.2.12.1, BA.4, and BA.5. This seems to be due to the ability of the Omicron variant and other variants of concern to escape immune responses induced by vaccination, although the timing of vaccination relative to exposure and number of doses also seems to play a role. Data from ten states in the United States as part of the VISION Network showed that vaccine effectiveness after the third dose of mRNA vaccine in preventing emergency department and urgent care visits due to COVID-19 during the period when early Omicron sublineages were circulating was 82% and prevention against hospitalization was 90%, compared with 94% vaccine effectiveness observed for preventing emergency department visits, urgent care visits, and hospitalizations during the period when the Delta variant predominated [20].

This waning immunity over time forms the basis for recommendations of booster vaccination, and available data suggest that booster vaccination does improve the effectiveness of protection against SARS-CoV-2, although the duration of this effect is not known. The efficacy of a BNT162b2 (Pfizer–BioNTech) booster in preventing symptomatic COVID-19 among clinical trial participants who never had COVID-19 and completed a primary series of the same vaccine at least 6 months prior was 95% with a median of 2.5 months of follow-up when Delta was the dominant strain [21].

Bivalent boosters began to be deployed by some countries starting in August 2022 and may offer additional protection over monovalent vaccine boosters. Bivalent boosters, the earliest of which encode both the spike protein of the original SARS-CoV-2 strain as well as that of one of the Omicron sublineages, are designed to improve waning immunity and reduce the potential for immune escape observed since the emergence of the Omicron variant and other variants of concern. In the fall of 2022, the US Food and Drug Administration (FDA) approved and the ACIP recommended bivalent mRNA booster vaccines encoding the spike protein of the Wuhan strain of SARS-CoV-2 and that of BA.4/BA.5 in people ages 5 and older who had completed a primary vaccine series at least two months prior [22–24]. Additionally, the FDA later authorized the bivalent mRNA booster for children as young as 6 months [25, 26].

The Impact of COVID-19 on Hospitalizations and Mortality

It is now well established that people with diabetes may have a worse clinical prognosis with COVID-19 [7]. One of the factors predisposing people with diabetes to severe COVID-19 is a chronic inflammatory state [3]. Individuals with diabetes are known to be prothrombotic at baseline. Endothelial injury from coronavirus can further increase the risk of thrombosis by activation of platelet and coagulation pathways [27, 28].

Additionally, the expression of ACE2 decreases after endocytosis of SARS-CoV-2 which affects pancreatic beta cell function and may play a role in worsened hyperglycemia, resulting in diabetic ketoacidosis or hyperosmolarity [27–29]. A paper in 2006 noted that hyperglycemia and diabetes were independent predictors of higher morbidity and mortality in patients with SARS [30]. Additionally, cases of new-onset diabetes have been reported to be associated with COVID-19 [27, 28].

Because diabetes mellitus disproportionately affects certain groups, and similarly COVID-19 has been demonstrated to have a greater impact on certain groups due to social and structural factors, the dual impact of diabetes and COVID-19 is not equally distributed. A study in England found that in persons with both type 1 and 2 diabetes (T2D), there was significantly higher mortality in people of Black and Asian race in comparison to those who identify as white; it was also noted to be higher for individuals reporting mixed ethnicity. The association with T2DM and mortality was higher in Black males compared to Black females [29]. However, an analysis of an urban cohort of over 4400 patients in the United States did not show increased mortality associated with race or ethnicity, although male gender and older age were associated [30]. Another study demonstrated that young people with diabetes have a higher excess relative mortality risk when compared to older individuals with diabetes as younger individuals are disproportionately impacted in terms of life years lost and can be at higher risk of exposure from being part of the workforce but agreed with other previous studies that there is a higher absolute risk of mortality in the elderly [31].

Early in the pandemic, the prioritization of groups to receive the vaccine was an issue as there was a limited supply [32]. Making recommendations for patients with diabetes was complicated by the fact that many early studies did not distinguish the risk between T1D and T2D [32]. However, there was some evidence that patients with T1D and T2D had a similarly higher risk of hospitalization [33] and death relative to those without diabetes [34]. One study reported increased rates of hospitalization in persons with T1D associated with a median Hemoglobin A1c (HbA1c) of 8.6% [35]. Another study in England found that in-hospital related deaths related to COVID-19 were higher in T1D [OR 2.86 (2.58–3.18)] over T2D when compared to those without diabetes [OR 1.80 (1.75–1.86)] [34]. Conversely, another study found individuals with T1D had less severe outcomes than those with T2D—although this might be because the T1D group on average was a younger population [36]. Another article concluded that there was no apparent difference in severity or mortality in SARS-CoV-2 infections between patients with T1D and T2D [37]. However, hyperglycemia in the setting of diabetes did not affect the quantity and durability of neutralizing antibodies against SARS-CoV-2 [38]. All of these observations have led many societies, including the Advisory Committee on Immunization Practices in the Centers for Disease Control and the WHO, as well as diabetes specialty societies such as the American Diabetes Association and Korean Diabetes Association, to recommend COVID-19 vaccination to patients with diabetes to reduce their risk of infection and severe disease [39–42]. The European Society of Endocrinology released a statement that patients with stable endocrine disorders should follow the same recommendations as the general population, stressing the recommendation for patients with both T1D and T2D [43].

Hospitalizations and Mortality in Pregnant Persons with Diabetes

COVID-19 has also been noted to contribute to unfavorable pregnancy course in women with diabetes. In severe COVID-19 infections in pregnancy, diabetes is one of the most common underlying conditions [44]. The full impact of vaccination in pregnant women with diabetes is unclear. For example, in a study of pregnant women with diabetes, pre-pregnancy diabetes mellitus was significantly associated with higher antenatal vaccine uptake, although pregnant women who had received at least one dose of vaccine experienced similar rates of adverse pregnancy outcomes, including stillbirth, fetal abnormalities, postpartum hemorrhage, cesarean delivery, small for gestational age, maternal intensive care admission, or neonatal intensive care unit admission compared with unvaccinated women [45]. Still, the abundance of evidence suggests that pregnant people with diabetes should be counseled about the benefit of COVID-19 vaccination to prevent SAR-CoV-2 infection during pregnancy, and these discussions should also be included in pre-pregnancy planning. While pregnant and lactating people were not included in initial vaccine trials, data from vaccinated pregnant and lactating people since demonstrates the safety of vaccination relative to the risks of infection, and breastfeeding does not need to be interrupted during vaccination [44].

Reasons for Vaccine Hesitancy and Strategies for Increasing Vaccine Confidence

Vaccine hesitancy is a complex issue that predates the COVID-19 pandemic and was identified by the WHO in 2019 as one of the top ten global health threats [46]. It is defined as a delay in acceptance or refusal of vaccination despite the availability of vaccination services [47]. Delays in intention to accept vaccination and ongoing refusal of vaccination represent significant challenges to achieving the full potential of vaccines to substantially control the transmission of SARS-CoV-2 and prevent the development of new variants. But the factors associated with vaccine hesitancy are multi-layered and complex as are the attitudes associated with higher rates of vaccine acceptance. A comprehensive approach to understanding population-specific reasons for skepticism about vaccines and addressing those reasons using evidence-based strategies is needed.

One study characterized varying levels of vaccine intent related to a broad range of sentiments to COVID-19 vaccination, with the lowest acceptance among those who held the sentiment of resistance due to firmly held beliefs such as the speed of vaccine production; prior adverse experiences with vaccination and skepticism about the severity of COVID-19; and those influenced by misinformation from myths, misconceptions, and falsehoods about the vaccine. However, higher levels of acceptance were seen in those who adopted a "wait and see" approach to gather more information from scientific data and the experiences of vaccine recipients, and readiness was observed in those who were already comfortable with accepting vaccination and endorsed willingness to share their experience with others [48]. Viewing vaccine-related intent as a continuum is a key step to understanding barriers to vaccine confidence and ultimately inequities in vaccine access and utilization.

One of the issues that has exacerbated COVID-19 vaccine hesitancy is the concept of an infodemic, which the WHO describes as the availability of too much information, including false or misleading information, during a disease outbreak [49]. Digital environments in particular allow for false information to be easily disseminated broadly to the general population as well as targeted to specific populations. This misinformation and disinformation can create confusion, sow mistrust in health authorities and institutions, and lead to attitudes and behaviors that can harm health [49]. A randomized controlled study conducted in the United States and the United Kingdom to measure the impact of exposure to online misinformation around COVID-19 vaccines on the intent to vaccinate prior to their widespread availability showed that exposure to misinformation about the vaccine resulted in a reduction of 6.2 percentage points in the United Kingdom and 6.4 in the United States among those who stated that they would definitely accept a vaccine compared with a control group who was shown scientifically accurate information about the vaccine [50]. Differences in exposure to certain media and online social networks can lead to political polarization of attitudes about vaccination. A US study analyzing changes in vaccine attitudes via online survey over the course of the COVID-19 pandemic found a decrease in the intention to receive a COVID-19 vaccine when one becomes available that was driven by participants who self-identified as Republicans and showed a negative trend in vaccine attitudes and intentions, whereas vaccine intention in participants who identified as Democrats remained largely stable [51].

In minoritized communities of color in the United States, particularly Black, Indigenous, and immigrant communities, the historical legacy of involuntary exploitative treatment and experimentation by the medical community as well as sometimes insufficient access to quality health care have led to mistrust of government and health-care institutions [48]. A cross-sectional survey of over 2500 US respondents showed that those reporting a past experience with racial discrimination had 21% increased odds of a higher level of COVID-19 vaccine hesitancy compared to those who did not report such an experience [52]. Additional reluctance about vaccination in minoritized communities stems from safety concerns about vaccine development and vaccine adverse effects and concerns that the vaccine development process did not take their needs into account [53]. Some immigrants may face barriers related to general vaccine knowledge and awareness and how to navigate the health system [54] and some undocumented immigrants may be reluctant to receive vaccination in order to avoid encounters with immigration authorities [55].

Vaccine hesitancy has also been observed in rural communities across the United States. A survey of 1000 adults in Tennessee focusing on beliefs about barriers to vaccination found that 54% indicated some hesitancy about COVID-19 vaccination; lack of evidence of vaccine effectiveness was cited as the leading reason for hesitancy, although fear of vaccination, conspiracy theories about vaccination, the influence of misinformation and disinformation, lower health literacy, and distrust in the medical establishment were all reasons for vaccine hesitancy [56]. Some rural communities may be particularly prone to targeted misinformation as they may be more likely to adapt to fear and conspiracy theories and have lower health literacy and vaccine awareness [55].

Vaccine acceptance around the world also varies widely. A study in Italy found that patients with chronic diseases were less willing to vaccinate and highly concerned about the side effects of vaccines [57]. But individuals with chronic conditions were found to have a relatively high willingness to receive a COVID vaccine in the United States, Canada, Uganda, and several European countries [58, 59].

One study noted that individuals who had received the influenza vaccine were 2.2 times more willing to receive a COVID-19 vaccine [58]. This protective factor was noted in several other countries including the United States, Canada, and several countries in Europe. Additionally, a study in Italy found that individuals who were less adherent with medical prescriptions and/or less concerned for their health had higher hesitancy [57]. These findings seem to suggest that individuals who maintain higher concerns about their health in general were more likely to receive COVID vaccinations.

In a study in Bangladesh, individuals with lower literacy were noted to have higher hesitancy, while a study in Oman found that individuals with low literacy were more willing to be vaccinated [60, 61]. A study in India found that lack of clarity about the vaccine was a detrimental factor in individuals with hesitance and/or resistance [62].

Vaccine Attitudes and Behaviors in People with Diabetes

A study in Oman found that individuals with diabetes were more likely to get vaccinated compared to patients with other chronic diseases [61]. This was theorized to be related to people with diabetes recognizing that they were at high risk for developing severe complications from COVID-19.

In contrast, a study in Malaysia found that individuals with diabetes were more hesitant to accept the vaccine [63]. Though vaccine hesitancy is not specific to diabetes, this study discussed that vaccine hesitancy was largely due to the perceived risk of vaccination as well as the perception that COVID-19 was not dangerous, religious reasons, belief in traditional remedies, fear of injection, and other cultural reasons.

A study in Bangladesh also reported that vaccine hesitancy was high in people with chronic disease (including diabetes) with an acceptance of 68.7% compared to 77.4% in those without chronic disease. The prevalence of vaccine acceptance in this study mirrored results from France, Denmark, Australia, Mexico, India, and Ireland. However, studies from China, Indonesia, Ecuador, and Brazil showed a higher prevalence of COVID-19 vaccine acceptance. The study also found that location of residence in Bangladesh (impoverished areas, semi-urban, rural), occupation, marital status, and confidence in the country's health-care system were also associated factors for vaccine unwillingness among the Bangladeshi population. The study suggests the hesitancy may be attributed to socioeconomic disadvantage and lack of knowledge about COVID-19 leading to low-risk perception for COVID-19. It was also pointed out in this study that rural areas in the United States had higher rates of vaccine hesitancy [60].

Strategies to Address Vaccine Skepticism and Build Vaccine Confidence

Because the health consequences of not vaccinating against COVID-19 are high, effective, evidence-based strategies must be employed to address vaccine hesitancy and build vaccine confidence. This requires the implementation of best practices at the organizational, interpersonal, and individual levels that have been developed and refined from experiences with previous vaccines [64].

First, it is necessary to remove access barriers to vaccination. This requires policy-level interventions, such as reducing out-of-pocket expenses for patients and requiring vaccination for child care and school and college attendance. Communities can also reduce barriers by offering vaccination programs in schools, child care centers, and through other community-based programs [64]. Professional organizations can help support these local, regional, and national efforts through engagement in advocacy.

Communication strategies that involve engaging trusted messengers have been demonstrated to help build vaccine confidence. In one study, perceived social norms correlated with vaccine intention, with participants who believed that "people close to you" wanting them to get vaccinated were more willing to get vaccinated [65]. Faith or community leaders are often viewed as trusted messengers in some marginalized communities and are an important part of educating individuals about vaccines to influence vaccine confidence. Health-care workers and medical experts can be the trusted messengers themselves, particularly when individuals perceive common identities and values, so engaging health-care workers from marginalized communities may be an effective strategy [48]. Also, in one study, highlighting common religious identity with medical experts led to increased vaccination intent in a population of unvaccinated Christian participants [66].

A comprehensive communication strategy also involves clear and transparent public health messaging on the safety and efficacy of COVID-19 vaccination and how historical and contemporary factors influence perceptions of the pandemic. This includes acknowledging forces such as structural racism and other types of discrimination as understandable reasons for the low acceptance of COVID-19 vaccines [65]. For example, in one study, an explanation of the FDA's vaccine approval process and an acknowledgment of the economic impacts of the pandemic increased participants' acceptance of vaccines [67].

Just as misinformation about COVID-19 has been targeted, vaccine education for specific populations can also be adapted to address identified needs more effectively. Events sponsored by trusted community leaders and local medical experts can provide comprehensive outreach to communities and engage community members in conversations that address their questions about COVID-19 vaccination, and surveys and interviews of local community members can help identify barriers to vaccine acceptance [55].

Adequate preparation of clinicians for conversations with patients about COVID-19 vaccination is also important. In one survey, respondents indicated a greater likelihood of accepting the COVID-19 vaccine if recommended by their clinician [68]. The CDC recommends clinicians use skills grounded in motivational interviewing in having conversations with patients at various levels of vaccine acceptance to positively influence their willingness to further consider vaccination [69].

More research is needed to better understand the complexity of vaccine hesitancy and to develop approaches to build vaccine confidence. However, making use of strategies that operate at multiple levels of influence and engaging stakeholders broadly will be most effective in building vaccine confidence [64].

Conclusion

Both pregnant and non-pregnant persons with diabetes are at increased risk for COVID-19-related morbidity, but vaccination is an effective strategy for preventing severe illness and complications. Ensuring persons living with diabetes are protected is necessary for success in managing the COVID-19 pandemic. This requires understanding barriers to vaccine intent and strengthening vaccine confidence.

References

1. Giacomelli A, Pezzati L, Conti F, Bernacchia D, Siano M, Oreni L, et al. Self-reported olfactory and taste disorders in patients with severe acute respiratory coronavirus 2 infection: a cross-sectional study. Clin Infect Dis. 2020;71(15):889–90.
2. Wang D, Hu B, Hu C, Zhu F, Liu X, Zhang J, et al. Clinical characteristics of 138 hospitalized patients with 2019 novel coronavirus-infected pneumonia in Wuhan, China. JAMA. 2020;323(11):1061–9.
3. Bashir S, Alabdulkarim N, Altwaijri N, Alhaidri N, Hashim R, Nasim E, et al. The battle against the COVID-19 pandemic—a perspective from Saudi Arabia. One Health. 2021;12:100229.
4. Casqueiro J, Casqueiro J, Alves C. Infections in patients with diabetes mellitus: a review of pathogenesis. Indian J Endocrinol Metab. 2012;16(Suppl 1):S27–36.
5. Li B, Yang J, Zhao F, Zhi L, Wang X, Liu L, et al. Prevalence and impact of cardiovascular metabolic diseases on COVID-19 in China. Clin Res Cardiol. 2020;109(5):531–8.
6. Fadini GP, Morieri ML, Longato E, Avogaro A. Prevalence and impact of diabetes among people infected with SARS-CoV-2. J Endocrinol Invest. 2020;43(6):867–9.
7. Huang I, Lim MA, Pranata R. Diabetes mellitus is associated with increased mortality and severity of disease in COVID-19 pneumonia – a systematic review, meta-analysis, and meta-regression. Diabetes Metab Syndr. 2020;14(4):395–403.
8. Huang Y, Yang C, Xu X, Liu SW. Structural and functional properties of SARS-CoV-2 spike protein: potential antivirus drug development for COVID-19. Acta Pharmacologica Sinica. 2020;3(41):1141–9.
9. Zhou P, Yang XL, Wang XG, Hu B, Zhang L, Zhang W, et al. A pneumonia outbreak associated with a new coronavirus of probable bat origin. Nature. 2020;579(7798):270–3.
10. Krammer F. SARS-CoV-2 vaccines in development. Nature. 2020;586(7830):516–27.
11. Alqassieh R, Suleiman A, Abu-Halaweh S, Santarisi A, Shatnawi O, Shdaifat L, et al. Pfizer-BioNTech and Sinopharm: a comparative study on post-vaccination antibody titers. Vaccines (Basel). 2021;9(11):1223.
12. Lampasona V, Secchi M, Scavini M, Bazzigaluppi E, Brigatti C, Marzinotto I, et al. Antibody response to multiple antigens of SARS-CoV-2 in patients with diabetes: an observational cohort study. Diabetologia. 2020;63(12):2548–58.
13. Karamese M, Tutuncu EE. The effectiveness of inactivated SARS-CoV-2 vaccine (CoronaVac) on antibody response in participants aged 65 years and older. J Med Virol. 2022;94(1):173–7.
14. D'Addio F, Sabiu G, Usuelli V, Assi E, Abdelsalam A, Maestroni A, et al. Immunogenicity and safety of SARS-CoV-2 mRNA vaccines in a cohort of patients with type 1 diabetes. Diabetes. 2022;71(8):1800–6.
15. Goldberg Y, Mandel M, Bar-On YM, Bodenheimer O, Freedman L, Haas EJ, et al. Waning immunity after the BNT162b2 vaccine in Israel. N Engl J Med. 2021;385(24):e85.
16. Rosenberg ES, Holtgrave DR, Dorabawila V, Conroy M, Greene D, Lutterloh E, et al. New COVID-19 cases and hospitalizations among adults, by vaccination status - New York, May 3-July 25, 2021. MMWR Morb Mortal Wkly Rep. 2021;70(34):1150–5.
17. Feikin DR, Higdon MM, Abu-Raddad LJ, Andrews N, Araos R, Goldberg Y, et al. Duration of effectiveness of vaccines against SARS-CoV-2 infection and COVID-19 disease: results of a systematic review and meta-regression. Lancet. 2022;399(10328):924–44.
18. Andrews N, Tessier E, Stowe J, Gower C, Kirsebom F, Simmons R, et al. Duration of protection against mild and severe disease by Covid-19 vaccines. N Engl J Med. 2022;386(4):340–50.
19. Yek C, Warner S, Wiltz JL, Sun J, Adjei S, Mancera A, et al. Risk Factors for severe COVID-19 outcomes among persons who completed primary COVID-19 vaccination series. MMWR Morb Mortal Wkly Rep. 2022;71(1):19–25.
20. Thompson MG, Natarajan K, Irving SA, Rowley EA, Griggs EP, Gaglani M, et al. Effectiveness of a third dose of mRNA vaccines against COVID-19-associated emergency department and urgent care encounters and hospitalizations among adults during periods of Delta and Omicron

variant predominance - VISION Network, 10 states, August 2021-January 2022. MMWR Morb Mortal Wkly Rep. 2022;71(4):139–45.

21. Moreira ED Jr, Kitchin N, Xu X, Dychter SS, Lockhart S, Gurtman A, et al. Safety and efficacy of a third dose of BNT162b2 Covid-19 vaccine. N Engl J Med. 2022;386(20):1910–21.

22. CDC recommends the first updated COVID-19 booster; 1 Sep 2022. https://www.cdc.gov/media/releases/2022/s0901-covid-19-booster.html. Accessed 9 Sep 2022.

23. Interim clinical considerations for COVID-19 vaccines: bivalent boosters. ACIP; 1 Sep 2022. https://www.cdc.gov/vaccines/acip/meetings/downloads/slides-2022-09-01/09-covid-hall-508.pdf. Accessed 9 Sep 2022.

24. Rosenblum HG, Wallace M, Godfrey M, Roper LE, Hall E, Fleming-Dutra KE, et al. Interim recommendations from the advisory committee on immunization practices for the use of bivalent booster doses of COVID-19 vaccines—United States, October 2022. MMWR Morb Mortal Wkly Rep. 2022;71(45):1436–41.

25. Coronavirus (COVID-19) update: FDA authorizes updated (bivalent) covid-19 vaccines for children down to 6 months of age; 8 Dec 2022. https://www.fda.gov/news-events/press-announcements/coronavirus-covid-19-update-fda-authorizes-updated-bivalent-covid-19-vaccines-children-down-6-months. Accessed 29 Dec 2022.

26. Puig-Domingo M, Marazuela M, Yildiz BO, Giustina A. COVID-19 and endocrine and metabolic diseases. An updated statement from the European Society of Endocrinology. Endocrine. 2021;72(2):301–16.

27. Rao GHR. Twindemic of coronavirus disease (COVID-19) and cardiometabolic diseases. Int J Biomedicine. 2021;11(2):111–22.

28. Yang JK, Feng Y, Yuan MY, Yuan SY, Fu HJ, Wu BY, et al. Plasma glucose levels and diabetes are independent predictors for mortality and morbidity in patients with SARS. Diabet Med. 2006;23(6):623–8.

29. Holman N, Knighton P, Kar P, O'Keefe J, Curley M, Weaver A, et al. Risk factors for COVID-19-related mortality in people with type 1 and type 2 diabetes in England: a population-based cohort study. Lancet Diabetes Endocrinol. 2020;8(10):823–33.

30. Myers AK, Kim TS, Zhu X, Liu Y, Qiu M, Pekmezaris R. Predictors of mortality in a multiracial urban cohort of persons with type 2 diabetes and novel coronavirus 19. J Diabetes. 2021;13(5):430–8.

31. McGovern AP, Thomas NJ, Vollmer SJ, Hattersley AT, Mateen BA, Dennis JM. The disproportionate excess mortality risk of COVID-19 in younger people with diabetes warrants vaccination prioritization. Diabetologia. 2021;64(5):1184–6.

32. Powers AC, Aronoff DM, Eckel RH. COVID-19 vaccine prioritisation for type 1 and type 2 diabetes. Lancet Diabetes Endocrinol. 2021;9(3):140–1.

33. Gregory JM, Slaughter JC, Duffus SH, Smith TJ, LeStourgeon LM, Jaser SS, et al. COVID-19 severity is tripled in the diabetes community: a prospective analysis of the pandemic's impact in type 1 and type 2 diabetes. Diabetes Care. 2021;44(2):526–32.

34. Barron E, Bakhai C, Kar P, Weaver A, Bradley D, Ismail H, et al. Associations of type 1 and type 2 diabetes with COVID-19-related mortality in England: a whole-population study. Lancet Diabetes Endocrinol. 2020;8(10):813–22.

35. O'Malley G, Ebekozien O, Desimone M, Pinnaro CT, Roberts A, Polsky S, et al. COVID-19 hospitalization in adults with type 1 diabetes: results from the T1D exchange multicenter surveillance study. J Clin Endocrinol Metab. 2021;106(2):e936–42.

36. Wargny M, Gourdy P, Ludwig L, Seret-Bégué D, Bourron O, Darmon P, et al. Type 1 diabetes in people hospitalized for COVID-19: new insights from the CORONADO study. Diabetes Care. 2020;43(11):e174–7.

37. Afshar ZM, Babazadeh A, Janbakhsh A, Mansouri F, Sio TT, Sullman MJM, et al. Coronavirus disease 2019 (Covid-19) vaccination recommendations in special populations and patients with existing comorbidities. Rev Med Virol. 2021;22:e2309.

38. Dispinseri S, Lampasona V, Secchi M, Cara A, Bazzigaluppi E, Negri D, et al. Robust neutralizing antibodies to SARS-CoV-2 develop and persist in subjects with diabetes and COVID-19 pneumonia. J Clin Endocrinol Metab. 2021;106(5):1472–81.
39. Dooling K, Marin M, Wallace M, McClung N, Chamberland M, Lee GM, et al. The advisory Committee on Immunization practices' updated interim recommendation for allocation of COVID-19 vaccine—United States, December 2020. MMWR Morb Mortal Wkly Rep. 2021;69:1657–60.
40. World Health Organization. WHO SAGE roadmap for prioritizing use of COVID-19 vaccines; 21 Jan 2022. https://www.who.int/publications/i/item/WHO-2019-nCoV-Vaccines-SAGE-Prioritization-2022.1. Accessed 29 Dec 2022.
41. American Diabetes Association applauds CDC decision to prioritize all people with diabetes for the COVID-19 vaccine; 30 Mar 2021. https://diabetes.org/official-statements/2021/ADA-applauds-CDC-decision-to-prioritize-all-pwd-for-covid-19-vaccine. Accessed 29 Dec 2022.
42. Hur KY, Moon MK, Park JS, Kim SK, Lee SH, Yun JS, Committee of Clinical Practice Guidelines, Korean Diabetes Association, et al. 2021 clinical practice guidelines for diabetes mellitus of the Korean Diabetes Association. Diabetes Metab J. 2021;45(4):461–81.
43. European Society of Endocrinology (ESE)'s statement concerning COVID-19 vaccination: 'follow the same recommendations for patients with stable endocrine disorders as for the general population'; February 2021. https://www.ese-hormones.org/news/ese-news/european-society-of-endocrinology-ese-s-statement-concerning-covid-19-vaccination-follow-the-same-recommendations-for-patients-with-stable-endocrine-disorders-as-for-the-general-population/. Accessed 15 Feb 2022.
44. Sculli MA, Formoso G, Sciacca L. COVID-19 vaccination in pregnant and lactating diabetic women. Nutr Metab Cardiovasc Dis. 2021;31(7):2151–5.
45. Blakeway H, Prasad S, Kalafat E, Heath PT, Ladhani SN, Le Doare K, et al. COVID-19 vaccination during pregnancy: coverage and safety. Am J Obstet Gynecol. 2022;226(2):236.e1–236.e14.
46. World Health Organization. Ten threats to global health in 2019. https://www.who.int/news-room/spotlight/ten-threats-to-global-health-in-2019. Accessed 7 Sep 2022.
47. MacDonald NE and the SAGE Working Group on Vaccine Hesitancy. Vaccine hesitancy: definition, scope and determinants. Vaccine. 2015;33(34):4161–4.
48. Marcelin JR, Swartz TH, Bernice F, Berthaud V, Christian R, da Costa C, et al. Addressing and inspiring vaccine confidence in Black, Indigenous and People of Color during the Coronavirus Disease 2019 pandemic. Open Forum Infect Dis. 2021;8(9):ofab417.
49. World Health Organization. Infodemic. https://www.who.int/health-topics/infodemic#tab=tab_1. Accessed 7 Sep 2022.
50. Loomba S, de Figueiredo A, Piatek SJ, de Graaf K, Larson HJ. Measuring the impact of COVID-19 vaccine misinformation on vaccination intent in the UK and USA. Nat Hum Behav. 2021;5(3):337–48.
51. Fridman A, Gershon R, Gneezy A. COVID-19 and vaccine hesitancy: a longitudinal study. PLoS One. 2021;16(4):e0250123.
52. Savoia E, Piltch-Loeb R, Goldberg B, Miller-Idriss C, Hughes B, Montrond A, et al. Predictors of COVID-19 vaccine hesitancy: socio-demographics, co-morbidity, and past experience of racial discrimination. Vaccines. 2021;9(7):767.
53. Hamel L, Lopes L, Muñana, C, Artiga S, Brodie M. Kaiser Family Foundation (KFF). Race, health and COVID-19: the views and experiences of Black Americans. Key findings from the KFF/undefeated survey on race and health. https://files.kff.org/attachment/Report-Race-Health-and-COVID-19-The-Views-and-Experiences-of-Black-Americans.pdf. Accessed 9 Sep 2022.
54. Painter JE, Viana De O, Mesquita S, Jimenez L, Avila AA, Sutter CJ, Sutter R. Vaccine-related attitudes and decision-making among uninsured, Latin American immigrant mothers of adolescent daughters: a qualitative study. Hum Vaccin Immunother. 2019;15(1):121–33.

55. Hildreth JEK, Alcendor DJ. Targeting COVID-19 Vaccine Hesitancy in Minority Populations in the US: Implications for Herd Immunity. Vaccines (Basel). 2021;9(5):489.
56. Gatwood J, McKnight M, Fiscus M, Hohmeier KC, Chisholm-Burns M. Factors influencing likelihood of COVID-19 vaccination: a survey of Tennessee adults. Am J Health Syst Pharm. 2021;78(10):879–89.
57. Scoccimarro D, Panichi L, Ragghianti B, et al. Sars-CoV2 vaccine hesitancy in Italy: a survey on subjects with diabetes. Nutr Metab Cardiovasc Dis. 2021;31(11):3243–6.
58. Al-Hanawi MK, Ahmad K, Haque R. Willingness to receive COVID-19 vaccination among adults with chronic diseases in the Kingdom of Saudi Arabia. J Infect Public Health. 2021;14(10):1489–96.
59. Bongomin F, Olum R, Andia-Biraro I, et al. COVID-19 vaccine acceptance among high-risk populations in Uganda. Ther Adv Infect Dis. 2021;9(8):20499361211024376.
60. Abedin M, Islam MA, Rahman FN, Reza HM, Hossain MZ, Hossain MA, et al. Willingness to vaccinate against COVID-19 among Bangladeshi adults: Understanding the strategies to optimize vaccination coverage. PLoS One. 2021;16(4):e0250495.
61. Al-Marshoudi S, Al-Balushi H, Al-Wahaibi A, et al. Knowledge, attitudes, and practices (Kap) toward the covid-19 vaccine in Oman: a pre-campaign cross-sectional study. Vaccines (Basel). 2021;9(6):602.
62. Umakanthan S, Patil S, Subramaniam N, et al. COVID-19 vaccine hesitancy and resistance in India explored through a population-based longitudinal survey. Vaccines (Basel). 2021;9(10):1064.
63. Syed Alwi SAR, Rafidah E, Zurraini A, Juslina O, Brohi IB, Lukas S. A survey on COVID-19 vaccine acceptance and concern among Malaysians. BMC Public Health. 2021;21(1):1129.
64. Rutten LJ, Zhu X, Leppin AL, Ridgeway JL, Swift MD, Griffin JM, et al. Evidence-based strategies for clinical organizations to address COVID-19 vaccine hesitancy. Mayo Clin Proc. 2021;96(3):699–707.
65. Bogart LM, Dong L, Gandhi P, Klein DJ, Smith TL, Ryan S, Ojikutu BO. COVID-19 vaccine intentions and mistrust in a National Sample of Black Americans. J Natl Med Assoc. 2022;113(6):599–611.
66. Chu J, Pink SL, Willer R. Religious identity cues increase vaccination intentions and trust in medical experts among American Christians. Proc Natl Acad Sci U S A. 2021;118(49):e2106481118.
67. Diament SM, Kaya A, Magenheim EB. Frames that matter: increasing the willingness to get the Covid-19 vaccines. Soc Sci Med. 2022;292:114562.
68. Reiter PL, Pennell ML, Katz ML. Acceptability of a COVID-19 vaccine among adults in the United States: how many people would get vaccinated? Vaccine. 2020;38(42):6500–7.
69. Centers for Disease Control. Talking with patients about COVID-19 vaccination. https://www.cdc.gov/vaccines/covid-19/hcp/engaging-patients.html. Accessed 9 Sep 2022.

Chapter 13

COVID-19 Vaccination in Persons with Diabetes: How they Work

Mahmoud Nassar, Anoop Misra, and Zachary Bloomgarden

Introduction

Coronavirus disease 2019 (COVID-19) is affecting global health systems. COVID-19 is characterized by a variety of symptoms and complications [1]. By October 2022, there will have been 626 million cases of COVID-19, causing 6.56 million deaths [2]. Although mortality rates (1.9%) are relatively low, patients with pre-existing conditions, such as diabetes, hypertension, cardiovascular disease, and metabolic syndrome, may have a fivefold (10%) increase in mortality [3]. Specifically, patients with diabetes have a high risk of developing severe infection and mortality when they contract COVID-19 [4]. Further, high fasting blood glucose levels are independently associated with mortality, even in patients not previously known to have diabetes [5, 6]. Poorly controlled diabetes and obesity are associated with a high risk of severe COVID-19 infection [7].

There were 592 articles in Embase and Medline using the search query "Diabetes Mellitus" AND "COVID-19 vaccine" by June 2022. We have reviewed

M. Nassar (✉)
Department of Medicine, Icahn School of Medicine at Mount Sinai/NYC Health + Hospitals, Queens, NY, USA
e-mail: Dr.Nassar@aucegypt.edu

A. Misra
Fortis-C-DOC Centre of Excellence for Diabetes, Metabolic Diseases and Endocrinology, Diabetes Foundation (India), National Diabetes Obesity and Cholesterol Foundation (NDOC), New Delhi, India

Z. Bloomgarden
Department of Medicine, Division of Endocrinology, Diabetes and Bone Disease, Icahn School of Medicine at Mount Sinai, New York, NY, USA

195

A. K. Myers (ed.), *Diabetes and COVID-19*, Contemporary Endocrinology, https://doi.org/10.1007/978-3-031-28536-3_13

this literature to address the following questions regarding patients with diabetes: What is the immune response to COVID-19? What is the response to the COVID-19 vaccine? Is it possible to administer the COVID-19 vaccine along with the usually recommended vaccines? What are the potential complications of the COVID-19 vaccines? What type of vaccine should be used? What is the expected effectiveness of the COVID-19 vaccine? What is the expected duration of COVID-19 immunity after vaccination? Is a booster dose of the COVID-19 vaccine needed? We present the following discussion based on scant data after the above search.

Diabetes and the Immune Response to COVID-19

Several factors contribute to the development of COVID-19 complications in patients with diabetes, including impaired innate/adaptive immunity following the onset of a state of chronic, low-grade inflammation referred to as metabolic inflammation. In addition, there is some evidence that chronic inflammation and dysfunctional adipose tissue associated with obesity may impair macrophage activation and impair cytokine production upon antigen exposure, which may explain impaired innate/adaptive immunity [8–10]. Antiviral-resistance and vaccine escape mechanisms may be present in patients with type 2 diabetes (T2D) due to this altered, obesogenic milieu. In addition, these patients also have compromised B and T cell responses, which contribute to an impaired immune response. In a small study of 31 patients with COVID-19, there was greater seronegativity at two weeks in those with diabetes when compared to those without diabetes [11]. In a study of 515 health-care providers in India, 57 people with T2D had a significantly lower seropositivity rate than those without (84.6 vs. 96.1%, $p = 0.002$) [12]. The dysregulation of the immune system may also be caused by an abnormal hormonal environment, such as an imbalance of adipokines and leptin levels [13]. In obese patients with T2D, pro-inflammatory proteins such as tumor necrosis factor (TNF)α, interferon (IFN)γ, interleukin-1 (IL-1)1β, IL-6, IL-12, and IL-18 are overexpressed, leading to defective innate and adaptive immunity [14]. These bioactive inflammatory proteins are responsible for increased susceptibility to developing COVID-19 complications [15]. An illustration of the pathophysiology of COVID-19 infection in patients with diabetes can be found in Fig. 13.1.

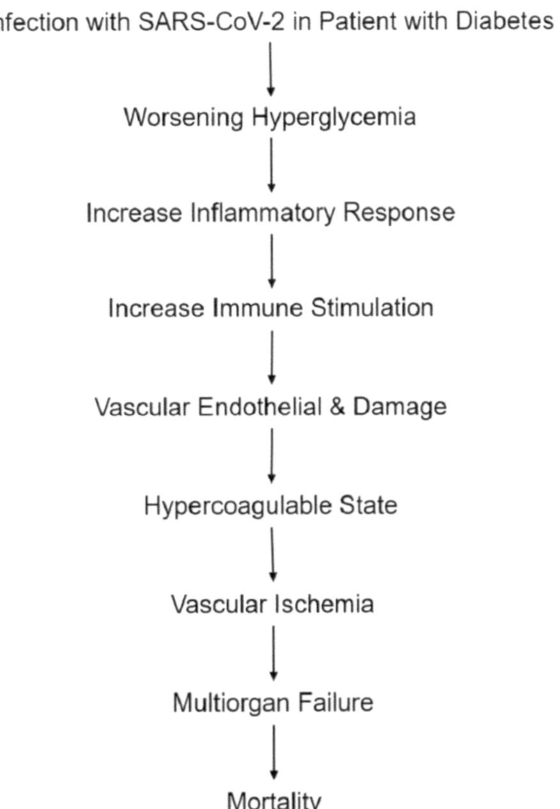

Fig. 13.1 Pathophysiology of COVID-19 infection in patients with diabetes

Vaccination and Immunity Against COVID-19

The COVID-19 vaccine has received media and public attention due to the emergence of new COVID-19 variants, booster doses, and new public policies and recommendations. As of June 2022, 203 vaccines had been studied in 714 vaccine trials in 75 countries. Of the 203 vaccines, 38 vaccines have been approved in at least one country [16]. The antibody response to the COVID-19 vaccine varies among COVID-19 vaccine types. Published data suggest that commonly used vaccines (Moderna, BNT162b2 Pfizer, Johnson & Johnson, AstraZeneca, CoronaVac, and Sputniks V) provide good immunity. Several COVID-19 variants have been identified, such as Alpha, Beta, Gamma, Delta, Epsilon, Eta, Iota, Kappa, Mu, Zeta, and Omicron. Several studies have shown that vaccines protect against severe diseases, hospitalization, and death from variants as well [17].

The five categories for COVID-19 vaccines are:

a. Inactivated virus vaccines are developed using inactivated whole virus particles, such as those for influenza and polio. The Sinopharm vaccine is one example of a COVID-19 vaccine that has been approved and is currently being used in China [18].
b. Viral vector vaccines use subparts of a virus delivered by a non-pathogenic viral vector to develop the immune response, such as Ebola and COVID-19 vaccines developed by Janssen, AstraZeneca, and CoronaVac.
c. Live attenuated vaccines, such as measles, mumps, rubella, and varicella, are not suitable for immunocompromised patients. Several trials have been conducted in rodents to develop a live attenuated COVID-19 vaccine [18].
d. Protein subunit vaccines contain isolated and purified viral proteins that are most useful for stimulating the immune system, such as hepatitis B and acellular pertussis vaccines. Novavax (NVX-CoV2373) contains harmless spike proteins (S protein). The spike protein found on the surface of SARS-CoV-2 is responsible for allowing the virus to enter human cells. Due to its location on the exterior of the virus, the immune system is able to identify it readily. In response to the S proteins, the immune system produces antibodies and defensive white blood cells that provide immunity to COVID-19 [19].
e. Messenger RNA (mRNA) to deliver instructions to the cell to produce specific proteins to encourage the body to develop immunity to it. BioNTech, Pfizer/BNT162b2, and Moderna have developed vaccines of this type.
f. A brief comparison of various vaccines is presented in Table 13.1. Only Moderna, Pfizer, Johnson and Johnson, and Novovax are approved for use in the United States [20].

A study from Denmark based on an analysis of 4 million RT-PCR-tests during the first and second surges revealed that exposure to COVID-19 resulted in developing antibodies for six months or more against reinfection by the same variant by 80% in adults under 65 years but in 50% of people over age 65 [27]. Based on the systematic review results, prior SARS-CoV-2 infection had a high protective effect on reinfection similar to that provided by vaccination, with a weighted reduction of 90.4% for reinfection [28]. Given the increase in the development of diabetes with aging, this adds to concern about measures to protect persons with diabetes against COVID-19 infection. Unfortunately, neither of these studies included a subgroup analysis for patients with diabetes.

Table 13.1 A brief comparison of currently available COVID-19 vaccines

Name	Type	Similar technology is used with other vaccines	Origin country	Studies included persons with diabetes	Number of doses required for immunity (excluding booster doses)	Efficacy after second dose	Time to maximal immunity
Moderna	mRNA	None	Moderna, USA	Yes	Two, 28 days apart	94% [21]	Two weeks after the second dose
BNT162b2 Pfizer	mRNA	None	Pfizer-BioNTech USA, Germany	–	Two, 21 days apart	95% [21]	Two weeks after the second dose
CoronaVac	Inactivated virus	Whooping cough, Rabies, Hepatitis A	Sinovac Biotech, China	–	Two, 14 days apart	83% [22]	Two weeks after second dose (estimated)
Covaxin	Inactivated virus	Whooping cough, Rabies, Hepatitis A	India	Yes	Two, four weeks apart,	78% [23]	–
Novavax	Protein subunit	Hepatitis B and acellular pertussis vaccines	India	–	Two, three weeks apart,	89% [24]	–
Johnson & Johnson	Viral vector (non-replication)	Ebola	Johnson & Johnson (Janssen Biotech, Inc.) USA	Yes	One	72% [21]	Two weeks after the first dose
AstraZeneca	Viral vector (non-replication)	Ebola	Oxford-AstraZeneca, England	Yes	Two, 12 weeks apart	70% [25]	Two weeks after the second dose
Sputnick V (GamCOVID-Vac)	Viral vector (non-replication, 2 Serotypes)	Ebola	Gamaleya, Russia	Yes	Two, 21 days apart	91% [26]	Two weeks after the second dose

COVID-19 Vaccination and Diabetes

Immune Response

In a small study from India, spike antibody response after Covaxin (Bharat Biotech, India) and Covidshield (AstraZeneca) vaccines were lower in patients with diabetes [12]. This same effect was not seen with patients with comorbidities including hypertension, ischemic heart disease, hypertension, or hyperlipidemia. A prospective study conducted on 262 patients (181 without diabetes and 81 T2D) to compare the effectiveness of BNT162b2 mRNA COVID-19 vaccination (Pfizer) between patients with diabetes and those without diabetes showed a high level of both SARS-CoV-2 IgG and neutralizing antibodies in both groups; however, people with T2D had lower SARS-CoV-2 neutralizing and IgG antibody titers than people without diabetes (79.7 ± 19.5% *vs.* 87.1 ± 11.6% and 138 ± 59.4 BAU/mL *vs.* 154 ± 49.1 BAU/mL, respectively). Despite these similar numeric values, authors questioned if the quality of the antibody response was adequate [3]. A recent systematic review included eight studies with a total of 64,468 patients; of these, 5156 (7.9%) had diabetes. As noted previously, the antibody response in patients with diabetes is lower than that of persons without diabetes in the short term (four weeks) [29]. Clearly, studies with longer follow-up are necessary.

Complications of COVID-19 Vaccines

The COVID-19 vaccine may lead to reactions localized at the injection site, such as pain, redness, or systemic effects such as tiredness, headache, muscle pain, chills, fever, or nausea. Several serious complications have been reported with low frequency, including myocarditis, rhabdomyolysis, vasculitis, and cutaneous adverse reactions [30–34]. Patients with diabetes may develop diabetic keto-acidosis (DKA) after contracting COVID-19 infection or being vaccinated with COVID-19 [35–37]. Although there have been few reports of DKA and hyperosmolar hyperglycemic syndrome (HHS) in patients with type 1 diabetes (T1D) after the second COVID-19 vaccine dose, their occurrence does not appear to be more common than in non-vaccinated persons with diabetes, although the evidence is limited [38, 39]. A recent study of 97 persons with T1D using a continuous glucose monitor (CGM) showed COVID-19 vaccination to be associated with lower time in range over the first week, particularly among those taking adjuvant metformin or sodium glucose transporter 1 inhibitors with insulin [37]. Severe hyperglycemia as manifested by HHS and/or DKA has also been reported three weeks after the first dose of an adenovirus-vector vaccine in two patients with a history of pre-diabetes [40]. After receiving the COVID-19 vaccine, hyperglycemia for a couple of days to a couple of weeks was reported in three cases of previously well-controlled T2D [41]. However, in a prospective multicentric study of 161 participants with T1D and T2D who were recently vaccinated, there were no changes with time in target two to three days after vaccination, except in those with T1D who had side effects [33]. The study was limited by the fact that only 74 participants had sufficient CGM data for analysis. In this context, the International Diabetes Federation (IDF) statement was as follows: "As with any vaccine you may have received in the past, the COVID-19 vaccine may cause your blood glucose levels to rise for a couple of days" [42]. A recent study suggests a potential caution in that vaccination of persons with diabetes having HbA1c >7% was associated with less virus-neutralizing antibody capacity than seen in normoglycemic persons and in T2D patients with good glycemic control [43].

Administration of the COVID-19 Vaccine Along with the Routine Vaccines for Patients with Diabetes

A randomized controlled trial in the UK demonstrated that the COVID-19 vaccine could be given simultaneously with the influenza vaccine without causing adverse events [44]. The Centers for Disease Control and Prevention (CDC) recommends the co-administration of the COVID-19 vaccine and influenza vaccine on the same day [45]. According to the CDC, the COVID-19 vaccine may be administered along with other vaccinations, but at different limbs [46]. The American Academy of Pediatrics (AAP) emphasizes the importance of maintaining regular vaccinations, particularly in light of the decrease in adolescent immunization during the pandemic. To address this issue and ensure timely COVID-19 vaccinations, the AAP supports providing routine childhood and adolescent vaccines concurrently with COVID-19 vaccines or closely before or after. This recommendation applies to children and adolescents who are due or overdue for vaccinations [47].

Vaccine Prioritization

Considering the initial limited supply of COVID-19 vaccines, prioritization of select groups to receive the vaccine is important. Therefore, the CDC prioritized this vaccine for first responders, adults 65 years and older, and those with comorbidities. People with diabetes are also among those with comorbid conditions for whom receiving the COVID-19 vaccine should be prioritized, given their high risk of severe complications [48].

COVID-19 Vaccine Booster Dose

COVID-19 vaccine booster doses are prepared using the same formula as the initial vaccine doses; however, Moderna COVID-19's booster dose is composed of half the original vaccine dose. There is not enough information about whether COVID-19 vaccines generate long-term immunity. Over time, immunity developed following vaccination may wane [49]. The fourth dose of the COVID-19 vaccine is effective in increasing antibody levels and cellular immunity above those attained after the third booster dose [50]. Even before receiving the fourth dose, individuals may have high antibody levels and a strong immune response. The CDC has authorized the bivariant COVID-19 vaccine, which includes the Omicron strain, for inclusion in the existing vaccine composition of BNT162b2 Pfizer and modern vaccines as of September 1, 2022 [51].

The CDC previously recommended that a COVID-19 booster dose be administered six months after receiving the primary dose to three high-risk groups: people over 65 years of age, residents of long-term care facilities, or those 50–64 years old with chronic diseases such as T1 or T2D, or obesity. However, the CDC has extended the booster dose to be administered five months after receiving the primary dose for those 12 years old or older [52]. Given that antibody response to primary doses may decline more quickly in patients with diabetes, the administration of booster dose assumes more significance.

Summary

Patients with diabetes are at high risk of developing severe infections and complications from SARS-CoV-2. Preliminary data indicate that immunity to vaccination declines faster in patients with diabetes than in persons without diabetes. Given the risks associated with COVID-19 infection, patients with diabetes should be prioritized for vaccination and for booster dose. COVID-19 vaccination appears to be safe in patients with diabetes.

References

1. Nassar M, Nso N, Alfishawy M, Novikov A, Yaghi S, Medina L, Toz B, Lakhdar S, Idrees Z, Kim Y, Gurung DO, Siddiqui RS, Zheng D, Agladze M, Sumbly V, Sandhu J, Castillo FC, Chowdhury N, Kondaveeti R, Bhuiyan S, Perez LG, Ranat R, Gonzalez C, Bhangoo H, Williams J, Osman AE, Kong J, Ariyaratnam J, Mohamed M, Omran I, Lopez M, Nyabera A, Landry I, Iqbal S, Gondal AZ, Hassan S, Daoud A, Baraka B, Trandafirescu T, Rizzo V. Current systematic reviews and meta-analyses of COVID-19. World J Virol. 2021;10:182–208. https://doi.org/10.5501/wjv.v10.i4.182.
2. COVID-19 coronavirus pandemic. 2021. https://www.worldometers.info/coronavirus/. Accessed 29 Dec 2021.
3. Ali H, Alterki A, Sindhu S, Alahmad B, Hammad M, Al-Sabah S, Alghounaim M, Jamal MH, Aldei A, Mairza MJ, Husain M, Deverajan S, Ahmad R, Cherian P, Alkhairi I, Alkandari A, Abubaker J, Abu-Farha M, Al-Mulla F. Robust antibody levels in both diabetic and non-diabetic individuals after BNT162b2 mRNA COVID-19 vaccination. Front Immunol. 2021;12:752233. https://doi.org/10.3389/fimmu.2021.752233.
4. Pal R, Bhadada SK, Misra A. COVID-19 vaccination in patients with diabetes mellitus: current concepts, uncertainties and challenges. Diabetes Metab Syndr. 2021;15:505–8. https://doi.org/10.1016/j.dsx.2021.02.026.

5. Wang S, Ma P, Zhang S, Song S, Wang Z, Ma Y, Xu J, Wu F, Duan L, Yin Z, Luo H, Xiong N, Xu M, Zeng T, Jin Y. Fasting blood glucose at admission is an independent predictor for 28-day mortality in patients with COVID-19 without previous diagnosis of diabetes: a multi-centre retrospective study. Diabetologia. 2020;63:2102–11. https://doi.org/10.1007/s00125-020-05209-1.

6. Huang Y, Guo H, Zhou Y, Guo J, Wang T, Zhao X, Li H, Sun Y, Bian X, Fang C. The associations between fasting plasma glucose levels and mortality of COVID-19 in patients without diabetes. Diabetes Res Clin Pract. 2020;169:108448. https://doi.org/10.1016/j.diabres.2020.108448.

7. Driggin E, Maddox TM, Ferdinand KC, Kirkpatrick JN, Ky B, Morris AA, Mullen JB, Parikh SA, Philbin DM Jr, Vaduganathan M. ACC health policy statement on cardiovascular disease considerations for COVID-19 vaccine prioritization: a report of the American College of Cardiology Solution Set Oversight Committee. J Am Coll Cardiol. 2021;77:1938–48. https://doi.org/10.1016/j.jacc.2021.02.017.

8. Lumeng CN. Innate immune activation in obesity. Mol Aspects Med. 2013;34:12–29. https://doi.org/10.1016/j.mam.2012.10.002.

9. Abu-Farha M, Al-Mulla F, Thanaraj TA, Kavalakatt S, Ali H, Abdul Ghani M, Abubaker J. Impact of diabetes in patients diagnosed with COVID-19. Front Immunol. 2020;11:576818. https://doi.org/10.3389/fimmu.2020.576818.

10. Nassar M, Daoud A, Nso N, Medina L, Ghernautan V, Bhangoo H, Nyein A, Mohamed M, Alqassieh A, Soliman K, Alfishawy M, Sachmechi I, Misra A. Diabetes mellitus and COVID-19: review article. Diabetes Metab Syndr. 2021;15:102268. https://doi.org/10.1016/j.dsx.2021.102268.

11. Pal R, Sachdeva N, Mukherjee S, Suri V, Zohmangaihi D, Ram S, Puri GD, Bhalla A, Soni SL, Pandey N, Bhansali A, Bhadada SK. Impaired anti-SARS-CoV-2 antibody response in non-severe COVID-19 patients with diabetes mellitus: a preliminary report. Diabetes Metab Syndr. 2021;15:193–6. https://doi.org/10.1016/j.dsx.2020.12.035.

12. Singh AK, Phatak SR, Singh R, Bhattacharjee K, Singh NK, Gupta A, Sharma A. Antibody response after first and second-dose of ChAdOx1-nCOV (Covishield(TM)(R)) and BBV-152 (Covaxin(TM)(R)) among health care workers in India: the final results of cross-sectional coronavirus vaccine-induced antibody titre (COVAT) study. Vaccine. 2021;39:6492–509. https://doi.org/10.1016/j.vaccine.2021.09.055.

13. Al-Suhaimi EA, Shehzad A. Leptin, resistin and visfatin: the missing link between endocrine metabolic disorders and immunity. Eur J Med Res. 2013;18:12. https://doi.org/10.1186/2047-783X-18-12.

14. Guest CB, Park MJ, Johnson DR, Freund GG. The implication of proinflammatory cytokines in type 2 diabetes. Front Biosci. 2008;13:5187–94. https://doi.org/10.2741/3074.

15. Tang Y, Liu J, Zhang D, Xu Z, Ji J, Wen C. Cytokine storm in COVID-19: The current evidence and treatment strategies. Front Immunol. 2020;11:1708. https://doi.org/10.3389/fimmu.2020.01708.

16. Vaccines candidates in clinical trials. 2021. https://covid19.trackvaccines.org/vaccines/#approved. Accessed 19 Nov 2021.

17. He X, Hong W, Pan X, Lu G, Wei X. SARS-CoV-2 omicron variant: characteristics and prevention. MedComm. 2020;2:838–45. https://doi.org/10.1002/mco2.110.

18. Okamura S, Ebina H. Could live attenuated vaccines better control COVID-19? Vaccine. 2021;39:5719–26. https://doi.org/10.1016/j.vaccine.2021.08.018.

19. Dunkle LM, Kotloff KL, Gay CL, Anez G, Adelglass JM, Barrat Hernandez AQ, Harper WL, Duncanson DM, McArthur MA, Florescu DF, McClelland RS, Garcia-Fragoso V, Riesenberg RA, Musante DB, Fried DL, Safirstein BE, McKenzie M, Jeanfreau RJ, Kingsley JK, Henderson JA, Lane DC, Ruiz-Palacios GM, Corey L, Neuzil KM, Coombs RW, Greninger AL, Hutter J, Ake JA, Smith K, Woo W, Cho I, Glenn GM, Dubovsky F, 2019nCoV-301 Study Group. Efficacy and safety of NVX-CoV2373 in adults in the United States and Mexico. N Engl J Med. 2021; https://doi.org/10.1056/NEJMoa2116185.

20. Overview of COVID-19 vaccines. 2022. https://www.cdc.gov/coronavirus/2019-ncov/vaccines/different-vaccines/overview-COVID-19-vaccines.html. Accessed 10 Oct 2022.
21. Mascellino MT, Di Timoteo F, De Angelis M, Oliva A. Overview of the main anti-SARS-CoV-2 vaccines: mechanism of action, efficacy and safety. Infect Drug Resist. 2021;14:3459–76. https://doi.org/10.2147/IDR.S315727.
22. Tanriover MD, Doganay HL, Akova M, Guner HR, Azap A, Akhan S, Kose S, Erdinc FS, Akalin EH, Tabak OF, Pullukcu H, Batum O, Simsek Yavuz S, Turhan O, Yildirmak MT, Koksal I, Tasova Y, Korten V, Yilmaz G, Celen MK, Altin S, Celik I, Bayindir Y, Karaoglan I, Yilmaz A, Ozkul A, Gur H, Unal S, CoronaVac Study Group. Efficacy and safety of an inactivated whole-virion SARS-CoV-2 vaccine (CoronaVac): interim results of a double-blind, randomised, placebo-controlled, phase 3 trial in Turkey. Lancet. 2021;398:213–22. https://doi.org/10.1016/S0140-6736(21)01429-X.
23. Vasireddy D, Vanaparthy R, Mohan G, Malayala SV, Atluri P. Review of COVID-19 variants and COVID-19 vaccine efficacy: what the clinician should know? J Clin Med Res. 2021;13:317–25. https://doi.org/10.14740/jocmr4518.
24. Novavax COVID-19 vaccine demonstrates 89.3% efficacy in UK phase 3 trial. 2021. https://ir.novavax.com/2021-01-28-Novavax-COVID-19-Vaccine-Demonstrates-89-3-Efficacy-in-UK-Phase-3-Trial. Accessed 10 Oct 2022.
25. Emary KRW, Golubchik T, Aley PK, Ariani CV, Angus B, Bibi S, Blane B, Bonsall D, Cicconi P, Charlton S, Clutterbuck EA, Collins AM, Cox T, Darton TC, Dold C, Douglas AD, CJA D, Ewer KJ, Flaxman AL, Faust SN, Ferreira DM, Feng S, Finn A, Folegatti PM, Fuskova M, Galiza E, Goodman AL, Green CM, Green CA, Greenland M, Hallis B, Heath PT, Hay J, Hill HC, Jenkin D, Kerridge S, Lazarus R, Libri V, Lillie PJ, Ludden C, Marchevsky NG, Minassian AM, McGregor AC, Mujadidi YF, Phillips DJ, Plested E, Pollock KM, Robinson H, Smith A, Song R, Snape MD, Sutherland RK, Thomson EC, Toshner M, Turner DPJ, Vekemans J, Villafana TL, Williams CJ, Hill AVS, Lambe T, Gilbert SC, Voysey M, Ramasamy MN, Pollard AJ, COVID-19 Genomics UK consortium; AMPHEUS Project; Oxford COVID-19 Vaccine Trial Group. Efficacy of ChAdOx1 nCoV-19 (AZD1222) vaccine against SARS-CoV-2 variant of concern 202012/01 (B.1.1.7): an exploratory analysis of a randomised controlled trial. Lancet. 2021;397:1351–62. https://doi.org/10.1016/S0140-6736(21)00628-0.
26. Di Valerio Z, La Fauci G, Solda G, Montalti M, Lenzi J, Forcellini M, Barvas E, Guttmann S, Poluzzi E, Raschi E, Riccardi R, Fantini MP, Salussolia A, Gori D. ROCCA cohort study: Nationwide results on safety of Gam-COVID-Vac vaccine (Sputnik V) in the Republic of San Marino using active surveillance. EClinicalMedicine. 2022;49:101468. https://doi.org/10.1016/j.eclinm.2022.101468.
27. Hansen CH, Michlmayr D, Gubbels SM, Mølbak K, Ethelberg S. Assessment of protection against reinfection with SARS-CoV-2 among 4 million PCR-tested individuals in Denmark in 2020: a population-level observational study. Lancet. 2021;397:1204–12.
28. Kojima N, Shrestha NK, Klausner JD. A systematic review of the protective effect of prior SARS-CoV-2 infection on repeat infection. Eval Health Prof. 2021;44:327–32. https://doi.org/10.1177/01632787211047932.
29. Soetedjo NNM, Iryaningrum MR, Lawrensia S, Permana H. Antibody response following SARS-CoV-2 vaccination among patients with type 2 diabetes mellitus: a systematic review. Diabetes Metab Syndr. 2022;16:102406. https://doi.org/10.1016/j.dsx.2022.102406.
30. Nassar M, Nso N, Gonzalez C, Lakhdar S, Alshamam M, Elshafey M, Abdalazeem Y, Nyein A, Punzalan B, Durrance RJ, Alfishawy M, Bakshi S, Rizzo V. COVID-19 vaccine-induced myocarditis: case report with literature review. Diabetes Metab Syndr. 2021;15:102205. https://doi.org/10.1016/j.dsx.2021.102205.
31. Liu BD, Ugolini C, Jha P. Two cases of post-moderna COVID-19 vaccine encephalopathy associated with nonconvulsive status epilepticus. Cureus. 2021;13:e16172. https://doi.org/10.7759/cureus.16172.

32. Waheed S, Bayas A, Hindi F, Rizvi Z, Espinosa PS. Neurological complications of COVID-19: Guillain-Barre Syndrome following Pfizer COVID-19 vaccine. Cureus. 2021;13:e13426. https://doi.org/10.7759/cureus.13426.
33. Kong J, Cuevas-Castillo F, Nassar M, Lei CM, Idrees Z, Fix WC, Halverstam C, Mir A, Elbendary A, Mathew A. Bullous drug eruption after second dose of mRNA-1273 (Moderna) COVID-19 vaccine: case report. J Infect Public Health. 2021;14:1392–4. https://doi.org/10.1016/j.jiph.2021.06.021.
34. Nassar M, Chung H, Dhayaparan Y, Nyein A, Acevedo BJ, Chicos C, Zheng D, Barras M, Mohamed M, Alfishawy M, Nso N, Rizzo V, Kimball E. COVID-19 vaccine induced rhabdomyolysis: case report with literature review. Diabetes Metab Syndr. 2021;15:102170. https://doi.org/10.1016/j.dsx.2021.06.007.
35. Alfishawy M, Nassar M, Mohamed M, Fatthy M, Elmessiery RM. New-onset type 1 diabetes mellitus with diabetic ketoacidosis and pancreatitis in a patient with COVID-19. Sci Afr. 2021;13:e00915. https://doi.org/10.1016/j.sciaf.2021.e00915.
36. Alhumaid S, Al Mutair A, Al Alawi Z, Rabaan AA, Alomari MA, Al Salman SA, Al-Alawi AS, Al Hassan MH, Alhamad H, Al-Kamees MA, Almousa FM, Mufti HN, Alwesabai AM, Dhama K, Al-Tawfiq JA, Al-Omari A. Diabetic ketoacidosis in patients with SARS-CoV-2: a systematic review and meta-analysis. Diabetol Metab Syndr. 2021;13:120. https://doi.org/10.1186/s13098-021-00740-6.
37. Heald AH, Stedman M, Horne L, Rea R, Whyte M, Gibson JM, Anderson SG, Ollier W. The change in glycaemic control immediately after COVID-19 vaccination in people with type 1 diabetes. Diabet Med. 2021:e14774. https://doi.org/10.1111/dme.14774.
38. Lee HJ, Sajan A, Tomer Y. Hyperglycemic emergencies associated with COVID-19 vaccination: a case series and discussion. J Endocr Soc. 2021;5:bvab141. https://doi.org/10.1210/jendso/bvab141.
39. Ganakumar V, Jethwani P, Roy A, Shukla R, Mittal M, Garg MK. Diabetic ketoacidosis (DKA) in type 1 diabetes mellitus (T1DM) temporally related to COVID-19 vaccination. Diabetes Metab Syndr. 2022;16:102371. https://doi.org/10.1016/j.dsx.2021.102371.
40. Edwards AE, Vathenen R, Henson SM, Finer S, Gunganah K. Acute hyperglycaemic crisis after vaccination against COVID-19: a case series. Diabet Med. 2021;38:e14631. https://doi.org/10.1111/dme.14631.
41. Mishra A, Ghosh A, Dutta K, Tyagi K, Misra A. Exacerbation of hyperglycemia in patients with type 2 diabetes after vaccination for COVID19: report of three cases. Diabetes Metab Syndr. 2021;15:102151. https://doi.org/10.1016/j.dsx.2021.05.024.
42. Diabetes & COVID-19 Vaccination and treatments. 07 Dec 2021. https://idf.org/our-network/regions-members/europe/europe-news/370-diabetes-coronavirus-vaccination.html. Accessed 1 Aug 2022, 2021.
43. Marfella R, D'Onofrio N, Sardu C, Scisciola L, Maggi P, Coppola N, Romano C, Messina V, Turriziani F, Siniscalchi M, Maniscalco M, Boccalatte M, Napolitano G, Salemme L, Marfella LV, Basile E, Montemurro MV, Papa C, Frascaria F, Papa A, Russo F, Tirino V, Papaccio G, Galdiero M, Sasso FC, Barbieri M, Rizzo MR, Balestrieri ML, Angelillo IF, Napoli C, Paolisso G. Does poor glycaemic control affect the immunogenicity of the COVID-19 vaccination in patients with type 2 diabetes: The CAVEAT study. Diabetes Obes Metab. 2022;24:160–65.
44. Toback S, Galiza E, Cosgrove C, Galloway J, Goodman AL, Swift PA, Rajaram S, Graves-Jones A, Edelman J, Burns F, Minassian AM, Cho I, Kumar L, Plested JS, Rivers EJ, Robertson A, Dubovsky F, Glenn G, Heath PT, 2019nCoV-302 Study Group. Safety, immunogenicity, and efficacy of a COVID-19 vaccine (NVX-CoV2373) co-administered with seasonal influenza vaccines: an exploratory substudy of a randomised, observer-blinded, placebo-controlled, phase 3 trial. Lancet Respir Med. 2021; https://doi.org/10.1016/S2213-2600(21)00409-4.

45. Interim guidance for routine and influenza immunization services during the COVID-19 pandemic. 2021. https://www.cdc.gov/vaccines/pandemic-guidance/index.html. Accessed 29 May 2022.
46. Administer the vaccine(s). 2021. https://www.cdc.gov/vaccines/hcp/admin/administer-vaccines.html#covid19-with-other-vaccines. Accessed 10 Oct 2022.
47. COVID-19 Vaccine Implementation in Pediatric Practices. Accessed: 3/26/2023, 2023. https://www.aap.org/en/pages/2019-novel-coronavirus-covid-19-infections/covid-19-vaccine-for-children/covid-19-vaccine-implementation-in-pediatric-practices/.
48. Dooling K, Marin M, Wallace M, McClung N, Chamberland M, Lee GM, Talbot HK, Romero JR, Bell BP, Oliver SE. The advisory Committee on Immunization practices' updated interim recommendation for allocation of COVID-19 vaccine - United States, December 2020. MMWR Morb Mortal Wkly Rep. 2021;69:1657–60. https://doi.org/10.15585/mmwr.mm695152e2.
49. Krause PR, Fleming TR, Peto R, Longini IM, Figueroa JP, Sterne JAC, Cravioto A, Rees H, Higgins JPT, Boutron I, Pan H, Gruber MF, Arora N, Kazi F, Gaspar R, Swaminathan S, Ryan MJ, Henao-Restrepo AM. Considerations in boosting COVID-19 vaccine immune responses. Lancet. 2021;398:1377–80. https://doi.org/10.1016/S0140-6736(21)02046-8.
50. Munro AP, Feng S, Janani L, Cornelius V, Aley PK, Babbage G, Baxter D, Bula M, Cathie K, Chatterjee K. Safety, immunogenicity, and reactogenicity of BNT162b2 and mRNA-1273 COVID-19 vaccines given as fourth-dose boosters following two doses of ChAdOx1 nCoV-19 or BNT162b2 and a third dose of BNT162b2 (COV-BOOST): a multicentre, blinded, phase 2, randomised trial. Lancet Infect Dis. 2022;22:1131.
51. CDC recommends the first updated COVID-19 booster. 2022. https://www.cdc.gov/media/releases/2022/s0901-covid-19-booster.html. Accessed 10 Oct 2022.
52. CDC expands booster shot eligibility and strengthens recommendations for 12–17 year olds. 2022. https://www.cdc.gov/media/releases/2022/s0105-Booster-Shot.html. Accessed 9 Jan 2022.

Chapter 14
Long-Haul COVID Symptoms in Persons with Diabetes

César Fernández-de-las-Peñas and Juan Torres-Macho

Introduction

The world has suffered a dramatic situation of catastrophic proportions due to the worldwide spread of the severe acute respiratory syndrome coronavirus 2 (SARS-CoV-2), the agent causing the coronavirus disease 2019 (COVID-19) [1]. Unfortunately, a second hidden, and sometimes ignored, crisis related to SARS-CoV-2 is here: the "long-haulers," that is, people experiencing symptoms after the acute phase far longer than it would be expected [2]. Since millions of people have been and will be infected, the number of "long-haulers" will dramatically increase [3]. This chapter will discuss current definitions of long COVID and how these symptoms are experienced in individuals with diabetes.

Long COVID

Long COVID is probably the first medical term referring to a condition to be collectively promoted by patients themselves through social media [4]. As a result of these efforts, long COVID has been recognized by the World Health Organization

C. Fernández-de-las-Peñas (✉)
Department of Physical Therapy, Occupational Therapy, Physical Medicine and Rehabilitation, Universidad Rey Juan Carlos (URJC), Madrid, Spain
e-mail: cesar.fernandez@urjc.es

J. Torres-Macho
Department of Internal Medicine, Hospital Universitario Infanta Leonor-Virgen de la Torre, Madrid, Spain

Department of Medicine, School of Medicine, Universidad Complutense de Madrid, Madrid, Spain

© The Author(s), under exclusive license to Springer Nature Switzerland AG 2023
A. K. Myers (ed.), *Diabetes and COVID-19*, Contemporary Endocrinology, https://doi.org/10.1007/978-3-031-28536-3_14

(WHO) as a worldwide health-care concern and an "emergency-use" ICD-10 code has been proposed: U09.9 post-COVID condition [5]. Overall, the term "long COVID" is generally used for describing the presence of symptoms far longer than it would be expected after recovering from acute SARS-CoV-2 infection, whereas the term "long-hauler" is proposed for people suffering from long COVID [6–9]. However, since long COVID–associated symptoms are highly heterogeneous, no consensus on its definition is available [10]. In fact, more than a hundred symptoms, affecting multiple systems, have been described [11].

Similarly, controversies on the naming of this condition are also present in the interchangeable use of different terms, for example, chronic COVID-19 syndrome, late sequelae of COVID-19, long COVID, long-term COVID-19, post-COVID-19 syndrome, post-acute COVID-19, and post-acute sequelae of COVID-19 (PASC). With the aim to get a consensus, an international Delphi study, supported by the WHO, has proposed the term "post-COVID-19" instead of long COVID with the following definition: "post-COVID-19 condition occurs in people with a history of probable or confirmed SARS-CoV-2) infection, usually 3 months from the onset of COVID-19 with symptoms that last for at least 2 months and cannot be explained by an alternative diagnosis. Common symptoms include fatigue, shortness of breath, and cognitive dysfunction (but also others) and generally have an impact on everyday functioning. Symptoms might be new onset after initial recovery from an acute COVID-19 episode or persist from the initial illness. Symptoms might also fluctuate or relapse over time" [12]. This definition is the first one to include the topic of the functional impact of these symptoms, supported by current data showing that individuals with post-COVID symptoms report worse self-perceived health-related quality of life [13]. However, this definition includes three topics discussed in the former literature of long COVID which should be considered.

First, the topic of "probable or confirmed infection" has been previously discussed by other authors questioning if a positive test for SARS-CoV-2 or the presence of positive antibodies should be always a prerequisite for the diagnosis of long COVID [14]. Being able to carry out such testing is much more difficult in those individuals infected with the initial Wuhan or Alpha variant, particularly those infected during the first wave of the pandemic when diagnostic tests were not available. In fact, it should be noted that most studies investigating the prevalence of different long COVID symptoms include patients infected during 2020 [15, 16]. This conflicting situation further raises concern since all diagnostic procedures, including RT-PCR or antibody tests, have some limitations, as patients may have a false negative result if they test prior to having symptoms [17].

Another issue is establishing the timeline needed to consider symptoms as post-acute or chronic [18]. Fernández-de-las-Peñas et al. originally proposed four phases depending on the period when a particular post-COVID symptom appears after the acute phase of the infection: transition phase, symptoms possibly related to COVID (up to 4–5 weeks after onset); phase 1, acute post-COVID symptom (weeks 5 to 12 after onset); phase 2, long post-COVID symptom (weeks 12 to 24 after); and phase

3, persistent post-COVID symptoms (more than 24 weeks after) [18]. These phases have been now adapted based on ongoing evidence, as using both *long* and *persistent* is redundant. As a result, phases have been renamed: (1) post-acute sequelae of COVID-19 (PASC) (from week 5 to week 12 after onset) and (2) chronic post-COVID (more than 12 weeks after) (see Fig. 14.1) [19]. The transition phase would still be the same, since the infectivity lasts about 14 days, the median incubation period around 5 days (total up to three weeks) [20], and the SARS-CoV-2 virus is still detectable up to 30 days after the resolution of symptoms in 10–15% of diagnosed individuals [21].

The third problem is that new symptoms may arise after the initial infection. This is included in the WHO definition: "symptoms might be new onset after initial recovery from an acute COVID-19 episode or persist from the initial illness" [12]. These two situations were previously defined as (1) delayed-onset (a new symptom not experienced by a patient at the acute phase of the infection but appears after a latency period) or (2) persistent (a new symptom experienced by a patient at the acute phase of the infection which persists without pain-free or remission periods) [22]. A third situation would be that a previous symptom would exacerbate (when a patient suffered from a particular symptom before infection and this symptom worsens after SARS-CoV-2) [22]. Nevertheless, the WHO definition [12] did not consider exacerbated COVID-19-associated symptoms. Based on current knowledge, we will use in this chapter the term "long COVID" for defining the condition of suffering any post-COVID symptomatology, and post-acute or chronic as the main stages of this fluctuating condition depending on the follow-up period where the symptoms appear.

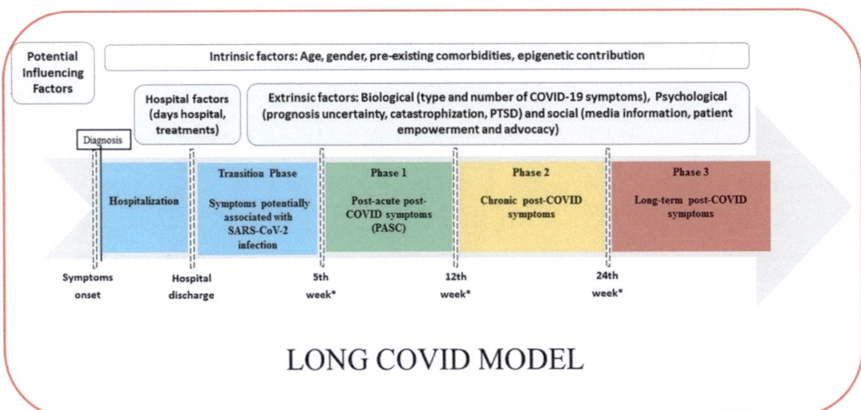

Fig. 14.1 Integrative model for long COVID showing transition phase (*blue*) and phases 1 (*green*), 2 (*yellow*), and 3 (*red*). PTSD: Post-traumatic stress disorder. In those individuals not requiring hospitalization, the phases would be the same but the transition phase would start two weeks after the symptom's onset

Symptoms Associated with Long COVID

Evidence has shown an unprecedented number of studies describing the presence of post-COVID symptoms in the past few years. More than 100 post-COVID symptoms affecting multiple systems, for example, respiratory, cardiovascular, neurological, and musculoskeletal, have been described (Fig. 14.2) [11, 23]. Different meta-analyses analyzing the prevalence of long COVID symptomatology have been published; however, the prevalence rate of each post-COVID symptom is highly heterogeneous and depends on the duration of time after the onset of infection [15, 16, 24–26]. Also, these meta-analyses are limited to studies with follow-up periods up to one year after infection [27, 28].

Current data supports that fatigue and dyspnea (Fig. 14.2) are the most prevalent post-COVID symptoms [15, 16, 24–28]. The WHO definition states "common symptoms including fatigue, dyspnea, and cognitive dysfunction" [12]. The inclusion of cognitive dysfunction as one of the most prevalent post-COVID

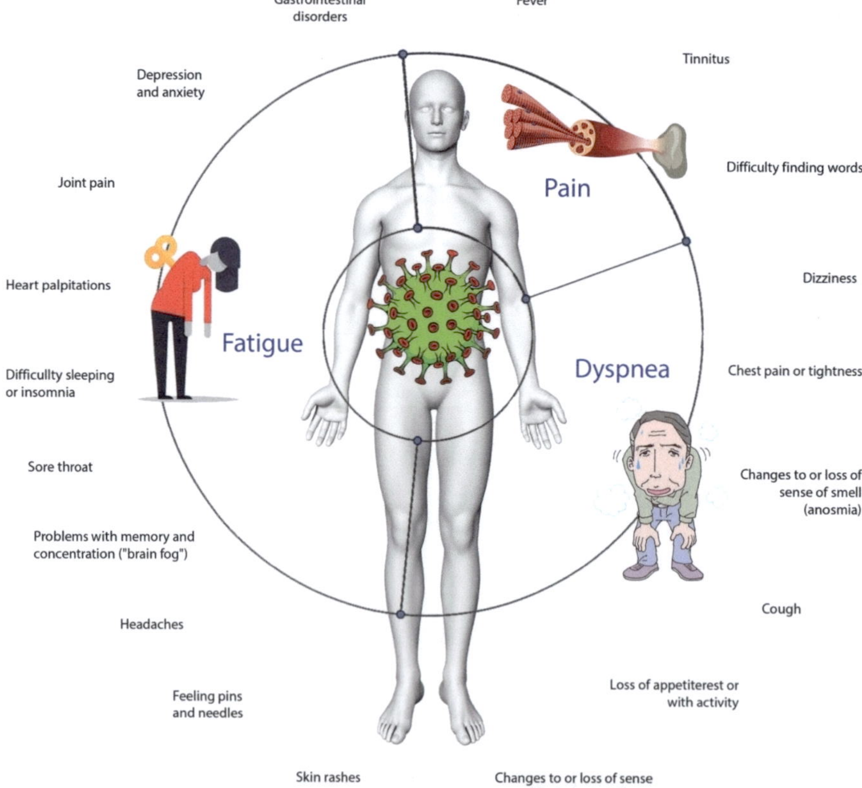

Fig. 14.2 Different post-COVID symptoms have been described. Fatigue, dyspnea, and pain are more prevalent. These symptoms seem to be similar in people with or without previous pre-existing comorbid diabetes

symptoms is restricting, because other symptoms, for example, headache or muscle/joint pain, are more prevalent after the infection [24–28]. Further, the prevalence of post-COVID symptoms could be different depending on the need for hospitalization. More importantly, the relapsing/remitting nature of post-COVID sequelae is variable since these patients exhibit fluctuations in their symptoms, with the potential for improvements of intensity and duration in some symptoms, but not in others [29]. Therefore, a single patient could present recurrent or persisting post-COVID symptoms. The erratic nature of post-COVID symptoms is supported by a meta-analysis showing a low prevalence of post-COVID symptoms 30 days after hospital discharge or onset, an increased prevalence 60 days after, but with another decrease > 90 days after [17]. This "roller coaster" state of post-COVID symptoms should be longitudinally monitored throughout weeks, months, or even years after SARS-CoV-2 infection. Accordingly, the assorted presentation of post-COVID symptoms reveals the need for prioritizing international studies of long COVID [30].

Diabetes and Long COVID

As noted in Chap. 3, individuals with pre-existing diabetes are at higher risk of complications during the acute phase of COVID-19 [31]. It is unclear if diabetes is also a risk factor for developing more severe long COVID. Accordingly, it has been suggested that the presence of pre-existing diabetes could lead to promote a more severe long COVID symptomatology [32].

Few studies have investigated the presence of long COVID symptoms in subjects with pre-existing diabetes. Mittal et al. also found that individuals with diabetes exhibited higher levels of post-COVID fatigue than those without diabetes [33]. They also noted that the fatigue correlated with glycemic control. Patients who had higher blood sugars after COVID-19 had worse fatigue than those with COVID-19 who had lower blood sugars (Average Postprandial Glucose: 200.9 ± 54.75 vs. 226.12 ± 67.57, $p = 0.05$). Other studies have not shown a difference in fatigue among those with and without diabetes. Akter et al. found that a higher proportion of patients with diabetes reported some symptoms such as pain, concentration loss, sleep disorders, and emotional problems, differences that were not significantly different between individuals with and without diabetes [34]. Additionally, the short-term follow-up period of this study (just four weeks after infection) did not allow researchers to determine if these symptoms are still related to the acute infection itself as it occurs just four weeks after symptoms onset. Like Akter, our case-control study found that diabetes was not a risk factor for post-COVID symptoms six months after the infection [35]. We observed that fatigue (66.2%), dyspnea on exertion (53.8%), and pain (44.8%) were the most prevalent long-term post-COVID symptoms in individuals with diabetes. Other post-COVID symptoms were sleep problems (37.9%), loss of memory (23.4%), anxiety and depressive levels (21%), or concentration loss (8.3%). Similar prevalence rates of these post-COVID symptoms were found in the control group without diabetes [35]. Based on available evidence, it seems that pre-existing diabetes itself does not represent a risk factor, for more severe manifestations of long COVID.

In a study looking at variables associated with greater rates of post-COVID symptoms, obesity and lipid disorder were associated with worse post-COVID symptoms, especially in those aged 46–60 [36]. Interestingly enough, diabetes was not found to have an association despite its common comorbidity with both lipid disorder and obesity. This association between obesity and post-COVID symptoms has been supported by a large population study showing that obesity is a risk factor (OR 1.25, 95% CI 1.08–1.44) for the development of long COVID [37]. Another study reported that obesity was associated with a systemic inflammatory state related to worse long COVID [38] and suggested that exercise may serve as a cure due to its anti-inflammatory effect [39].

Vaccines and Long COVID

It should be noted that the effect of vaccines on long COVID symptoms is conflicting. Some studies have reported that people with long COVID who had received vaccination experienced neither improvement nor worsening of their symptoms [40]. On the contrary, others reported that vaccines are able to reduce the odds of developing long COVID by 45% [41]. No data exists about the effect of vaccines on long COVID in people with diabetes.

Conclusion

This chapter presents the current controversies about the definition and characteristics of long COVID as well as its association, or lack of, with diabetes. Current evidence suggests that long COVID manifestations are similar in patients with diabetes when compared with those without diabetes, but future longitudinal population-based studies are needed. Other comorbidities associated with diabetes, such as hypertension or obesity, should be also considered when evaluating or treating long haulers with diabetes. Vaccination has been associated with potentially decreasing the chance of long COVID, but it remains unknown if vaccination can decrease long COVID in persons with diabetes.

References

1. Zhu N, Zhang D, Wang W, Li X, Yang B, Song J, Zhao X, Huang B, Shi W, Lu R, Niu P, Zhan F, Ma X, Wang D, Xu W, Wu G, Gao GF, Tan W, China Novel Coronavirus Investigating and Research Team. A novel coronavirus from patients with pneumonia in China, 2019. N Engl J Med. 2020;382:727–33.

2. Marshall M. The lasting misery of coronavirus long-haulers. Nature. 2020;585:339–41.
3. Rubin R. As their numbers grow, COVID-19 "Long Haulers" stump experts. JAMA. 2020;324:1381–3.
4. Callard F, Perego E. How and why patients made Long Covid. Soc Sci Med. 2021;268:113426.
5. World Health Organization. Emergency use ICD codes for COVID-19 disease outbreak. https://www.who.int/standards/classifications/classification-of-diseases/emergency-use-icd-codes-for-covid-19-disease-outbreak.
6. Mahase E. COVID-19: what do we know about "long COVID"? BMJ. 2020;370:m2815.
7. Nabavi N. Long COVID: how to define it and how to manage it. BMJ. 2020;370:m3489.
8. National Institute for Health and Care Excellence (NICE), Royal College of General Practitioners, Healthcare Improvement Scotland SIGN. COVID-19 rapid guideline: managing the long-term effects of COVID-19. London: National Institute for Health and Care Excellence; 2020. www.nice.org.uk/guidance/ng188. Accessed 30 Dec 2020.
9. Akbarialiabad H, Taghrir MH, Abdollahi A, Ghahramani N, Kumar M, Paydar S, Razani B, Mwangi J, Asadi-Pooya A, Malekmakan L, Bastani B. Long COVID, a comprehensive systematic scoping review. Infection. 2021;49:1163–86.
10. Baig AM. Chronic COVID syndrome: need for an appropriate medical terminology for long-COVID and COVID long-haulers. J Med Virol. 2021;93:2555–6.
11. Hayes LD, Ingram J, Sculthorpe NF. More than 100 persistent symptoms of SARS-CoV-2 (Long COVID): a scoping review. Front Med. 2021;8:750378.
12. Soriano JB, Murthy S, Marshall JC, Relan P, Diaz JV, WHO Clinical Case Definition Working Group on Post-COVID-19 Condition. A clinical case definition of post-COVID-19 condition by a Delphi consensus. Lancet Infect Dis. 2022;22:e102–7.
13. Amdal CD, Pe M, Falk RS, Piccinin C, Bottomley A, Arraras JI, Darlington AS, Hofsø K, Holzner B, Jørgensen NMH, Kulis D, Rimehaug SA, Singer S, Taylor K, Wheelwright S, Bjordal K. Health-related quality of life issues, including symptoms, in patients with active COVID-19 or post COVID-19; a systematic literature review. Qual Life Res. 2021;30:3367–81.
14. Raveendran A. Long COVID-19: challenges in the diagnosis and proposed diagnostic criteria. Diabetes Metab Syndr. 2020;15:145–6.
15. Lopez-Leon S, Wegman-Ostrosky T, Perelman C, Sepulveda R, Rebolledo PA, Cuapio A, Villapol S. More than 50 Long-term effects of COVID-19: a systematic review and meta-analysis. Sci Rep. 2021;11:16144.
16. Fernández-de-las-Peñas C, Palacios-Ceña D, Gómez-Mayordomo V, Florencio LL, Cuadrado ML, Plaza-Manzano G, Navarro-Santana M. Prevalence of Post-COVID-19 symptoms in hospitalized and non-hospitalized COVID-19 survivors: a systematic review and meta-analysis. Eur J Int Med. 2021;92:55–70.
17. Deeks JJ, Dinnes J, Takwoingi Y, Davenport C, Spijker R, Taylor-Phillips S, Adriano A, Beese S, Dretzke J, Ferrante di Ruffano L, Harris IM, Price MJ, Dittrich S, Emperador D, Hooft L, Leeflang MM, Van den Bruel A, Cochrane COVID-19 Diagnostic Test Accuracy Group. Antibody tests for identification of current and past infection with SARS-CoV-2. Cochrane Database Syst Rev. 2020;6:CD013652.
18. Fernández-de-las-Peñas C, Palacios-Ceña D, Gómez-Mayordomo V, Cuadrado ML, Florencio LL. Defining post-COVID symptoms (post-acute COVID, long COVID, persistent Post-COVID): an integrative classification. Int J Environ Res Public Health. 2021;18:2621.
19. Fernández-de-las-Peñas C. Long COVID: current definition. Infection. 2022;50:285–6.
20. Lauer SA, Grantz KH, Bi Q, et al. The incubation period of coronavirus disease 2019 (COVID-19) from publicly reported confirmed cases: estimation and application. Ann Intern Med. 2020;172:577–82.
21. Ikegami S, Benirschke R, Flanagan T, Tanna N, Klein T, Elue R, Debosz P, Mallek J, Wright G, Guariglia P, Kang J, Gniadek TJ. Persistence of SARS-CoV-2 nasopharyngeal swab PCR positivity in COVID-19 convalescent plasma donors. Transfusion. 2020;60:2962–8.

22. Fernández-de-las-Peñas C, Florencio LL, Gómez-Mayordomo V, Cuadrado ML, Palacios-Ceña D, Raveendran AV. Proposed integrative model for post-COVID symptoms. Diabetes Metab Syndr. 2021;15:102159.
23. Nalbandian A, Sehgal K, Gupta A, Madhavan MV, McGroder C, Stevens JS, Cook JR, Nordvig AS, Shalev D, Sehrawat TS, Ahluwalia N, Bikdeli B, Dietz D, Der-Nigoghossian C, Liyanage-Don N, Rosner GF, Bernstein EJ, Mohan S, Beckley AA, Seres DS, Choueiri TK, Uriel N, Ausiello JC, Accili D, Freedberg DE, Baldwin M, Schwartz A, Brodie D, Garcia CK, Elkind MSV, Connors JM, Bilezikian JP, Landry DW, Wan EY. Post-acute COVID-19 syndrome. Nat Med. 2021;27:601–15.
24. Michelen M, Manoharan L, Elkheir N, Cheng V, Dagens A, Hastie C, et al. Characterising long COVID: a living systematic review. BMJ Glob Health. 2021;6:e005427.
25. Nasserie T, Hittle M, Goodman SN. Assessment of the frequency and variety of persistent symptoms among patients with COVID-19: a systematic review. JAMA Netw Open. 2021;4:e2111417.
26. Chen C, Haupert SR, Zimmermann L, Shi X, Fritsche LG, Mukherjee B. Global prevalence of post COVID-19 condition or long COVID: a meta-analysis and systematic review. J Infect Dis. 2022;226:1593–607.
27. Taha RM, Kashour Z, Kashour T, Berbari EF, Alkattan K, Tleyjeh IM. Prevalence of post-acute COVID-19 syndrome symptoms at different follow-up periods: a systematic review and meta-analysis. Clin Microbiol Infect. 2022;28:657–66.
28. Han Q, Zheng B, Daines L, Sheikh A. Long-term sequelae of COVID-19: a systematic review and meta-analysis of one-year follow-up studies on post-COVID symptoms. Pathogens. 2022;11:269.
29. Mahase E. Long COVID could be four different syndromes, review suggests. BMJ. 2020;371:m3981.
30. Carson G, Long Covid Forum Group. Research priorities for Long COVID: refined through an international multi-stakeholder forum. BMC Med. 2021;19:84.
31. Huang I, Lim MA, Pranata R. Diabetes mellitus is associated with increased mortality and severity of disease in COVID-19 pneumonia—a systematic review, meta-analysis, and meta-regression. Diabetes Metab Syndr. 2020;14:395–403.
32. Raveendran AV, Misra A. Post COVID-19 syndrome ("Long COVID") and diabetes: challenges in diagnosis and management. Diabetes Metab Syndr. 2021;15:102235.
33. Mittal J, Ghosh A, Bhatt SP, Anoop S, Ansari IA, Misra A. High prevalence of post COVID-19 fatigue in patients with type 2 diabetes: a case-control study. Diabetes Metab Syndr. 2021;15:102302.
34. Akter F, Mannan A, Mehedi HMH, Rob MA, Ahmed S, Salauddin A, Hossain MS, Hasan MM. Clinical characteristics and short-term outcomes after recovery from COVID-19 in patients with and without diabetes in Bangladesh. Diabetes Metab Syndr. 2020;14:2031–8.
35. Fernández-de-las-Peñas C, Guijarro C, Torres-Macho J, Velasco-Arribas M, Plaza-Canteli S, Hernández-Barrera V, Arias-Navalón JA. Diabetes and the risk of long-term post-COVID symptoms. Diabetes. 2021;70:2917–21.
36. Fernández-de-las-Peñas C, Torres-Macho J, Elvira-Martínez CM, Molina-Trigueros LJ, Sebastián-Viana T, Hernández-Barrera V. Obesity is associated with a greater number of long-term post-COVID symptoms and poor sleep quality: a multicentre case-control study. Int J Clin Pract. 2021;75:e14917.
37. Loosen SH, Jensen BO, Tanislav C, Luedde T, Roderburg C, Kostev K. Obesity and lipid metabolism disorders determine the risk for development of long COVID syndrome: a cross-sectional study from 50,402 COVID-19 patients. Infection. 2022;50:1165–70.
38. PHOSP-COVID Collaborative Group. Clinical characteristics with inflammation profiling of Long-COVID and association with one-year recovery following hospitalisation in the UK: a prospective observational study. Lancet Respir Med. 2022;10:761–75.

39. Florencio LL, Fernández-de-las-Peñas C. Long COVID: systemic inflammation and obesity as therapeutic targets. Lancet Respir Med. 2022;10:726–7.
40. Arnold DT, Milne A, Samms E, Stadon L, Maskell NA, Hamilton FW. Are vaccines safe in patients with Long COVID? A prospective observational study. medRxiv. https://doi.org/10.1101/2021.03.11.21253225.
41. Senjan SS, Balhara YP, Kumar P, et al. Assessment of post COVID-19 health problems and its determinants in North India: a descriptive cross section study. medRxiv. https://doi.org/10.1101/2021.10.03.21264490.

Index

K
Ketogenesis, 128
Kidney transplantation, 71

L
Lactate dehydrogenase (LDH), 5
Leptin, 101
Lipolysis, 128
Live attenuated vaccines, 198
Long hauler, 212

M
Mean absolute relative difference (MARD), 164, 165
Messenger RNA (mRNA), 198
Metformin, 143
Moderna, 199
Molnupiravir, 10
Monoclonal antibodies, 10

N
Neuropathy, 81
Neuropilin 1, 24
New-onset diabetes, 36, 37
Nirmaltrevir-Ritonavir, 10
Nonsteroidal anti-inflammatory drugs (NSAIDs), 139
Novavax, 199

O
Obesity, 93, 94, 102
Oral antidiabetic agents (OAD), 116
Outpatient setting, 142

P
Pancreatitis, 24, 25
Personal protective equipment (PPE), 128, 164
Persons with diabetes (PWD), 111
Point of care (POC), 129, 165
Post-COVID, 208, 210–212
Prediabetes, 34, 37, 39
Prolonged insulin resistance, 28
Protein subunit vaccines, 198
Proteinuria, 70
Pseudomonas aeruginosa, 54
Pulmonary embolism, 52

R
Randomized control trial (RCT), 125
Receptor for advanced glycation end-products (RAGE), 49
Remdesivir, 10, 141
Remote patient monitoring, 168
Renin-angiotensin system (RAS), 48

S
Severe acute respiratory syndrome coronavirus 2 (SARS-CoV-2), 3, 20, 21, 35, 48, 70, 84, 93, 98, 118, 124, 125, 137, 181, 185, 207, 208
Severity, 33, 38, 40
Sodium-glucose cotransporter-2 inhibitors (SGLT2i), 68, 116, 144
Steroid-induced hyperglycemia, 115, 116
Subcutaneous insulin, 126, 129, 130
Sulfonylureas, 145

T
Telehealth, 85, 87, 158
Telemedicine, 168
Thiazolidinediones, 145
Thromboprophylaxis, 11
Time below range (TBR), 162
Total daily dose (TDD), 116
Transferrin receptor (TFRC), 24, 36
Transmembrane serine protease 2 (TMPRSS2), 36
Tubuloglomerular feedback, 66
Tumor necrosis factor-alpha (TNF-α), 27, 50, 94, 97
Type 1 diabetes (T1D), 37, 45, 127
Type 2 diabetes (T2D), 112, 127, 196

V
Vaccine, 180, 182, 185, 188
   hesitancy, 185–188
   prioritization, 201
Variants of concern (VOC), 3
Variants of high consequences (VOHC), 3
Variants of interest (VUI), 3
Variants under monitoring (VUM), 3
Venous thromboembolism (VTE), 52

W
Waning immunity, 182, 183